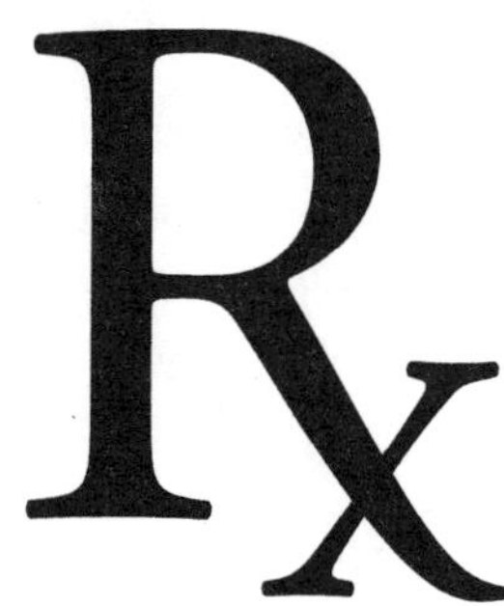

EXERCISE Rx

The Lifetime Prescription for Reducing Medical Risks and Sports Injuries

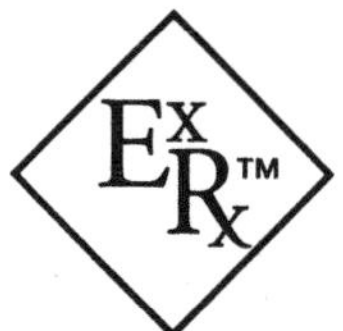

GARY YANKER

AND A TEAM OF LEADING MEDICAL EXPERTS

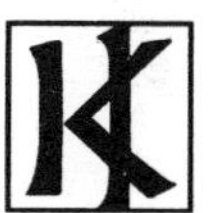

New York • Tokyo • London

Dedicated to Virginia Rice—
We miss you very much, Ginny

Other Books by Gary Yanker

Walkshaping

Walking Medicine

The Complete Book of Exercisewalking

Gary Yanker's Walking Workouts

America's Greatest Walks

The Walking Atlas of America Series

California Walking Atlas

Mid-America Walking Atlas

New England Walking Atlas

Kodansha America, Inc.
575 Lexington Avenue, New York, New York 10022, USA

Kodansha International Ltd.
17-14 Otowa 1-chome, Bunkyo-ku, Tokyo 112-8652, Japan

Published in hardcover in 1999 by Kodansha America, Inc.
First paperback edition 2002

Library of Congress Cataloging-in-Publication Data
Yanker, Gary.
Exercise Rx : the lifetime prescription for reducing medical risks and sports injuries / Gary Yanker, and a team of leading medical experts.
p. cm.
Includes index.
ISBN 1-56836-247-1
1-56836-317-6 (pbk.)
1. Exercise. 2. Sports injuries—Prevention. I. Title.
RA781.Y36 1999 99-18092
613.7'1—dc21 CIP

Printed in the United States of America

02 03 04 05 06 10 9 8 7 6 5 4 3 2 1

CONTENTS

PREFACE

The idea for *Exercise Rx* grew out of the numerous questions students have asked me over the last ten years at my exercise clinics throughout the United States, Germany, and Japan. These questions were most often related to sports injuries, illnesses, aging, or obesity. For those students who had already experienced serious medical problems or physical injuries, a preventive walking approach was too late. They were already experiencing symptoms, such as joint and back pain, breathing trouble, stress, and weight problems, which prevented them from exercising regularly. At first, I sent these students to doctors, feeling I could not give them the specific advice they needed. I gradually realized, however, that most doctors were unfamiliar with exercise techniques and were not comfortable prescribing exercise regimens. Many could only advise their patients to "exercise more" or "exercise regularly." Working with doctors and physical therapists to develop a series of exercise programs for common medical problems is the central idea and origin of this book.

The Epidemiological Model of Health

The genetics revolution is upon us. We are just a few paces away from completing the human genome, the puzzle-map locating the 100 thousand genes on our twenty-three chromosomes. We can already identify genes that forecast the probability of contracting Alzheimer's disease, arthritis, and breast cancer. Scientists foresee the day when most major diseases will be traced to a gene or combination of genes. Identifying genes for diseases, however, is still a long way from preventing or curing them.

Until that day comes, therefore, we must work with the epidemiological model to understand our personal health profile. Epidemiology and comparative epidemiology (the studies of disease as it affects groups of people) along with sports medicine injury statistics, allow us to predict with some degree of accuracy the prevalence of diseases and injuries based on sex, age, occupation, social class, marital status, geography, ethnicity, health habits (e.g. smoking, overeating, alcohol consumption), and so forth. From this, we can identify those people most likely to either contract a disease or incur an injury and, by extrapolation, the chances of whether we, ourselves, will get the same disease or injury. Each disease has risk factors, which are conditions that increase the probability of developing that disease. Family health history, including our own health history and that of our siblings, parents, and grandparents, is perhaps the most accurate predictor of our health future. It is also important to be aware of the top ten or twenty diseases that affect between one-third and one-half of the population as a whole. While predicting the probability of future afflictions is beneficial, the power to transform our own health fate through the actions we take should never be underestimated. Central to this action is exercise.

What Is Exercise?

Exercise is a concentrated form of physical activity that repeats the same movements over and over again, so that the overall body or an individual body part becomes stronger or more flexible.

Since Hippocrates' time, medical doctors have known that exercise is the best medicine for keeping your body healthy. The body needs to grow and rebuild itself constantly to survive and thrive. A consistent exercise program conditions the body to function more efficiently. This includes not only the muscles but also the chemical and nervous-system components of the body. Exercising your whole body and specific body areas stimulates tissue growth and regeneration. It also promotes blood and fluid flow. In a body that is inactive, blood and fluids slow down their natural flows and can "pool" allowing bacteria to grow and other waste products to deposit. Inactive muscles and bones can grow weak, leaving them subject to tearing and breaking. Without support, the body's infrastructure—the skin, skeleton, muscles, and tendons that hold it together—begins to sag and compress under the pull of gravity. This compression may be felt in the form of pinched nerves and pain signals sent back to the brain. As the condition worsens, the associated pain can become unbearable, and the lack of physical well-being can infiltrate the mind and psychological health in the form of chronic tension. Metabolic and nervous-system functions also slow down and become dysfunctional.

When under stress, you are more prone to rely on external aids: illicit and prescription drugs, nicotine to make you feel more alert and to stimulate thinking, or alcohol to relax you and make you feel more confident. Inactivity itself provides you the feeling of rest and freedom from stress. With the help of these aids, stress symptoms are temporarily relieved. In the long run, however, the use of these temporary "fixes" weakens the body and inhibits its ability to combat disease and physical deterioration.

An eight-year study conducted by the Cooper Institute for Aerobic Research looked at the death rates among exercising and nonexercising populations. It concluded that a complete lack of exercise is as dangerous to your health as smoking or having high cholesterol. The Cooper Institute study and other exercise, longevity, and health studies add to the growing body of medical and scientific evidence that physical inactivity poses a threat to your life. In addition to this evidence, many studies show that moderate-intensity exercises have fewer health risks and greater medical benefits than vigorous exercise. Conversely, other studies claim that vigorous activity may provide even greater health benefits. All agree, however, that increasing the amount of exercise and physical activity that you do produces positive health benefits for almost all of us. A study of Harvard alumni reported that respondents who exercised vigorously lived longer than those who exercised moderately or not at all. A twelve-year study (the Honolulu Heart Program) of 8,000 men of Japanese descent living in Hawaii between sixty-one and eighty-one years of age, found that a daily walk of two miles reduced their death rate almost by half. It also kept older people healthier by reducing their rates of heart disease and cancer.

The way you *now* exercise, however, *will not* necessarily reduce your medical risks and, even worse, may be hazardous to your health. That's because many chronic injuries or disabilities are the all-too-common effects of competitive sports and high-impact exercises. These outmoded methods of exercise result in unbalanced body development and can lead to physical injuries that can eventually (if they haven't already) reduce the quality of your life.

Exercise Rx treats exercise as a **medical prescription,** an integral part of a health care program, linking it to the prevention and treatment of aging, arthritis, heart disease, obesity, high blood pressure, depression, and many other medical ailments. Designed for the lay person, *Exercise Rx* takes sports and exercise out of the competitive domain of sports training, and into the realm of preventive and rehabilitative medicine.

Gary Yanker
New York City and Tucson, Arizona
January, 1999

Special Warning

For Prevention Therapy and Rehab Patients and Their Caregivers

Warning: Before beginning any exercise program, check with your doctor. **EXERCISE RX™** is not designed as a substitute for medical evaluation or medical care. Seek prompt medical attention, if you are experiencing any serious or recurring medical symptoms. If you are over thirty-five years of age or have not done any regular physical exercise for three months, you need a medical checkup before starting or restarting any exercise program. After starting the **EXERCISE RX™ PROGRAM**, if you experience any sustained pain or discomfort, stop exercising and check again with your doctor. Any exercise program, including walking, has inherent risks which you must assume. Exercise caution, stay focused, and concentrate on what you are doing. Above all, do not exercise with an untreated injury or during an acute illness or when you are fatigued or when you are under excessive stress.

STOP EXERCISING IMMEDIATELY or **DO NOT START EXERCISING** if you or your child or patient experience or feel any of the following: abnormal joint or muscle pain, chest pain, dizziness, lightheadedness, nausea, excessive fatigue, excessive shortness of breath, heart palpitations, joint swelling, or severe pain of any kind.

STOP AND SEEK MEDICAL ATTENTION if you or your child or patient experiences or feels: fever, joint immobility, severe joint swelling or red, painful, hot joints or chest pain or severe injury pain, or tingling or numbness in an arm or leg.

If you have had a stroke, spinal cord injury, or any other disease or surgery that can cause a contracture, do not start exercising again until your doctor has determined that your joints have normal function and your doctor or physical therapist has administered passive assisted exercise Phase I.

ACKNOWLEDGMENTS

Illustrations by Scott Cohn
Associate Editors/ Researchers: Susan Jeffers Casel, Richard Levine, Wendy Mackenzie, Jennifer Marshall, Julie Miller, Herb Sandhu, Amy Spenrath

Many thanks to the following health professionals who reviewed all or large parts of the Ex Rx manuscript.

Advisors and Contributors

Mark Arnett, Ed.D., University of Arizona
Detlef Boeckenhauer, M.D., University of Lubeck
Susan Bovre, M.A., Vassar College, University of Arizona
Diana Dickey, P.T., Kansas City, Missouri
Susan Fish, M.A., P.T., New York University
Barry Franklin, Ph.D., Professor, Wayne State University, Director of Cardiac Rehabilitation, William Beaumont Hospital, Royal Oak, Michigan
Gwen Hyatt, M.S., Exercise Science, University of Arizona
Sam Kiem, M.D., Assoc. Professor, Emergency Medicine, University of Arizona College of Medicine
Mark La Porta, M.D., Northwestern University Medical School
Mark Landry, D.P.M., M.S. Biomechanics, Ohio College of Pediatric Medicine
Jack Redekop, M.D., Medical Director of the Extended Care Center and Staff Geriatrician, Hineg Veterans Administrator Hospital, Himes, Illinois
Jack Stern, M.D., University of Maryland Medical School
James Thomas, M.D., Harvard Medical School, Director of Cardiovascular Imaging, Department of Cardiology and Professor of Medicine and Biomedical Engineering, Cleveland Clinic Foundation, Ohio
Robert Tomkins, D.O., Anesthesiology and Pain Management, University of Miami
Shelley Whitlach, M.S., Director, Tucson Medical Center FitCenter, University of Arizona
Elliot Wineburg, M.A., M.D., Life Fellow of the American Psychiatric Association

Contributors

Many thanks to the following health professionals for reviewing specific chapters and sections of the manuscript or being interviewed on special topics.

Edmund Burke, Ph.D., Exercise Physiology, University of Colorado, Colorado Springs
Deepak Chabra, M.D., U.C., Davis Medical School
Joseph Citron, M.D., Opthalmologist
James Joseph DeLauney, B.S., University of Houston, Manager, The Excelsior Athletic Club, New York City
Rafael Escamilla, Ph.D., C.S.C.S., Duke University Medical Center, Department of Orthopedic Surgery
Pedro Escobar, M.D., Tucson, Arizona

Jeffery Fisher, M.D., F.A.C.C., Clinical Associate Professor of Medicine, New York Presbyterian Hospital–Weill Medical College of Cornell University

Robert Friedman, M.D., New York City

Avrum Froimsom, M.D., Tulane University Medical School, Director of Orthopedics at Mount Sinai Medical Center, Cleveland, Ohio

Stephen Gambert, M.D., Columbia University College of Physicians, Director of the Center for Aging, New York Medical College

Gary Giangola, M.D., Assistant Professor of Surgery, New York University Medical Center

Sabine von Glinski, M.D., Kaiser Permanente Orthopedic Program, University of Colorado HSC, Denver

Joseph Gulyas, D.C., New York Chiropractic College

Lloyd Hines P.T., New York City

Damien Howell, M.S., P.T., O.C.S., University of Pennsylvania and Medical College of Virginia

Annie Lee Jones, Ph.D., Staff Clinical Psychologist for Geriatrics, Brooklyn Veterans Administration Medical Center, New York

Joseph Kansao, D.C., New York City

Marc Kitrosser, D.P.M., P.A.

Robert Lang, M.D., Albany Medical College

Arthur S. Leon, M.D., Henry L. Taylor, Professor and Director of the Laboratory of Physiological Hygiene and Exercise Science in the Division of Kinesiology, University of Minnesota and Chief Cardiologist in the Heart Disease Prevention Clinic

Ruth Lerner, Ph.D., Clinical Psychology, California School of Professional Psychology, Los Angeles

Tim Lohman, Ph.D., University of Arizona

Morton Malkin, D.D.S., New York University

Ralph Martin, D.O., College of Osteopathic and Surgery Medicine, Des Moines, Iowa

Terri Merritt, M.S., San Francisco, California

Marliee S. Niehoff, Ph.D., Illinois State University

Todd Pelleschi, D.P.M., Ohio College of Podiatric Medicine

J. Edward Pickering, M.D., University of Kansas, Associate Professor of Medicine, Thomas Jefferson University, Philadelphia

Robert L. Pincus, M.D., University of Michigan, Associate Professor of Otolarynsology, New York Medical College

Ron Pochak, T., Back Treatment and Learning Center, New York City

Henry Ramsey, D.D.S., New York City

Robert G. Rhode, Ph.D., Assistant Professor of Clinical Family Practice, Psychiatry, University of Arizona

Albert Rosen, M.D., P.A., Staff Member, Pediatrics, Columbia Presbyterian Medical Center, New York City

Elaine Rosen, P.T., New York City

Rick Rother, P.T., New York City

Gary H. Rusk, M.D., Clinical Assistant Professor of Psychiatry and Assistant Attending Psychiatrist, New York Hospital, Cornell Medical Center

Neil Scheffler, D.P.M., Baltimore, Maryland

Allen Selner, D.P.M., Los Angeles, California'

Terry Spilken, D.P.M., New York College of Podiatric Medicine

Steve Syrop, D.D.S., Director of Temporomandibular Disorders, Facial Pain Clinic, and Associate Professor of Columbia University's School of Dental and Oral Surgery

Lawrence Turtil, M.D., New York City

Chris Eugene Vance, D.P.M., Northwest Foot and Ankle Specialists, Washington State

Andrew Wasserman, D.C., C.C.S.P., team chiropractor, Florida Panthers, National Hockey League

Arthur Winter, D., F.C.S., Director of the New Jersey Neurological Institute

Mark Young, M.D., Physical Medicine and Rehabilitation at John Hopkins School of Medicine, Baltimore, Maryland

INTRODUCTION

HOW *EXERCISE Rx*™ WORKS

Although *Exercise Rx* began with my efforts to treat injuries from high-impact exercises and sports, and to find safer ways to exercise in order to avoid injury and gain the benefits of an active lifestyle, it evolved, over time, into a series of specific exercise prescriptions aimed at rehabilitating diseased, injured, or damaged body areas and managing the symptoms they incur. The exercises outlined here are based on a rehabilitation or "first do no harm" model rather than the high-performance sports training model of "fix 'em up to play again." Our program covers over 1,000 diseases and injuries, many of which have never been connected to any exercise prescription.

In *Exercise Rx*, you will read motivational stories about patients who have overcome serious diseases and injuries or may have slowed down the aging process to add as much as five to twenty-five years to their lives. Not all stories are dramatic: some are just about everyday coping. But all share the common thread of exercise and will inspire you to take action to preserve your own health. Even if you are not seriously ill, reading about someone who was ill or injured and who came back to a healthy state should motivate you to start and stick with a balanced, moderate, low-impact exercise program such as those featured in *Exercise Rx*.

Regular and safe exercise is probably the most important health habit for preventing disease and injury, and in the long run is as important as surgery, medication, or any other medical treatment for rehabilitating injuries and controlling painful symptoms. Being physically active thirty minutes or more, three to five days a week, is as essential as maintaining good nutrition, quitting smoking, and fighting alcohol or drug addictions. Without a doubt, exercise has a direct effect on such conditions as aging, arthritis, osteoporosis, diabetes, high blood pressure, obesity, and indirect effects on most other diseases. Although exercise cannot always cure or slow down a disease, exercise can do something as equally important: it can help manage and control the aches, pains, and chronic symptoms that go hand-in-hand with aging, disease, injuries, or depression. Exercise is the body's natural antidote to these symptoms.

Modern medicine is not directed so much at healing as it is at managing the symptoms of disease. Exercise can play a similar role by helping you avoid or reduce your pain and discomfort and improve the quality of your life. Moderately sick and seriously ill people need to be as fit as they can be to stop the side effects of disease from further damaging their bodies and undermining their mental health.

How Exercise Works on Diseases and Disorders

From an exercise perspective, our health has two components: body area health and body system health. A particular **body area** includes one or more such body parts as an elbow joint and the surrounding muscles or an internal organ and the surrounding tissue that holds the organ in place. A **body system** is a group of body parts that together performs a body function. For example, the nervous system is the brain and nerve network controlling your muscle movement and sensory organs. The metabolic system is comprised of the digestive organs, endocrine glands (e.g. thyroid and adrenals), and the natural chemicals or hormones that communicate messages within the system.

Exercise plays two major roles in the maintenance, prevention, and rehabilitation of injured or broken body parts and disrupted body systems caused by injury, disease, and other disabling physical conditions. First, exercise keeps your overall body systems physically fit and hardy. Second, exercise helps you avoid or control painful and disabling physical symptoms. Your exercise program can target a specific body part that has grown weak, such as thin bones, painful joints, low-breathing capacity, or constipated bowels. Weak spots can slow down or interrupt a body-system function and begin a deterioration process or weakening of the whole system.

For example, if you are laid up by a broken bone or a torn muscle, your heart and lung functions can grow weaker. In their decline, there is a slowing of blood and fluid flow to your internal organs. Poor blood or lymphatic flow can reduce nutrients, which in turn allows germs and bacteria to pool, and which can cause infection and lead to further weakening of your body system. Decreased metabolic activity leads to a slowing of essentially all body systems. Physical weakness can also affect your mind and disturb your emotions.

In some cases, the effect of exercise is immediate; in others, it is felt over a period of days, weeks, months, or even years. Exercise can also have an indirect effect on diseases and symptoms by helping to repair the damage of a disease and restore your body to its normal function. Exercise, for example, may not prevent lung cancer, but it can help rehabilitate your lungs after cancer surgery. And, it can help restore a weakened cardiovascular system after chemotherapy or a long bed rest.

In Part One, you'll identify specific weak spots and disabling physical symptoms upon which exercise can impact directly or indirectly.

The "Best" Exercises

For most people, **walking** may still be the single best form of exercise and the most medicinal activity of all exercises and sports. For others, swimming and stationary cycling may be better because of the greater body coverage obtained with these exercises. But walking has set the highest standard for how exercise should be practiced—namely with a low-impact, moderate-intensity, balanced approach. Walking is still the best preventive exercise for such common ills as lower back pain, lower leg circulatory problems, and for long-term cardiovascular (blood vessel) health. Walking is also the safest body-weight-bearing exercise for strengthing bones, and the prevention and rehabilitation of osteoporosis. However, many health problems, such as those involving internal muscles and organs, require other kinds of moderate exercise to help remedy them faster and more efficiently. Stretching, strengthening, range-of-motion exercises, as well as various sports, taken together, can be more effective than walking. *Exercise Rx* modifies the basic moves of athletic activities and redefines how they should be practiced for health benefits. In Part Two, you'll learn not only the safer forms of exercise but also why your exercise choices have been narrowed down to certain types of warm-up, stretching, strengthening, continuous movement, and relaxation exercises. Additionally, you'll learn why the exercises outlined in this book can be alternatives to surgery or medication.

What is not included in this book are many such popular exercises as yoga, tai chi, jogging, inline skating, cross-country skiing, and rowing. Each of these activities has special advantages and can be practiced as either a supplemental exercise or enjoyed for play and leisure. Please note, however, that it is the moderately active people, those who fall between the "super jocks" and the "couch potatoes," who have the least amount of medical problems. Practitioners of such low-impact exercises as walking, stationary cycling, and water exercises don't suffer from disabling aches, pains, injuries, or inabilities caused by vigorous exercise.

How To Use This Book

Exercise Rx is not a typical medical encyclopedia for identifying and solving symptoms. It is really an exercise how-to manual providing specific exercise remedies as well as overall, long-term health solutions that you can follow according to your medical risk priorities. The exercise prescriptions are based not only on gender, age, fitness level, and activity preference, but also on family health history and the propensity for medical risks and physical weaknesses or disabilities. *Exercise Rx* provides five separate health and exercise prescriptions that correspond to the following five major health systems:

1. **Age ExRx™** is the overall prescription that applies to any and all age groups. It also helps prevent and rehabilitate atrophy and damage to the nervous and sensory-motor systems caused by aging.
2. **MuSkel (Musculoskeletal) ExRx™** is the prescription for optimum bone, skin, and muscle health.
3. **Meta (Metabolic) ExRx™** is the prescription for metabolic health and includes reducing and maintaining your weight as well as managing the symptoms of diabetes. **Meta** also refers to the internal organs of the lower trunk including those used for digestion, excretion, and reproduction.
4. **Cardio (Cardiovascular) ExRx™** is the prescription that applies to preventing, managing, or reversing the single greatest health risk factor: cardiovascular (heart

and arterial) disease. It also applies to cardio respiratory (heart and lung) disease.

5. **Psyche-Immune (Psychological and Immune) ExRx™** is the prescription for psychological health and helps with anxiety, depression, stress, and other potentially destructive thoughts and feelings. Because of the connection between mental state and the immune system **psyche-immune** also includes immune disorders, especially those with inflammatory conditions such as rheumatoid arthritis.

Each of these five prescriptions are divided into two types: preventive (Part Two) and rehabilitative (Part Three). Prevention ExRx will provide direction as to how to delay—or prevent altogether—the onset of diseases, symptoms, and injuries. Rehabilitation ExRx will help reduce or reverse the pain symptoms after diseases and disabilities have occurred, and repair and restore health to injured body parts and systems. Consequently, more than 80% of the 1,000-plus diseases and disabilities that can kill, disable, or injure you, are given a health prescription.

Therapeutic Exercises

The therapeutic exercises cover the in-between problem areas. Sometimes, physical symptoms or weaknesses are not as severe and can be helped or managed with Prevention ExRx. Other times, symptoms may be moderate to very severe and will require Rehabilitation ExRx. You and your doctor will have to make the choice between these two. The health risk questionnaires in Chapters Two to Six will assist you in making an informed choice.

If you think you are healthy and have been at least moderately active for the last year (i.e. physically active one to two days a week), use the preventive exercises and follow the recommendations for Age ExRx. If you have a specific health weakness, such as heart disease, weak joints, obesity, or stress, use one of the other four health prescriptions. If you have multiple problems, use the health prescription for the most severe condition or you may combine various health prescriptions. All health prescriptions intersect and each one will build on the successes you have achieved in other areas.

Where To Start

First, read through Part One to help you establish your ExRx profile. Rate your five body health systems on a scale of 1 (least severe) to 5 (most severe). Then, apply your health-risk rating by concentrating on one or more prevention exercises while practicing the overall Prevention ExRx Program in Part Two. If you are already physically disabled from a disease, injury, or disorder, use the disease and injury index, p. 473, to identify a specific exercise prescription in Part Three for your ailment. If nothing seems to be wrong, use Part One to establish areas of vulnerability and apply your health-risk rating to determine the amount and types of exercise you should do in Part Two (e.g. warm-ups, stretching, strengthening, aerobic, cool down, and so on).

PART ONE

LINKING PREVENTION AND REHABILITATION

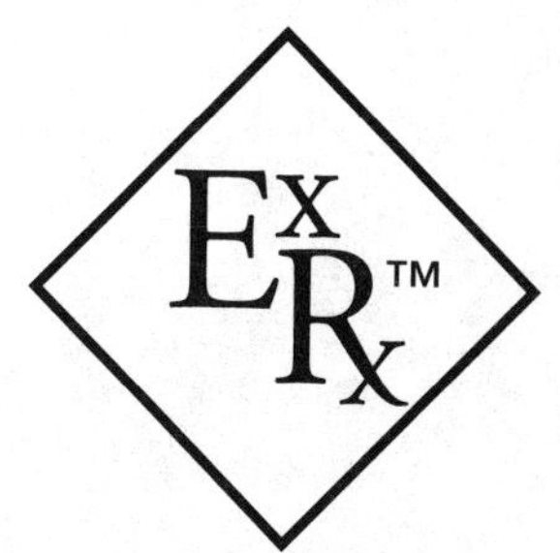

CHAPTER 1

What Can Go Wrong with Your Health and When

Assessing Your Medical Risks and Determining Your Health Profile

EXERCISE PRIORITIES

To determine what your exercise priorities are, you will be rating your ten medical risk factors (see Medical Profile Questionnaire, page 24). Your total score on major risk factors will determine which health system needs more preventive work. Risk factors in specific body systems will determine those specific exercise routines that will be necessary. If you already have a disease or injury or have undergone surgery, your exercise priorities will shift from prevention to rehabilitation.

MEDICAL RISK FACTORS

Because there is no absolute certainty about the cause of many diseases, experts have assigned a series of probable factors that are present in those persons who already have that disease. Infectious and genetic diseases are, of course, the exceptions. For most people, age is the number-one risk factor. Sports injuries often have a single or limited number (two or three) of contributing causes. But other factors can also play important roles. It is difficult to rate the value or ranking of any particular risk factor. For some, all factors can play a role; for others, a single element will predominate.

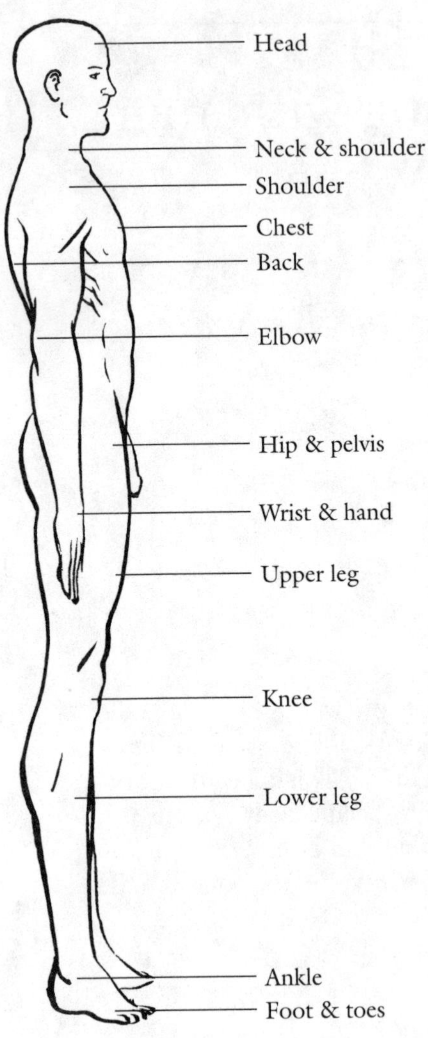

TEN MAJOR RISK FACTORS

Risk Factor 1: Age

Diseases and injuries are more apt to occur in certain groups. Exercise can help you turn back your body's biological clock from five to twenty years. Your body will look, feel, and function—inside and out—like a body that belongs to someone five to twenty years younger. This phenomenon holds true over most of your life, even though the body's natural aging process will continue. Atrophied muscles have not disappeared, but can be brought back with stretching and strengthening exercises. Even though your heart and lung capacities may have dwindled, they can be revived with a gradual increase in your exercise intensity. Even if your body is disease-ridden with arthritis or atherosclerosis, exercise will rejuvenate you. The few exceptions to this rule can be found in Part Three—Rehabilitation ExRx.

Risk Factor 2: Gender

Increasingly, men and women are sharing the same diseases, disabilities, and symptoms. For example, heart disease, at one time much more prevalent in men, is now the number-one killer of women who smoke or who are employed in a stressful workplace—usually located in a big city. Eating disorders, once attributed to young females almost exclusively, are now found in young men as well as among men and women in the middle- and older-age categories. There are, however, differences in the types and severity of diseases that women and men suffer.

Although men and women share the diseases of aging and the psyche on an almost equal basis, women have a higher incidence of those autoimmune disorders as well as severe musculoskeletal problems and other side effects, including osteoporosis (90% are found in females), lupus (80%), rheumatoid arthritis (75%), and multiple sclerosis (60%). Females also experience a slight increase in the number of psychological disorders: depression (50%+) and eating disorders (90%). Additionally, over a lifetime, women need to do more weight-bearing exercises to strengthen their bones. For a more complete list of predominantly female diseases, see Table 1.1.

One major area of concern for preadolescent and adolescent females is the relationship of poor eating habits to menstrual problems and bone stress fractures. As with crash dieting, too much or too vigorous physical activity can reduce body fat to dangerously low levels (i.e. below 17%). When body-fat content is diminished to very low levels, such menstrual irregularities as **amenorrhea** (menstrual cessation) or **oligomenorrhea** (cycle irregularity) begin to occur. These conditions, in turn, can lead to a reduction of estrogen production, a necessary component for bone rebuilding. Irregular periods can pose the danger of premature osteoporosis or reduced bone density (i.e. up to 20% bone density loss). The irreversible effects of these disorders can lead to stress fractures of weight-bearing bones (e.g. back, hip, pelvis, lower leg, and foot) in younger women and broken bones and fractures later in life.

Another pitfall for many young women is the focus on exercise as a form of weight loss. This can lead to an obsession with being thin, rather than being healthy. This obsession is a major reason why the rate of eating disorders among female athletes—especially gymnasts, divers, ballet dancers, and figure skaters—is fifteen to sixty times higher than in the general female population.

Of particular importance to women, the natural body weight and exercise standards found in Meta Rx should be combined with wholesome, well-balanced eating habits.

TABLE 1.1
COMMON OR PREDOMINANTLY FEMALE DISEASES

Age

Nervous System

multiple sclerosis (60% women)

myasthenia gravis (60% women)

trigeminal neuralgia (women, age 40+)

MuSkel

Muscle and Bone Disorders

carpal tunnel syndrome (primarily women ages 30–60)

hammer toe (narrow-toed high heels)

osteoporosis (age 50+, 80% women)

Cardio

Lung and Breathing

sarcoidosis (66% women, ages 20–40)

lung embolisms

Heart and Blood Vessel

cardiomyopathy (enlarged heart) (women, age 30+ or who have had two or more pregnancies)

high blood pressure (age 50+)

migraine (vascular) headaches (75% menstruating women; 3× more than men)

pulmonary hypertension (women, ages 20–40, high mortality rate in pregnant women)

Raynaud's disease (puberty to age 40)

varicose veins

Meta

Digestive Disorders

colitis (peak ages 55–60)

lactose intolerance

rectal prolapse (75% women, usually around age 45)

gallstones (85% women, ages 20–50; thereafter about equal to men)

Kidney and Urinary Disorders

acute pyelonephritis (most common kidney infection)

bladder infections

lower urinary tract infections (cystitis and urethritis)

Gynecological Disorders (all)

amenorrhea, secondary (absence of period 3 months or more)

inflammation of vulva and vagina (can occur at any time or be aggravated by intense exercise)

cardiovascular disease in pregnancy

diabetes complications during pregnancy

Sexual Disorders

vaginal spasms

Hormone and Gland Disorders

inflammation of the thyroid

Cancer

breast (ages 35–59)

cervical (ages 30–50)

lung (men ahead, women closing gap fast)

ovarian

thyroid (66%)

uterine (postmenopausal women, ages 50–65)

vulvar (mid-60s)

Psyche-Immune

Immune

chronic fatigue syndrome (mostly women, under age 45)

rheumatoid arthritis (more women, peak onset, ages 30–60)

scleroderma (more women, ages 30–50)

Psychological

agoraphobia (66% women)

major depression

pain disorder (more women, ages 30–50)

systemic lupus (88% women)

Common Injuries

hip injuries (related to osteoporosis)

The first major area of concern for men is their cardiovascular respiratory system—heart and lung disease, in particular. Far more men have heart attacks, chronic bronchitis, and emphysema than women.

Another major concern for men is muscle imbalance and inflexibility. Balanced muscle development and flexibility exercises will not only reduce sports injuries, but will enable many men in their forties and fifties to maintain a cardio exercise program.

Many male health problems are not biologically inherent, but arise either because of the traditionally male consumption habits of eating and drinking (alcohol), smoking cigarettes, or the ways in which men practice competitive sports. Namely, men give little attention to warm-ups and stretching—and they tend to overuse certain body areas such as knees, shoulders, and ankles.

TABLE 1.2
COMMON OR PREDOMINANTLY MALE DISEASES

Age

Nervous System

cluster headaches (90% men)

amyotrophic lateral sclerosis (Lou Gehrig's disease) (75% men)

Parkinson's disease (60% men)

peripheral nerve degeneration (men, ages 30–50)

MuSkel

Muscle and Bone

bone tumor (35–60)

gout (men, age 30+)

herniated disk (men, under age 45)

Paget's disease (mostly men, age 40+)

Eye Disorders

retinal detachment (66% males; caused by traumatic injuries)

Cardio

Heart, Lung, and Vessel Disorders

aortic aneurysms (80% men)

arterial occlusive disease

Buerger's disease (men, ages 20–40; smokers; Jewish)

coronary artery disease (no longer exclusively men)

heart attack

chronic bronchitis/emphysema

legionnaires' disease

high blood pressure (men, under age 50)

Meta

Digestive Disorders

alcoholism

cirrhosis of the liver (66% men)

diverticulosis (men, age 40+)

groin hernia (60% men)

pilonidal disease (hairy men, ages 18–30)

Kidney and Urinary

enlarged prostate (most men, age 50+)

kidney cancer (66% men)

kidney stones

Sexual Disorders

impotence

Cancer

bladder (men, age 50+)

bone tumor (men, ages 35–60)

brain tumor (slightly more men than women)

kidney (66% men)

larynx (voice box) (90% men, ages 50–65)

leukemia, chronic lymphocytic (most all men, age 50+)

liver (more men, particularly age 60+)

lung (men ahead, women closing in fast)
malignant lymphomas (66%–75% men)
multiple myeloma (mostly men, age 40+)
pancreatic (mostly men, ages 35–70)
prostate (men, age 50+)
smoking-related
squamous cell (white men, age 60+)
stomach (men, age 40+, 66% male)
testicular (young to middle-age men, ages 20–40)
throat (pharynx) (66% male)
tongue (85%)

Psyche-Immune

Immune

Reiter's syndrome (polyarthritis; young men, ages 20–40)

Common Injuries

shoulder injuries (related to sports play)
knee injuries (related to sports play)

Risk Factor 3: Genetics—Your Family Health Tree

After your age, activity level, and gender, your genes could be the next biggest risk factor in your overall health and longevity. Diseases that occur earlier than normal are often those with a strong familial or genetic component. Conversely, a genetic history that shows an absence of early onset may provide you with some comfort. If a disease or disorder has a familial component it means the disease runs in families. If a disease runs in your family, your probability of contracting this disease is greater than average. This is not because you are just genetically prone, but is the result of a combination of genes and environment. Some of the major familial-component diseases are:

- alcoholism
- Alzheimer's
- arteriosclerosis
- breast cancer
- colon and rectal cancers
- diabetes
- emphysema
- hypertension (60% genes, 40% environment)
- migraine headaches
- obesity
- prostate cancer
- psoriasis

A variety of other disorders are also suspected of being hereditary, including duodenal ulcers, bronchial asthma, uterine and stomach cancers, schizophrenia, and osteoarthritis.

A little research into the health history of your grandparents, parents, and siblings will increase your awareness of other aspects of your health and its vulnerabilities. For example, you may have acquired habits from your parents, such as eating fatty foods or smoking cigarettes, which now put you at greater risk of obesity, heart disease, or lung cancer. Being injury- and accident-prone may also have a familial component (e.g. body size and structure, weak backs, knees, ankles, and flat feet). Race, culture, and prior or current diseases and are additional factors that should also be considered.

Knowing your family health history may motivate you to take early action to avoid, prevent, or slow down the progress of a disease that may now be in its early stages, or to just improve your basic physical condition. What's more, certain diseases such as coronary artery disease, lung cancer, and osteoporosis may be curtailed by strengthening the body system far ahead of the time when these conditions usually first appear. Knowing those impediments that lie in the path of your health is like knowing the weather forecast *and* being able to alter it.

Risk Factor 4: Health Habits and Addictions

Your health habits can carry either minimal or great weight as predictors. If you are prone to heart disease, your health habits can impact greatly on your life expectancy. If you have musculoskeletal problems, health habits may play only a moderate role in determining your health future.

Some diseases are not only delayed, but perhaps avoided altogether because of more culturally determined health habits. The members of certain religious groups, for example Mormons, orthodox Jews, Amish, and Buddhists often lead long, healthy, and active lives, avoiding most major diseases because of such health habits as vegetarianism or moderation in all things.

In drawing up a family health history, don't take everything at face value. A highly stressful job may have contributed to a relative's heart attack—not a familial or genetic component.

Risk Factor 5: Personality Traits

These are the mental and emotional qualities that define you as a person and include the way you react to situations and relate to others.

The Type A Personality—an aggressive, frenetic, and hostile temperament—ranks as a major risk factor for heart disease. Otherwise, personality traits that relate to how we cope with stress show how much our immune system is under threat. Personality traits play a role in many of the conditions in the psyche-immune health system.

Risk Factor 6: Environment

Environmental risk factors can adversely affect each of your five health systems. Living alone can cause you to be more sedentary and thus accelerate the aging process. A physically demanding job can put you at risk of musculoskeletal injury. Smog and excessive heat and humidity can raise blood pressure and weaken the lungs. Contaminated food and overcrowded living can wreak havoc on the metabolic system. Noise pollution (e.g. living near an airport) and a cluttered living space can affect your psyche-immune health.

Risk Factor 7: Diseases, Disorders, and Injuries

Diseases, disorders, and injuries you already have are risk factors for potential diseases you may still get. Some aspects about each of these are:

Disease can be a deep-seated type, such as cancer, or a superficial type, such as a cold. The deep-seated diseases can permanently damage or destroy organs; the ailment-type (superficial) disease, although not destructive unless it is left untreated, can become chronic, however.

A **disorder** can be as serious as a disease, but usually involves an upset in a body function that is not necessarily caused by an unhealthy or diseased organ. Exercise can improve the outlook of some diseases and disorders by reducing the number and intensity of symptoms and by healing the physical damage that both have caused to the body.

Physical **injuries** your body has suffered from accident, disease, or bad health habits are often good indicators of what lies ahead for your health. One serious organ, joint, or bone injury can weaken a body area permanently. When the injury count piles up, pain and discomfort from the injury can become chronic. Injuries can also be caused by surgery, or drug/alcohol abuse. Perhaps the worst injury is infarction or tissue death. When 10% of your heart muscle is destroyed by a heart attack, it can permanently reduce your heart capacity and be a risk factor and predictor of future heart attacks.

Because the five health systems are linked to one another, failure in one system can lead to failure in another. As a result, some diseases and disorders (e.g. diabetes) are risk factors for other diseases. Alcoholism **(Meta)** can lead to osteoporosis **(MuSkel)**. Diabetes **(Meta)** can lead to circulatory **(Cardio)** and skin **(MuSkel)** problems. Being overweight **(Meta)** can contribute to high blood pressure **(Cardio)**.

Risk Factor 8: Symptoms

There are hundreds of **symptoms,** pains, discomforts, and signals that our bodies give us to indicate the state of our health. One or two infrequent aches or pains may not carry any weight nor be symptomatic of any disease or disorder . . . however, they may be the harbingers of more serious problems down the road. A **syndrome** is a number of symptoms occurring together, which characterizes a specific disease or condition.

Exercise helps relieve symptoms by improving blood flow to a painful area and by relaxing muscles in the vicinity that have grown tense in response to the pain. As soon as the pressure is off the nerves, the pain begins to subside. Exercise also stimulates the release of hormones (e.g. endorphins), which act as natural painkillers.

Overall, many major symptoms are shared by many diseases. They are the common aches and pains that signal a breakdown is coming or has already begun in a body area or body system. Of course, a single symptom does not necessarily a disease make. Additionally, symptoms require a doctor's evaluation before a disease or disorder can be diagnosed. The following is a list of the major mental and physical symptoms upon which exercise has a direct and significant impact:

- aches/pains (in specific body areas)
- breathlessness (in response to exertion)
- cramps (including tremors and spasms)
- depression or anxiety
- discomfort (itching, irritability)
- fatigue (overall weariness or a weak body organ)
- imbalances (outer body: clumsiness; inner body: nutritional imbalance)
- immobility (outer body: your whole body or a specific body part; inner body: a sluggish colon)
- loss of function/control (a body part stops working correctly)
- sensitivities increased or decreased

Some symptoms become part of a disease; others stand alone and remain as the aches, pains, and discomforts of daily life. Whether or not an ache or pain is a symptom of a disease or disorder, exercise can still help you get relief. Many times, this is the best you can hope for from any medical treatment because most serious diseases cannot be cured. Conversely, even if a disease is cured or reversed or put into remission, the symptoms may persist. Again, exercise may relieve these symptoms as well.

Risk Factor 9: Physical Condition

Physical condition refers to the current state of your body, rather than a specific disease. It's similar to a physical fitness rating. Physical condition is also based on your build and bone type, age, anatomic abnormalities, body fat, muscle, and stress. It determines your ability to exercise and the strength and hardiness of your body system. You can either take a test or you can rate yourself.

Your score or rating is used to determine the level at which you should start to do an exercise and, if you have a health weakness, to what level you should progress.

The core of your medical health is measured on basic strength. How flexible are your lower back and hamstring muscles? How strong are your abdominals, arms, and shoulders? Bone strength is also measured. Leg strength is determined as part of your ability to do leg-based cardio exercise. Your cardio fitness level is your ability to perform continuous motion exercises, such as walking, jogging, bicycling, or swimming. These exercises test your heart muscles, your lung capacity, and your muscles' ability to use oxygen pumped into the blood from your heart.

Risk Factor 10: Exercise and Activity Level

For many, **inactivity** can be the biggest risk factor for disease and disability. In this way, inactivity shares similar characteristics with aging.

Studies show that the cumulative amount of physical activity is more important for your health than the intensity of the exercise. That is, if you are mildly to moderately active every day of your life, you are in better shape than if you are vigorously active for six months out of every year. Your health is more damaged by the days of inactivity than it is helped by the days of high activity. Over a lifetime, thirty minutes of moderate physical activity a day is the best prescription for basic health.

WHERE DO YOU START?

In Chapters Two through Five you will be evaluating the health problems for each of your five body systems—Age, MuSkel, Cardio, Meta, and Psyche-Immune. Determine those systems that are the weakest by scoring your risk factors, major diseases, symptoms, and injuries. You will also evaluate the weakest body parts or areas in each system. With this information, you will be able to design your own body map and plot out your own personal ExRx, which you can then use when going on to Part Two or Three.

CHAPTER 2

Saving Your Life through Exercise

What Exercise Can and Can't Do to Slow Down the Aging Process

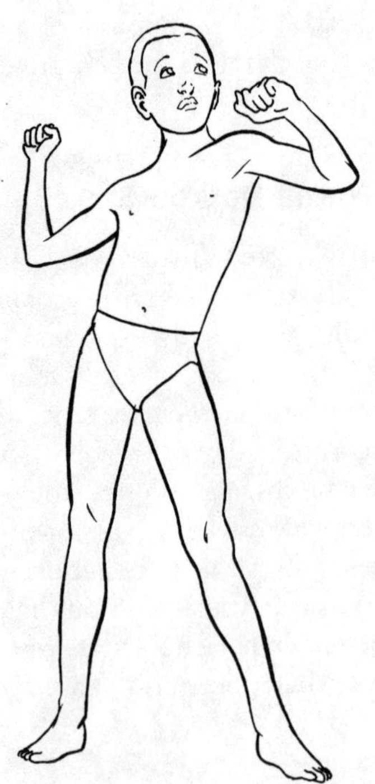

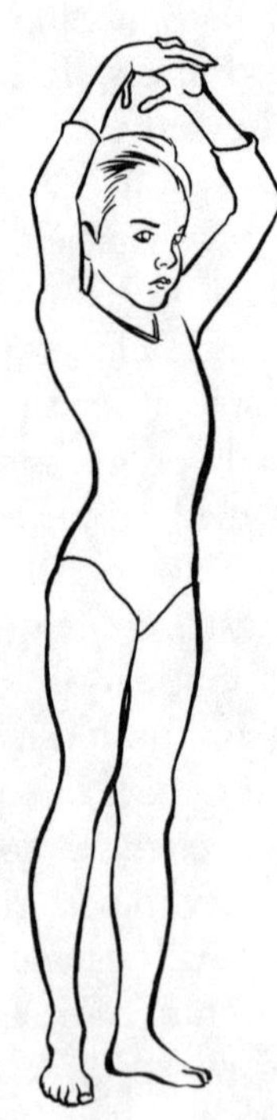

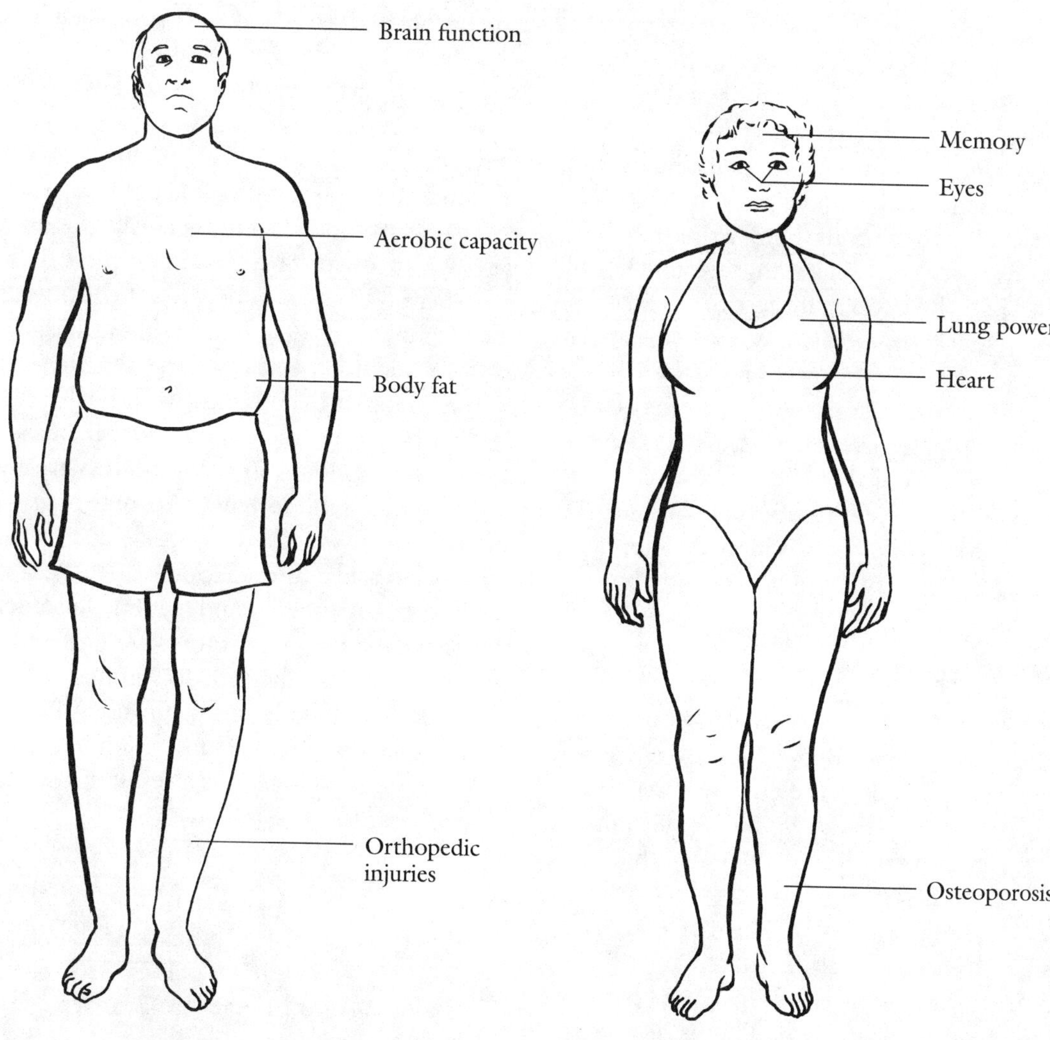

The Aging Process

The natural aging process occurs in two phases. Phase 1 is the **growth phase** when the body develops (i.e. muscles grow larger, bones grow denser, and organs mature). This phase lasts until age 25 to 35. Phase 2 is the **decline phase** when muscles weaken and bones thin down. From age 30 to 70, 1% of the body's physical capacity is lost annually. (If you are sedentary, it's 2% or more; if you are highly active, it is only a small fraction of a percent.) By age 70, your physical capacity has decreased by 40%. Consequently, the older you become, the more likely you are to contract one or more diseases or incur injuries. This decline translates into the loss of muscle strength, endurance, flexibility, coordination, agility, and balance. This can be measured by a reduction in your maximum heart rate and its stroke volume, the amount of weight you can lift, the range of motion of your joints, and the circumference of your bones. There are also internal declines, for example, high blood pressure results from a loss in flexibility of the arteries. (See risk factors, pages 4–11.)

About half of the changes in the decline phase are inevitable and cannot be helped by exercise (e.g. thinning hair, wrinkling skin, hearing loss, and weakening eyesight). The other half, however, can be slowed down or even *reversed* by exercise. With regular exercise, you can significantly arrest the decline phase by increasing your cardiovascular health through the strengthening and expansion of your lungs and heart. You can also increase the size and strength of your muscles and bones, so that there is more development to chip away from during the decline phase.

PREMATURE AGING

Premature aging is an acceleration of the aging process caused by disuse, overuse, or misuse of our bodies, the effects of which can be devastating. Disease, injury, environment (e.g. sun exposure), and poor health habits (e.g. alcoholism) can be factors as well. But, by far, the fastest way to age your body is by being physically inactive. Inactivity will hasten the rate of aging just as increased physical activity will slow it down. That is, it is possible to look and feel like a fifty-year-old while you are still in your thirties. In exercise terms, age can provide a standard for our physical condition or the physical shape that we're in.

AGES OF DISEASE ONSET

Almost all diseases have an age component (i.e. they worsen with age, or rather, the older you become the more likely you will get them) but certain diseases, especially those that attack your brain and nervous system, are associated with old age itself—namely, Alzheimer's and Parkinson's disease.

Age affects more than just one system. It is also a standard by which we measure almost any disease—age, gender, genetic, lifestyle (human-made)—whether you get it earlier or later than the norm. This is called the **average age of onset of a disease,** which is the time period when most people get the disease. Throughout Part One, you will use the age of onset standard to measure the severity of a disease in order to determine your health risk.

Although most diseases can strike at any age, and, in most cases, hit both men and women, they tend to have a "center of gravity" (i.e. the average age of onset) as to when they begin and continue. Some diseases, such as infectious diseases and genetic disorders may appear when a person is young. A select few strike particular ethnic groups. Many other diseases (e.g. lung cancer) are primarily human-made, caused by lifestyle choices such as cigarette smoking, or as a result of occupational hazards.

TABLE 2.1
YOUTH DISEASE ONSET: AGES 0–19

Babies: Ages Prenatal to 2 Years

Lungs and Breathing Disorders

croup (3 months to 3 years)

infant respiratory distress (newborns, 28–37 weeks)

sudden infant death syndrome (SIDS) (4 weeks to 7 months)

Muscle, Bone, and Joint Disorders

Down syndrome

hemophilia

Nervous System Disorders

cerebral palsy (premature infancy through childhood)

fluid on the brain (prenatal to birth)

spinal cord defects (5% of pop.; 12,000 infants per year)

Digestive System Disorders

gastroenteritis (affects all ages; life-threatening in young children and elderly)

groin hernia (all ages, but most common in male infants)

Nutritional Disorders

protein-calorie malnutrition (infant 6–18 months, usu. 1 year of age)

vitamin E deficiency

Kidney and Urinary Disorders

urinary reflux (infants, males)

Cancers

brain tumor (before age 1)

Immune Disorders

infection

juvenile arthritis (peak onsets 1–3 and 8–12)

polio

haemophilus influenzae (50% before age 1, other 50% by age 3)

respiratory syncytial virus infection (most children under 4)

Children: Ages 2–5 Years

Heart and Blood Vessel Disorders

rheumatic fever (ages 5–15)

Nervous System Disorders

attention deficit disorder (ADD) (diagnosed ages 4–5)

Lungs and Breathing Disorders

adenoid enlargement

epiglotiditus (ages 2–8)

Infectious Diseases

chicken pox (ages 2–8)

German measles (ages 5–9, also adolescents and young adults)

measles (ages 2–5, but also adolescents and adults)

mumps (ages 5–9)

Cancer

brain tumor (ages 2–12)

leukemia (ages 2–8)

melanoma (child to youth)

Muscle and Bone Disorders

muscular dystrophy (Duchenne's) (ages 3–5; succumbs by ages 9–12)

muscular dystrophy (Becker's) (ages 5–15; succumbs by age 40)

osteomyelitis (boys)

juvenile scoliosis (ages 4–8)

hammer toe

Kidney and Urinary Disorders

kidney reflux (girls, ages 3–7; inherited)

Metabolic Disorders

galactosemia (any age)

high cholesterol (33% are children as young as 3)

protein malnutrition (any age)
vitamin A or B deficiency
vitamin K deficiency (cystic fibrosis)

Kids: Ages 6–12

Heart and Blood Vessel Disorders

Raynaud's disease (females, puberty to age 40)
cocaine-induced stroke

Muscle and Bone Disorders

adolescent humpback (ages 12–16)
adolescent scoliosis (girls, ages 10 to maturity)
loose bodies in elbow joint (ages 12–17)
nursemaid's elbow

Immune Disorders

asthma (50% of all cases under age 10)
juvenile arthritis (peak onset ages 1–3 and 8–12)

Accidents/Sports Injuries

avulsion fracture in the pelvic area
collar bone fracture (any age)
dislocated shoulder (any age)
elbow fracture (any age)
Little League elbow (ages 6–12)
osteochondritis dissecans of the knee (ages 10–12)
scaphoid (wrist) bone fracture (any age; young athletes)
stress fracture of top of thigh bone (death of hip joint) (children running long distance)

Teens: Ages 13–19

Digestive Disorders

colitis (more in women, ages 15–20 and 55–60)

Gynecological Disorders

amenorrhea/oligomenorrhea (can start at age 18; excessive dieting and exercise)
dysfunctional uterine bleeding (sexually mature teenage girls)
painful menstruation (leading cause of school absences; 40% of high school girls each month, and 140 million of lost work hours per year)

Cancer

Hodgkin's disease (ages 15–38 and over age 50)
lung cancer (when smoking begins before age 15 and smokes 1 pack a day for next 20 years)

YOUTH: BABIES, CHILDREN, KIDS, AND TEENS

Disease- and disorder-wise, youth (prenatal to nineteen years of age) is largely a period of physical injury, predominantly caused by accidents sustained in sports and play. Sports injuries in children and young teens can damage growth mechanisms in the body and stunt physical body development. It's up to parents and coaches to equip children and teens with responsible attitudes and safer movement techniques that they can take with them into adulthood and use to set their courses for proper, lifelong health.

Even though it's best to start exercising as early in life as possible, it may be difficult to sell this idea to all children. Some will be very active in sports; others won't. Indeed, adult health is now often better than the health of our young people. One-third of children under age seven have high cholesterol, and half are overweight.

Health education in school plays a major role in motivating children and teens, but ultimately, parents are responsible for the health and health habits of their children. As parents, even if you are not athletic, you should lead the way by your own example and by making sure that your kids learn the basic skills of posture, and practice such individual sports and exercises as walking, stretching, calisthenics, swimming, and bicycling. After you have mastered the exercises in Part Two, you can teach them to your children, which will help make exercise as easy and accessible as such basic movement skills as brushing your teeth or walking, rather than as complex and inaccessible as many such higher profile sports as gymnastics, basketball, and aerobic dancing.

The key is to start while your child is an infant by influencing their basic motor skills. Hold your baby's feet and hands and pump his or her legs and arms, moving them in different directions through a full and natural range of motion. Massage your baby to stimulate circulation and muscle toning. At three months, help your baby to sit up by holding his or her head until he or she has learned to sit up without your help. From seven to nine months, promote movement by giving your child verbal encouragement as well as space to crawl and slide across the floor in the seated position. At ten to eleven months, gently encourage your child to stand. During the eleventh or twelfth month, your child should be able to walk with your help, and by twelve to fourteen months should be able to walk alone. During months fifteen to seventeen, your child will develop the ability to walk sideways and backward, and by seventeen to twenty-four months should be able to walk upstairs and downstairs with your help, and then gradually to walk unassisted in all directions.

From ages one to six, concentrate on walking, posture, range of motion, and balancing skills. Show your child different arm and leg movements to maintain balance. Make exercise into a game of follow the leader.

The growth spurt years are from ages six to twelve, and your child's body is growing in all its parts: muscles, bones, and so forth. Diseases are rare to this age group, the most common being asthma. The greatest concern is the introduction of either too much exercise (associated with growth rate problems) or too little exercise (associated with early development of fat cells).

From ages thirteen to nineteen, most boys and girls experience puberty and the maturing of their reproductive systems and organs. The greatest danger to their health, however, is drug experimentation. Whatever the drug—alcohol, cocaine, marijuana—children can permanently endanger their physical and emotional health by casual use and experimentation.

By the age of twenty, a youth begins to see that by growing older the natural, youthful shape of his or her body will not "hold together" unless given exercise, and careful attention is paid to diet. The more exercise that is done during your teens and young adulthood, the stronger your body will be at its peak when your heart, muscles, and lungs reach their full strength and capacity and the greater your functional capacity will be when you reach middle and old age.

As age 27 approaches, you begin a countdown that takes you to the big "three-oh." A year, now, seems shorter than it seemed during your teens. At thirty, your life takes on a different rhythm. You measure time not in years, but in decades: your thirties, forties, fifties, and so on. As you approach middle age, you may be more interested in maintaining an exercise program to regain your youthful shape and vigor.

TABLE 2.2
YOUNG ADULT DISEASE ONSET: AGES 20–29

Heart and Vessel Disorders

Buerger's disease (Ages 20–40)

pulmonary hypertension (pregnant women, ages 20–40; high mortality)

sarcoidosis (women, blacks; ages 20–40)

Nervous System Disorders

Huntington's disease (ages 25–55)

multiple sclerosis (ages 20–40)

myasthenia gravis (ages 20–40)

Digestive Disorders

Crotin's disease (ages 20–40; may be familial)

hemorrhoids (common ages 20–50)

gallstones, and gallbladder and bile duct diseases (ages 20–50)

liver diseases (begin ages 20–30)

Kidney and Urinary Disorders

renal hypertension (more common under age 30 and age 50+)

Gynecological Disorders (Young Women)

premenstrual syndrome (PMS) (ages 25–45)

Sexually Transmitted Diseases

AIDS

gonorrhea (prevalent during ages 19–25)

Immune Disorders

Goodpasture's syndrome (mostly men, ages 20–40)

Infectious Diseases

infectious mononucleosis (young adults and children)

TABLE 2.3
MIDDLE-AGE DISEASE ONSET: Ages 30–39

Nervous System Disorders

Guillain-Barré syndrome (ages 30–50)

Muscle and Bone Disorders

bone tumor (mostly men, 35–60)

bursitis (usually occurs in middle age from repeated injury or inflammatory joint disease) (85% women, until age 50)

carpal tunnel syndrome (primarily women, ages 30–60)

gout (men, average age 30)

pectoral muscle insertion inflammation (age 40+; tennis, golf, swimming)

Kidney and Urinary Disorders

kidney stones (ages 30–50)

Gynecological Disorders (Women)

dysfunctional uterine bleeding

failure to ovulate (women, late 30s to early 40s)

endometriosis (ages 30–40; especially women who postpone childbearing)

Hormone and Gland Disorders

Graves' disease (most often between ages 30–40)

Ear, Nose, and Throat Disorders

Meniere's disease (vertigo, ringing, and hearing loss) (ages 30–60)

Cancer

bowel (ages 35–65)

cervical (women, ages 30–50)

pancreatic (mostly men, ages 35–70)

pituitary tumors (ages 30–50)

Immune Disorders

psoriatic arthritis (ages 30–35)

rheumatoid arthritis (ages 30–60, 6.5 million annually, mostly women)

scleroderma (ages 30–50, more women)

MIDDLE AGE

Middle age (ages thirty to fifty-nine) is characterized by the presence of muscle and joint pain caused either by the loss of overall physical strength and endurance or by harbingers of familial diseases. These symptoms affect the cardiovascular system, the metabolic system, or the musculoskeletal and skin system. The diseases of the psyche-immune and nervous system play a smaller role. If you experience these symptoms before your peers do, you are probably aging prematurely.

At about age thirty, the blood flow to your back muscles decreases, your bone-growth rate reaches its peak and begins to decline. These effects can lead to more physical symptoms such as back and knee pain after exertion. Your stomach and hips may expand and your muscles may stiffen after playing weekend sports. Your mental processes also reach their peak with the challenge—and stress—of added mental and emotional problems. Your brain begins to pull away from the cortex, shrinks slightly, and loses some of its cells. This can contribute to slower reaction times, increased absentmindedness, memory loss, and sleeplessness. As you pass from your thirties into your forties the effects of aging become more outwardly obvious: graying hair and wrinkling skin as the result of reduced blood circulation of nutrients and loss of moisture and elasticity.

In your forties, you become aware of such fatal diseases as cancer and heart disease, because your older friends and family members are contracting them. At this age most of us can now be persuaded to change our lifestyles and eating habits, and to get more exercise and medical checkups because we want to live longer and avoid disabling illnesses.

Men age more slowly (perhaps ten years slower) in their musculoskeletal and skin system than women do. A man's bones are thicker and stay thicker longer; his skin looks younger and less wrinkled because it's thicker and contains more oils. His shape retains a more youthful appearance longer because it contains up to one-third less body fat than a woman's body. And, historically, men are more physically active throughout their early lives.

On the other hand, women maintain their cardiovascular respiratory health longer.

A woman will get heart and artery disease ten years later than a man will. She will also die from a heart attack or stroke at a more advanced age than a man. But these male-female differences are being blurred as men and women are sharing the major diseases more equally, showing that many so-called "inherent differences" can be erased by doing the same amount of physical activity, eating the same foods, and working the same jobs.

Middle age also presents some of the biggest challenges of your life: parenting your children, caring for your aging parents, growing work-related stress from greater job responsibilities. Middle age is also the time when most diseases and disorders begin to surface.

In your fifties, you will probably begin to look at your alcohol and caffeine consumption, conclude it's too much and, maybe, cut back or quit altogether. You also begin to take cholesterol and/or blood pressure medicines and make more frequent visits to doctors. Some of your male and female friends (who smoke) will probably die young from a heart attack, stroke, or cancer.

TABLE 2.4
OLDER MIDDLE-AGE DISEASE ONSET: AGES 40–59

Ages 40–49

Nervous System Disorders

brain tumor (slightly more men, ages 40–60)

glaucoma (age 40+)

legionnaires' disease (middle-age to elderly men)

amyotrophic lateral sclerosis (Lou Gehrig's disease) (ages 40–70)

Parkinson's disease (30% men, under age 50)

Muscle and Bone Disorders

herniated disk (men, age 45)

osteoarthritis (age 45+)

Digestive Disorders

diverticulosis (men, age 40+)

rectal prolapse (men, under age 40+)

Heart, Lung, and Blood Vessel Disorders

pulmonary hypertension (ages 20–40)

Hormone and Gland Disorders

diabetes mellitus type II, non-insulin-dependent (starts around age 40, especially with obesity)

Cancer

basal cell (skin) (age 40+)

brain tumor (mostly ages 40–60+)

colon (risks higher age 40+)

kidney (2% of all cancers; 66% men, usually age 40+)

lung (smokers, age 40+)

multiple myeloma (bone marrow) (mostly age 40+)

stomach (men 40+)

Immune Disorders

chronic fatigue syndrome (mostly women, under age 45)

Ages 50–59

Heart and Blood Vessel Disorders

aortic aneurysms (80% men, ages 50–80)

high blood pressure onset (women, 50+)

Nervous System Disorders

Parkinson's disease (60% men, age 50+)

Muscle and Bone Disorders

gout (women, past menopause)

Digestive Disorders

colitis (women, ages 55–60)

cirrhosis of the liver

Kidney and Urinary Disorders

enlarged prostate (most men, age 50+)

prostatitis (inflammation of the prostate)

Kidney and Urinary Tract Infections

renal (kidney artery) hypertension (more common under age 30 and age 50+)

Cancer

bladder (men, age 50+)

breast (mostly women, often age 50+)

Hodgkin's disease (age 50+ and ages 15–38)

laryngeal (voice box) (men, ages 50–65)

malignant melanoma (peaks ages 50–70)

prostate (men, age 50+)

OLDER AGE

Older age (sixty to one hundred-ten years—particularly from sixty to seventy-five years of age—called "young-old" by gerontologists) is the age range when fatal and serious diseases surface (e.g. cancer, diabetes, glaucoma, heart disease, heart attack, and stroke). Exercise, even if you start later on in life, will take the edge off both the symptoms and the trauma and stress of managing these diseases. Lifelong exercisers will now receive a payoff; their diagnoses are often not as serious, not now and maybe never, as they might have been.

In your sixties, counting yourself lucky to be among the survivors, you continue trying to control your weight while nursing the wounds caused by major diseases such as emphysema, cancer (lung, prostate, or breast), or heart disease. More of your male friends and relatives have died from their second heart attack or from cancer. If you are not living under a death watch, you may be experiencing a crippling physical disability or chronic pain caused by the early onset of rheumatoid arthritis, Parkinson's or Alzheimer's disease. In fact, the ultimate disease of old age is Alzheimer's: more than 10% of adults ages 65 and older may have some form of it and about 50% of these are sixty-five to eighty-five years old—the other 50% are over 85.

This period of your life is the time when your nervous system and psyche-immune system suffer the greatest challenges: depression, retirement, loss of spouse, and the realization of growing old. Exercise can add structure to your life and help you cope and develop a positive attitude. For many, an exercise break takes the place of a drink.

TABLE 2.5
OLDER-AGE DISEASE ONSET:
Ages 60–69

Nervous System Disorders

Alzheimer's disease (age 65+, 5% have severe dementia; 12% have mild dementia)

Parkinson's disease (1 in 100 age 60+, 60,000 cases per year)

Cancer

liver (age 60+, more men; women's incidence increases with age)

squamous cell (white men, age 60+)

TABLE 2.6
OLD-AGE DISEASE ONSET:
Ages 70+

Nervous System Disorders

Alzheimer's disease (age 85+)

Eye Disorders

macular degeneration (age 70+)

cataracts (age 70+)

In your seventies, you will attend the funerals of your friends who have succumbed to congestive heart failure or prostate cancer, just as you once attended their birthday and anniversary parties. Don't think you can rest on the laurels of a strong constitution because there are more obstacles yet to overcome. And it's still not too late to make changes. Weight control is probably not a problem. Now it's just the opposite: Feeling fragile with thinning bones and muscles, you're concerned with either maintaining or gaining weight and preventing falls. The feeling of frailty and, perhaps, helplessness continues through your eighties and nineties as you probably become a patient or client of a care giver, whether living at home or in a nursing facility.

Diseases of the nervous system also define this "older age" group. These involve diseases of the nerve fibers in the brain that interfere with the transmission of nerve impulses. Systematically, these diseases affect sensory perception and motor control including balance and coordination, sight, hearing, gait, bone density, and muscle size and strength. Your whole body can become a smaller or weaker version of your former self. These musculoskeletal weaknesses are the areas most correctable, even reversible, through exercise. This is particularly true for seniors. With the proper effort, you can regain the strength and vigor of someone up to twenty years younger if you are between sixty and seventy-five years old; if you are between seventy-five and ninety years old, you could regain five to ten years of strength and vigor. The self-confidence that grows from being more fit will help you cope with the more debilitating diseases, including those of the nervous system. Many older Americans have lost their mobility and independence and they also have a fear of injury from accidents. Increased strength and vigor can help them regain their independence, confidence, and ability to function.

The drying out or stiffening effects of age also affects your blood vessels and arteries. **Atherosclerosis,** or "hardening of the arteries," is a disease characterized by slower blood flow and higher blood pressure resulting from increased friction in clogged and brittle arteries. Blood pressure seems to go up as you age, even without the presence of a particular disease. Atherosclerosis compounds this problem.

In any case, exercise—especially of the cardiovascular or continuous motion variety (e.g. bicycling, swimming, and walking)—reverses the "hardening" process by opening up narrowed arteries and thereby increasing blood flow, reducing the viscosity (or thickness) of blood, and, ultimately reducing blood pressure. It's difficult to measure, but exercising the arteries may also make them more flexible and supple, much the same as stretching and strengthening your muscles and tendons. Increased blood flow from cardio exercise acts like a massage to the artery walls and also leads to the formation of more blood vessels that help carry the blood to and from your organs and muscles.

If that isn't enough to sell you on its merits, then listen to this: Exercise burns off excess fat that reduces the relative work load of your heart and lowers your blood pressure, too. (Being overweight is another major cause of high blood pressure.)

SLOWER BLOOD FLOW

The slowing of blood flow to muscles and organs is a natural part of the aging process. When blood flow slows and decreases, the flow of nutrients and oxygen also slows. This may, in turn, slow down the functions and cell regeneration process of a particular body part or area. In this book, you've already read that slower blood flow to the back area in men over age thirty-five leads to more pain and less flexibility in those muscles. Did you also know that decreased blood circulation is linked to varicose veins, phlebitis, and intermittent claudication (i.e. calf cramps from inadequate blood and oxygen flow to lower limbs)? Reduced blood flow in reproductive organs is also linked to the decline in fertility in women over age thirty-five.

For middle-age women, exercise can also prevent complications and reduce the side effects of pregnancy. Stronger stomach and lower back muscles and a fitter heart, lungs, and circulatory system can prepare a woman for middle-age childbirth and help avoid such complications as diabetes, hypertension, heart disease, while also reducing the need for a cesarean section. Stronger muscles can also reduce some of the side effects and symptoms of severe premenstrual syndrome (PMS) and menopause.

For men, exercise also has an effect on the reproductive system, particularly during middle and old age. Moderate exercise can increase the level of testosterone and, in turn, enhance sexual performance. It also strengthens resistance to physical fatigue and stress—two major causes of impotence and the ability to maintain an erection.

YOUR AGE—NERVOUS SYSTEM PROFILE

After reading about these various scenarios, don't you wish you had a crystal ball to tell you how your own life might turn out? Well, you have one—of sorts. You have the knowledge of the general risks of aging prematurely, as well as the personal risks of your family health history. From the age-risk factors, you have learned what the average person can expect at the various stages or decades of life. From genetic (family) and gender-risk factors, you have discovered more specifically what you as a man or woman can expect as the descendant of your parents and grandparents.

To determine how much age exercise you should be doing, rate your age health and weaknesses using the Age–Nervous System Profile. If you rate I, II, or III, practice the Age Preventive Exercises in Part Two. If you rate IV or V, practice the Age Rehab program in Part Three. By taking the extra time to answer the medical questionnaires which follow each of the next four chapters, you will be able to find out which body areas and systems are your weakest. Armed with this knowledge, you can then move on to creating an exercise prescription to 1) help you head off problems entirely, 2) prevent existing conditions and symptoms from getting worse, and/or 3) manage the symptoms associated with a vast array of diseases and disorders.

Your Medical Profile Questionnaire

For the Aging System Profile below and the four health system profiles that follow in Chapters Three through Six, circle each of the major risk factors that apply to you and multiply the number of these factors by the number of point values assigned to each category. Total up your points for the category before continuing on to the next category. You may also use this questionnaire to evaluate the medical risk factors of a child or adult under your care and supervision. The final score will determine which of the five health systems are the weakest. These are the areas on which you should concentrate your Exercise Rx program.

The average score for each health system, serious disease, or disorder can range from 1 to 5. A score of 1 or 2 points is low risk, 3 points shows a moderate risk, and 4 to 5 points illustrates a high risk. Scores of 4 or 5 require a rehabilitative exercise. Scores of 1 to 3 may only require a preventive or therapeutic solution (Exercises are found in Part Two).

If your risk factor is highest in the Age–Nervous System—an Age ExRx Comprehensive will help you turn back your biological clock and alleviate such physical symptoms as lack of balance and coordination that are the result of being out of shape.

First, rate each of your five systems by answering the questions at the end of Chapters Two through Six. Next, enter your five health system scores and ratings below. Then add your total score and divide by five to convert your average score to an overall health rating. You now have an overall rating as well as a system-specific rating to start your Exercise Rx.

	Score	***Rating***
1. Age System	_____	_____
2. MuSkel System	_____	_____
3. Meta System	_____	_____
4. Cardio System	_____	_____
5. Psyche-Immune System	_____	_____

Total Score ______ /5 systems = Overall Health Rating ______

Age–Nervous System Profile

Compute your age-risk factor by rating the severity of your diseases, symptoms, and physical weaknesses on a scale of 1 point (least severe) to 5 points (most severe). Average your points and convert your averages to an overall rating that corresponds to the intensity or difficulty level for which you will begin your prevention or rehabilitation exercises. Please note: No answer equals a score of 0.

1. Rate your age-risk factor
Score: ____

Fill in the blank with the point value that corresponds to your age or that of your child/patient.

Age Group	*Point Value*
0–19 yrs.	1
20–29	2
30–39	3
40–59	4
60+	5

2. Rate your gender-risk factor by adding, averaging, and rating the two figures asked for below.
Average Score: ____

a. Rate your early onset gender disease-risk factors
Average Score: ____

Circle the gender-specific aging diseases you already have (or have had), and then circle their corresponding point value. The average onset age is shown in parentheses after each disease. Example: amyotrophic lateral sclerosis (Lou Gehrig's Disease) (ages 40–70). For those illnesses without an average age, score the level of disability from 1 (least severe) to 5 (most severe).

Disease Onset	*Point Value*
Later than norm	1
Within the norm	2
Up to 5 yrs. before	3
5–10 yrs. before	4
10+ yrs. before	5

Common or Predominantly Male Diseases					
brain tumor (40–50)	1	2	3	4	5
cerebral palsy (boys at birth)	1	2	3	4	5
amytrophic lateral sclerosis (Lou Gehrig's disease) (40–70)	1	2	3	4	5

Parkinson's disease	1	2	3	4	5
peripheral nerve degeneration (30–50)	1	2	3	4	5

Common or Predominantly Female Diseases

multiple sclerosis (20–40; avg. 27)	1	2	3	4	5
myasthenia gravis (20–40)	1	2	3	4	5
trigeminal neuralgia (age 40+)	1	2	3	4	5

Total Score ____ ÷ # of Items (that apply to you) ____ = Average Score ____

b. Rate your life expectancy (optional)
Average Score: ____

This category may be difficult to research because of the dispersion of families and lack of access to death records. Nevertheless, if the information is available, it can help you predict life expectancy. Circle how many premature (before age 60) deaths occurred among same sex, close blood relations. (Please note: Only count grandparents, parents, and their siblings, and your siblings).

Death By Early Onset Of Disease	***Point Value***
No early deaths	1
1–2 deaths	2
3 deaths	3
4 deaths	4
5+ deaths	5

3. Rate your age-related genetic, inherited disease-risk factors
Average Score: ____

Circle and score the severity of any inherited age-related diseases that you already have (or have had) or that a close relative may have (or have had). (Only count grandparents, parents, their siblings, and your siblings related by blood.) Next, circle the corresponding point value. The average onset age is shown in parentheses after each disease. Example: Alzheimer's (65+). For those illnesses without an average onset age, score the level of disability from 1 (least severe) to 5 (most severe).

Disease Onset	*Point Value*
Later than norm	1
Within the norm	2
Up to 5 yrs. before	3
5–10 yrs. before	4
10+ yrs. before	5

Alzheimer's disease (65+)	1	2	3	4	5
glaucoma (40+)	1	2	3	4	5
migraines (early childhood or adolescence)	1	2	3	4	5

Total Score ____ ÷ # of Items (that apply to you) ____ = Average Score ____

4. Rate your age-related health habits- and addiction-risk factors
Average Score: ____

Circle and score the severity of age-related habits and addictions from 1 (least severe) to 5 (most severe).

hygiene neglect	1	2	3	4	5
reckless driving	1	2	3	4	5

List and rate any others

______________________	1	2	3	4	5
______________________	1	2	3	4	5
______________________	1	2	3	4	5

Total Score ____ ÷ # of Items ____ = Average Score ____

5. **Rate your age-related personality trait-risk factors**
Average Score: ____

Circle and score your unhealthy age-related personality traits from 1 (least severe) to 5 (most severe).

absentmindedness	1	2	3	4	5
accident proneness	1	2	3	4	5
attention deficiency	1	2	3	4	5
carelessness	1	2	3	4	5

List and rate any others

____________________	1	2	3	4	5
____________________	1	2	3	4	5
____________________	1	2	3	4	5

Total Score ____ ÷ # of Items (that apply to you) ____ = Average Score ____

6. **Rate your age-related environmental risk factors**
Average Score: ____

Circle and score the unhealthy environmental risk factors that apply from 1 (least severe) to 5 (most severe).

cluttered living space	1	2	3	4	5
living alone	1	2	3	4	5

List and rate any others

____________________	1	2	3	4	5
____________________	1	2	3	4	5
____________________	1	2	3	4	5

Total Score ____ ÷ # of Items (that apply to you) ____ = Average Score ____

7. Rate your age-related diseases- and injuries-risk factors
Average Score: ____

Circle any of the major aging diseases and injuries you may have experienced, and then circle the corresponding point value. The average onset age is shown in parentheses after each disease. Example: Alzheimer's (65+). For those illnesses without an average age, score the level of disability from 1 (least severe) to 5 (most severe).

Disease Onset	***Point Value***
Later than norm	1
Within the norm	2
Up to 5 yrs. before	3
5–10 yrs. before	4
10+ yrs. before	5

Nervous System					
Alzheimer's (65+)	1	2	3	4	5
cerebral palsy (early age)	1	2	3	4	5
epilepsy (any age)	1	2	3	4	5
headaches	1	2	3	4	5
memory problems (50)	1	2	3	4	5
migraines	1	2	3	4	5
stroke (65)	1	2	3	4	5

Sensory, Balance, Ear, and Nose					
hearing loss	1	2	3	4	5
middle ear infection	1	2	3	4	5
Meniere's disease (vertigo, ringing, hearing loss)	1	2	3	4	5
motion sickness	1	2	3	4	5
nose bleeds	1	2	3	4	5

Eyes

macular degeneration (71+)	1	2	3	4	5
cataract (71+)	1	2	3	4	5
vision loss	1	2	3	4	5

Total Score ____ ÷ # of Items (that apply to you) ____ = Average Score ____

8. Rate your age-related symptoms-risk factor
Average Score: ____

Circle and score the severity of the symptoms of aging already present from 1 (least severe) to 5 (most severe).

inability to concentrate	1	2	3	4	5
poor posture	1	2	3	4	5
poor balance	1	2	3	4	5
poor coordination	1	2	3	4	5
poor mobility	1	2	3	4	5

List and rate any others

____________________	1	2	3	4	5
____________________	1	2	3	4	5
____________________	1	2	3	4	5

Total Score ____ ÷ # of Items ____ = Average Score ____

9. Rate your physical condition- and fitness-risk factor (e.g. biological vs. chronological age)
Average Biological Age: ____

You will have to wait until you complete the MuSkel and Cardio system profiles (in Chapters Three and Five) to determine biological age because it is based on ratings you will determine there. Average the test scores for muscle strength and flexibility (MuSkel) and aerobic endurance (Cardio).

muscle strength age (MuSkel ques. #9f, page 56): ____

flexibility age (MuSkel ques. #9g, page 57): ____

exercise endurance age (Cardio ques. #10, page 116): ____

Total Age ____ ÷ 3 Items ____ = Average Biological Age ____

Now, compare the average biological age to chronological age, and compute the difference in number of years (plus or minus) and choose one of the following ratings:

Rating

1 Excellent fitness—10–20 yrs. more fit than age group.

2 Very good fitness—5–10 yrs. more fit than age group.

3 Good fitness—Fit for age to 5 yrs. more fit than age group.

4 Fair fitness—5–10 yrs. less fit than age group.

5 Poor fitness—10–30 yrs. less fit than age group.

10. Rate your lifetime exercise- and activity level-risk factor
Average Score: ____

Circle and score your lifetime exercise level from age thirteen to the present. Exercise includes any physical activity done for more than twenty minutes. Ideally, this should be a subjective measurement of the normal activity level for 75% of your life or more. If less than 75%, reduce this rating by one point for every segment of your life where you were inactive for five or more consecutive years.

Lifetime Activity	***Score***
exercise 5+ days/wk.	1
exercise 3–5 days/wk.	2
exercise 1–3 days/wk.	3
exercise 1 day/2 wks.	4
rarely exercise	5

PROFILE SUMMARY

Take the time to compute the average score for each category, then convert it to a risk rating (which you will use later) as follows:

Average Score	*Risk Rating*
0.0–1.4	I
1.5–2.4	II
2.5–3.4	III
3.5–4.4	IV
4.5–5.0	V

Write in the average scores and converted ratings for all ten risk factor categories, then compute your overall average aging score:

Risk Categories	*Average Score*	*Converted Rating*
1. Age	_____	_____
2. Gender	_____	_____
3. Genetic	_____	_____
4. Habits and addictions	_____	_____
5. Personality traits	_____	_____
6. Environment	_____	_____
7. Diseases and injuries	_____	_____
8. Symptoms	_____	_____
9. Physical condition and fitness	_____	_____
10. Exercise and activity	_____	_____

Total Score ____ ÷ 10 ____ = Average Age System Score ____

CHAPTER 3

One Wrong Move Can Cost a Lifetime

Why Thicker Bones Are Better than Thinner Thighs

Musculoskeletal and Skin System

The **musculoskeletal and skin system (MuSkel)** is the body's frame and shield against disease and injury and is also the system most susceptible to disease and injury. It contains the largest number of parts—more than 650 muscles, over 100 tendons, more than 200 bones, and over fifty joints, all covered by the largest organ of the body: the skin. The skin's role is to protect the body against external infections, to protect the blood vessels, and to hold organs and fluids inside your body. But, as you will see, the major features of the MuSkel system are the joints of the arms, shoulders, back, hips, and legs, and the cartilage and bones that make up these joints.

MuSkel health is not about athletic prowess: It's about building up bone density and muscle mass. At one time, the traditional, competitive approach to sports training included such exercises as weight lifting and running to condition athletes for competition on the playing field (and prior to that, the battlefield). This sports training eventually became exercise training and evolved into long-distance running for cardiovascular conditioning, and calisthenics and bodybuilding for body shaping. Along the way, the basic body strengthening and conditioning was left behind. Our health concerns then followed this new path, for example, sports medicine emphasized quickly fixing broken bones, rather than keeping them from breaking. In this highly charged, competitive environment, many sports enthusiasts stopped playing sports and turned into

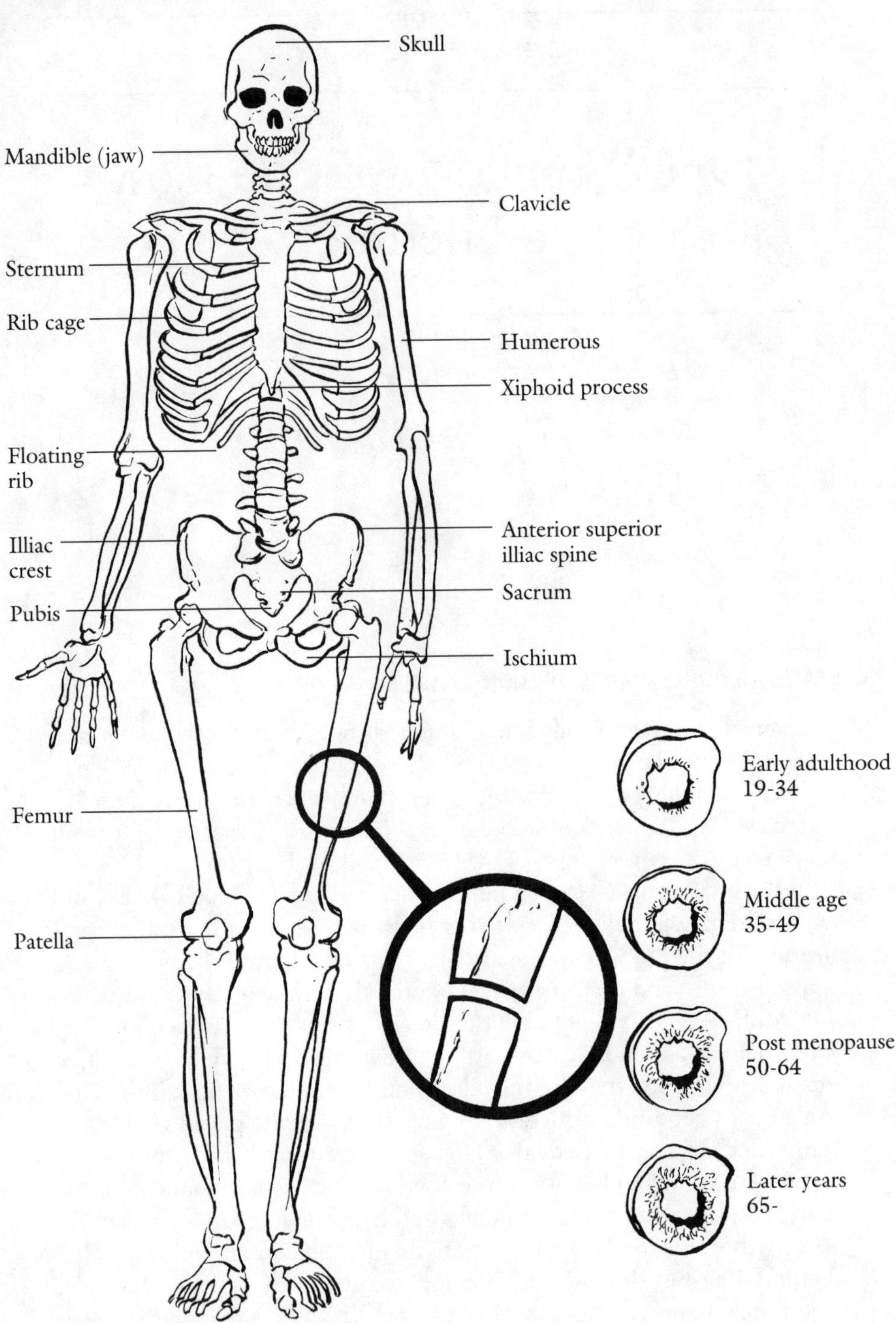

Human Skeletal System (front)

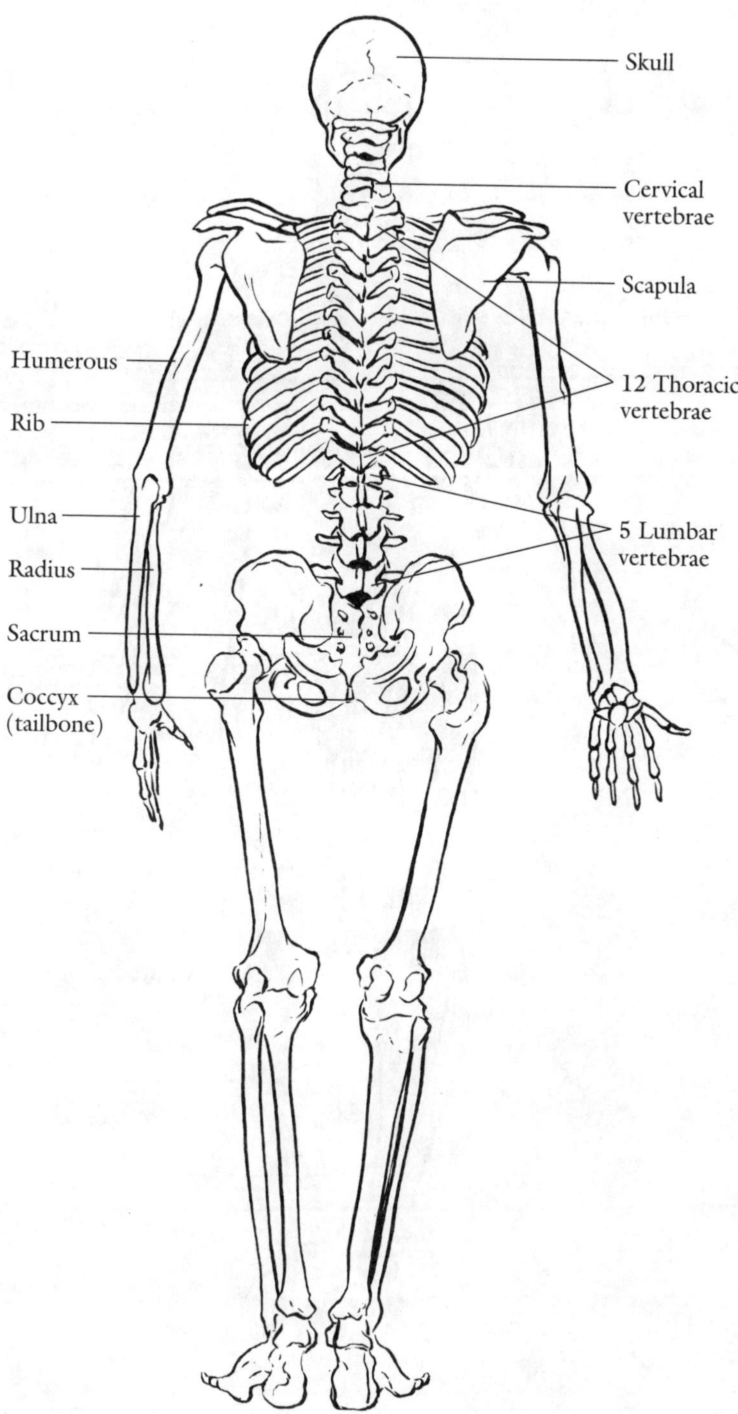

Human Skeletal System (back)

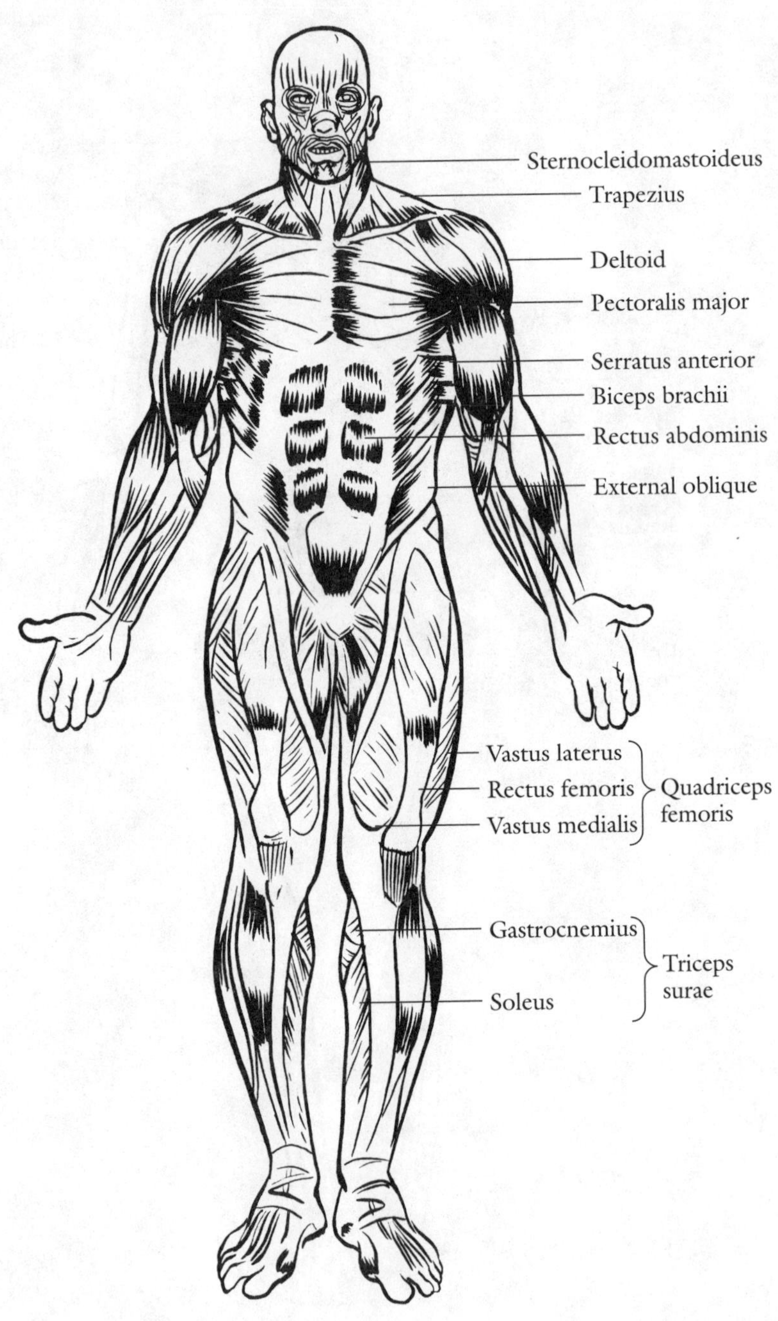

Human Muscle Groups (front)

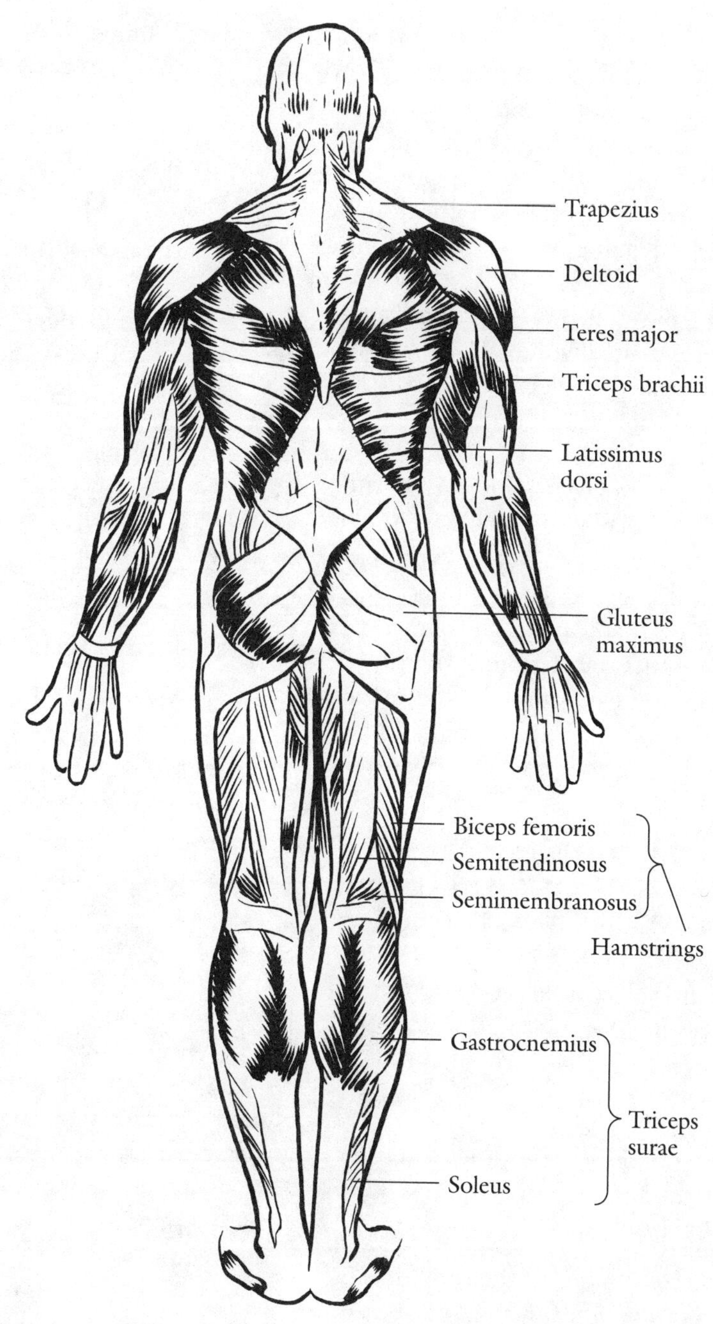

Human Muscle Groups (back)

spectators. We are evolving into a nation of injured athletes and couch potatoes, both types at great risk of compromising their health. The injured athlete has chronic pain from broken bones and pulled tendons that have never healed properly. The couch potatoes have let their bones and muscles grow thin. The body shapers may also have let their bones grow thin by neglecting weight-bearing exercises in favor of floor and mat exercises. All have neglected the basics of building a body frame and health system that will last a lifetime.

The *Exercise Rx* approach for strengthening the musculoskeletal body system does more good than harm and causes the fewest injuries by finding the safest limits on the amount of stress that you put on your working body. These limits translate into the number of repetitions you can safely do, the amount of work load you can perform, in addition to an evenly balanced body coverage of exercise.

TABLE 3.1
MAJOR MUSCULOSKELETAL AND SKIN DISEASES AND INJURIES

For Men: Mainly wear and tear to their joints (women who lead athletic/active lifestyles are equally susceptible to joint injuries):

- impact and stress injuries to the weight-bearing joints, such as knees, back, hips, and ankles
- overuse injuries to the shoulders, wrists, and arms, which make men more susceptible to osteoporosis, soft tissue conditions such as tendinitis, impingement, and bursitis.
- osteoarthritis

For Women: Mostly bone thinning, which makes them susceptible to:

- osteoporosis (men who are alcoholics or lead sedentary lives are also threatened)
- rheumatoid arthritis

For Both Genders: Lower back pain, which both sexes get from back strain caused by increased body weight that is supported by weakened back muscles; extra weight carried during pregnancy can also contribute to women's lower back pain.

MuSkel Symptoms and Injuries

The musculoskeletal and skin system is composed of two types of interconnected body tissue: (1) **fibrous** or **connective tissues,** which include muscles, tendons, ligaments, skin, and bones, and (2) **cushioning materials,** which include joints, bones, cartilage, and fluid sacs.

Exercise can build, stretch, and nourish the system tissues, prevent or reduce pain symptoms caused by injury and disease, and promote tissue and cellular regeneration. Musculoskeletal symptoms are not just the early signs of conditions, disorders, and diseases, but also are indicative of body weaknesses that exercise can help correct.

Muscles, tendons, and joints also express early symptoms of overexertion or misuse by becoming achy, sore, or tender to the touch. These are early signs that you should stop and rest for a while and stretch or massage the achy or sore area(s). Often, stretching or massaging will alleviate the temporary discomfort—as will the conditioning or hardening effect of a regular exercise program. If symptoms persist, however, they may be a sign that you are doing too much and are not within the safety limits of your exercise program. If this is the case, drop down a level. **A general rule: If any symptoms (i.e. pain, soreness, tenderness) persist more than five days, you should consult a physician.**

Moreover, if you are too sore and achy to move easily the following day, you probably did too much; after a day of rest, you should exercise again but at a lower level. Whatever you do, don't regress into a life of inactivity!

Symptoms caused by inactivity can become more serious the longer you are inactive. At the low end of the symptoms scale are those that arise upon the start of an exercise program. If you build up your activity gradually (in increments of no more than 10% per week) these symptoms will remain minimal and will eventually disappear as your body strengthens. If you overexert yourself by increasing the speed, intensity (i.e. work load), or duration of your activity, then your body will signal its objection with immediate "hot-spots": joint and muscle soreness accompanied by such cardio symptoms as breathlessness and overheating (see Chapter Four for more details.) These symptoms indicate that it is time to stop and rest, or perhaps to cut back on your activity level to avoid more serious pain or injury. Contrary to the "jock" approach to sports and exercise, **you should never work through pain.**

SYMPTOMS: A CLOSER LOOK

Each of the five parts of your musculoskeletal system—joints and bones, muscles, tendons, ligaments, and skin—can develop symptoms. Because the parts are connected, the symptoms are often related. The following three lists are: (1) the symptoms and injuries to joints and bones, (2) symptoms and injuries to muscles and connective tissues; and (3) the benefits of exercise to the MuSkel system. The first two lists are ranked in order from least severe (e.g. 1 or 2) to most severe (e.g. 13 or 14).

Joints and Bones Symptoms and Injuries

1. Cartilage depletion (least severe)
2. Bone fraying
3. Bone calcification
4. Bone spur formation
5. Joint inflammation
6. Joint swelling
7. Bursitis
8. Disk flattening
9. Disk herniation
10. Disk rupture
11. Bone chipping
12. Bone break
13. Joint break
14. Bone stress fracture (most severe)

Muscle and Connective Tissue Symptoms and Injuries

1. Skin softening and/or hot-spots (least severe)
2. Skin tenderness to touch
3. Muscle stiffness and/or soreness
4. Muscle tenderness to touch
5. Muscle cramp

6. Tendinitis (inflammation)
7. Tendon strain
8. Muscle strain
9. Tendon pull
10. Muscle pull
11. Muscle spasm
12. Tendon tear
13. Ligament tear
14. Muscle tear (most severe)

What Kind of MuSkel Exercises Are the Most Effective?

The best overall exercises for the MuSkel system are those performed with the least impact and least "shearing" (i.e. sideways) forces levied against the joints. The best *preventive* exercises are arm, leg, and torso movements, which use resistance, and are done slowly through the full range-of-joint motion. This translates into posture, stretching, and strengthening exercises. The best *rehabilitative* exercises are balancing, range-of-motion, isometric and slow-motion strengthening exercises. All of these exercises should be performed with proper body alignment (called **posture training**) to allow for full range of motion, balanced muscle and bone development, and the least amount of stress on joints and tendons.

The best rehabilitative, continuous exercises include "water exercise," sliding machines, bicycling and walking, all of which involve forces that do not exceed one and a half times your body weight. Initially, these continuous exercises are performed with greater body weight support (e.g. in water or with seat support), gradually progressing to

MUSKEL BENEFITS OF EXERCISE

1. Exercise strengthens the whole system—skin, muscle, bones, ligaments, joints, tendons, cartilage, vertebrae, and disks—by bringing a fresh flow of blood, nutrients, and fluids (i.e. water and lubrication by way of synovial fluid), and by washing away waste products and infectious organisms.
2. Lifelong exercise thickens bones, which counteracts the natural thinning process caused by aging.
3. Weight-bearing and resistance exercise strengthens and regenerates thin bones.
4. Stretching and range-of-motion exercise improves the function, reaction time, and mobility of the entire MuSkel system.
5. Muscle strengthening exercise improves strength, balance, coordination, and stability.
6. Well-conditioned muscles are less susceptible to cramping, spasms, and strain.
7. Well-lubricated, stronger joints and more flexible tendons and ligaments are less apt to be injured or to stiffen or become inflamed.

increase the weight load on arms, legs, and hips. As muscles and bones grow stronger, the exercise position changes to upright with full body-weight support.

The worst exercises are those that involve any force that exceeds more than one and a half times your body weight or that involve repeated, high-impact movement. The running, jumping, and bumping moves that are prevalent in jogging, basketball, football, tennis, and other running and contact sports are examples; injuries sustained in these sports can cause weeks and even months of downtime when it is difficult to move—let alone exercise. This does not mean that you should give up sports play, but, rather, you should stop thinking of sports as an exercise regimen in and of itself. The best way to use sports to stay healthy is to practice sports in moderation only after you have started conditioning your body with regular exercise. Moderation means not playing too much of such high-impact sports as football or running, and varying the sports you play to avoid putting too much stress on one body area, for example, elbow joints in tennis or shoulder joints in baseball.

Remember that the forces of impact are not only created by collisions with the ground, other players, or from batting or kicking a ball, they are also caused internally by the muscles working against joints during the course of playing sports. For example, although the overall impact of a running step on the hip and ankle joints is two to three times greater than that of a walking step, it has six times more impact on the knees. This is a result of the additional force exerted by the quadriceps to raise and lower your body two to three feet off the ground as you bend and straighten your legs to jump off the ground and land on each foot and leg. Both these impact and shear forces can be reduced with safer running techniques (see page 229).

Of course, strengthening and stretching the muscles that surround the joints helps to cushion them against impact. Muscles provide only a limited cushioning effect, however; they fatigue after repeated movements and become less resilient, requiring more of your body weight to be supported by your joints.

Using a stationary bicycle offers many of the same cardiovascular benefits and lower body range-of-motion effects as jogging, but decreases the weight on your legs and hips by at least half by letting the bicycle seat, rather than your body, support your weight.

The term "water exercise" means stretching, strengthening, range-of-motion, and walking exercise performed in water. Swimming and water exercise cut the weight-bearing effects even further by letting the water support your body. This lack of weight does decrease the stimulation your bones receive, however, and presumably also reduces the degree to which bones grow stronger, but it makes for effective and safe rehabilitative exercises. When joints, muscles, or bones have been damaged and are painful and inflamed, such low-weight-bearing exercises as swimming and stationary bicycling makes exercise possible without bringing the full body weight to bear on a damaged area.

Although walking is one of the best preventive exercises for strengthening the muscles of the lower back and those that surround the hip, knee, and ankle joints, it is not as effective as stretching and strengthening exercises for rehabilitating those same areas after they have been damaged. This is because the impact of walking on muscle groups is generalized and not specific to a particular joint.

THE MAJOR WEAK SPOTS

With age, our muscles shorten, causing reduced strength and range of motion. Aches, pains, and stiffness in your muscles and joints will multiply and make you prone to joint and muscle injuries. If not properly rehabilitated, injured areas can easily be injured again.

After becoming weakened, your body is far less prepared to deal with physical exertion and the side effects and complications of major diseases. Joints, muscles, tendons, and bones are not only threatened by overuse and high impact, but also by such major diseases as arthritis (especially osteoarthritis), rheumatoid arthritis, osteoporosis, multiple sclerosis, and Parkinson's disease. **Rheumatoid arthritis** inflames the joints; **osteoarthritis** is the breakdown of cartilage around bone resulting from the normal aging process and is aggravated by falls, injuries, or **osteoporosis,** which is the thinning and weakening of bones caused by loss of calcium and phosphates. Such nervous system diseases as **Parkinson's disease** and **multiple sclerosis** cut off nerve impulses to muscles, disabling and causing them to become rigid and spastic. These dysfunctional muscles make movement difficult and reduce the physical activity needed to keep bones and joints healthy. Lifelong exercise can help you lessen the effects of any of these diseases by delaying their onset and slowing their progress. Even after a disease strikes, you can use rehabilitative exercises to regain a substantial amount of mobility.

BONE LOSS

Because the hips, wrists, and backbone contain the highest percentage of the more porous **trabecular** bone, rather than the denser **cortical** bone, they are the bones usually involved in osteoporosis.

Women are at a greater risk for osteoporosis than men because their initial bone mass is smaller; also traditionally, women have been less athletic throughout life, giving them less opportunity to build up bones. In addition to this factor, after menopause, women lose bone mass at three times the rate they did before. Such unhealthy habits and addictions such as alcoholism and overexercising can also damage bones. Alcoholic men and young athletic women increasingly run the same risk as older women when it comes to premature bone thinning.

Remember: Bones do not have to break completely to cause damage. Often bones remain intact but develop hairline fractures that can weaken the bone's structure and can also be very painful. For example, many bone pain complaints arise from stress fractures in the vertebrae of the spinal column.

Your spinal column is composed of vertabrae that are bones. But the bones that constitute the rest of your musculoskeletal system, namely your hips, pelvis, thighs, shins, and ankles, are also at risk from weakening caused by lack of physical activity and to the natural bone-thinning process that accompanies aging. Next in line is your rib cage, which can crack as easily as your spine as soon as bone thinning has reached a dangerous level.

BONE EXERCISE PRINCIPLES

Scientists now know that bones can only be kept strong by activity and exercise. Even though calcium tablets and eating foods rich in calcium is a good idea, that calcium will not be absorbed into the body without an accompanying exercise program.

When it comes to your medical health, bone strengthening is even more important than muscle strengthening. Indeed, strong muscles tug on the bones they are attached to and stimulate their regeneration. By exercising regularly over a lifetime, you can build up your bone mass to counteract the natural bone-thinning process.

The best exercises to prevent bone thinning are performed while standing to give the bones of your lower body the added resistance of your own body weight. This way, the stimulation effect is increased each time your foot touches the ground. Such high-impact exercises as jogging and dancing can also stimulate bone growth, but do so at the risk of causing joint damage and stress fractures.

To rehabilitate a broken bone or stress fracture, begin with slow to moderate range-of-motion exercises accompanied by moderate cardio exercises performed by the parts of your body that are still whole. This will increase blood flow to the damaged bone and stimulate the healing process. After the bone has healed sufficiently, you can begin to add more steps to stimulate the bone healing and regeneration process.

Muscles and Tendons

Lack of use reduces the blood flow to muscle tissue, and, hence muscles tend to atrophy and weaken. Reduced blood flow causes both reduced oxygen and nutrients and leads to undernourishment of muscle and tendon tissue.

Although muscles and tendons are the body areas that are least vulnerable to disease, they are usually among the first to be damaged by sports injuries. Muscles themselves are very nearly invulnerable, however, the tendons that attach the muscles to the bones can easily fall prey to overstretching and inflammation. **Tendinitis** occurs with overreaching, overstretching, and overusing muscles in repeated exercise and sports movements. Overuse and misuse are the greatest sources of most sports injuries. Tendinitis can be healed with rest, but repeated attacks of tendinitis will permanently damage tendon tissue that must then be surgically removed. A tendon or muscle can also be ruptured, ripped, or detached from its bone connection.

The best way to avoid muscle strains, tendinitis, and muscle damage is by not overloading or overusing any muscle and by not stretching it beyond its natural limits. To keep muscles and tendons healthy, condition them gradually with stretching and strengthening exercises, working against moderate resistance through a full range of natural motion. Only manageable amounts of stress will increase the strength and flexibility of muscles and tendons.

Joints

Your joints, the same as your car, have a limited warranty. If you abuse or overuse them, they will not fully recover. Instead, you'll bring on an earlier onset of osteoarthritis—also known as the "wear and tear" disease. A gradual disease, osteoarthritis is a combination of the natural aging process (i.e. "wear"), joint injuries from falls and blows caused by accidents and contact sports, and overuse injuries including those from high-impact exercises (i.e. "tear").

If you are fortunate to live long enough, you will probably get osteoarthritis (by age sixty-five, 80% of the population shows signs of osteoarthritis), which is a degenerative disease that strikes your hips, knees, ankles, and spine. It causes painful symptoms such as stiff, swollen, and aching joints, and the most debilitating lower back pain. (You can produce these same symptoms by injuring your joints and back while playing contact sports or doing high-impact exercises.) Osteoarthritis is a fraying of your bone ends resulting from the depletion of the smooth rubbery substance in your joints known as **cartilage.** When joint bones rub together, they form jagged lumps called **spurs.**

The exercise solution to preventing or delaying the onset of osteoarthritis is to work joints at a moderate pace with low-impact and continuous, smooth movement rather than jerking motions. Exercising your joints safely through a full range of motion will build up the flexibility of the muscles and tendons that surround your joints. This can be accomplished by safer stretching and strengthening exercises as well as walking, bicycling, and water exercise. Such high-impact and jerking movements as aerobic dancing and tennis are murder on joints.

Easy, smooth exercises will slow down cartilage depletion and promote its repair or replacement by the body. You can't preserve your joints by not exercising or moving them. Joints need movement to stimulate the flow of blood and nutrients to them and to wash away waste products. Movement also stimulates the secretion of synovial fluid that acts as a lubricant. This process is similar to getting an oil, grease, and lube job for your car. The stretching and strengthening exercises for your muscles in Part Two are organized around the key joints.

Just as cartilage acts as a cushion, strong and flexible muscles act as shock absorbers, diffusing the forces of impact before they reach the joints. However, muscles must be strengthened in a balanced way or they, too, can put too much pressure on a joint. For example, a runner's overdeveloped quadriceps muscle can pull her knee joints too far in one direction; and a bodybuilder's overdeveloped chest muscles can pull his shoulder joints too far forward.

After joint deterioration, **joint dislocation** is the second most common form of joint damage caused by sports injuries and falling accidents. Bones pop out of their joint sockets when they are subject to too much lateral or twisting stress caused by sharp turns to the body and hard contact; activities associated with lateral or twisting stress include dancing, baseball, karate, and gymnastics.

Finally, the **bursa,** located in all limb joints (i.e. arms, legs, hips), is a small, fluid-filled sac that, along with the cartilage, cushions joints against injury. Repeated joint motion can inflame the bursa, causing a condition known as **bursitis.**

BACK AND NECK

Back health is synonymous with total musculoskeletal health. It is often difficult to identify a simple cause for back pain; usually it involves a complex set of causes. Spinal abnormalities are not usually the cause. More common causes are aging or damaged disks. As you age, disks lose their water content and elasticity. Also such small joints as those in the hands become stiff and sore from arthritis. Other causes include stress fractures, ligament strains, and muscle spasms. A herniated or squeezed disk can press on or pinch a nerve and cause a radiating pain down one leg. This condition is called **sciatica.** When pain radiates down into both legs, it's usually from a condition that commonly occurs in older people called **spinal stenosis** (narrowing of the space within the spinal cord). Stenosis pain usually worsens when standing or walking. A rarer case of back and leg pain is **spondylolisthesis,** which is an instability of a section of the spine that slips backward and forward. It can worsen when you are lying down and even disturb your sleep and bowel and bladder functions. (Problems with bowel and bladder in a person with back pain may be the sign of a true emergency.)

Protecting the back is similar to protecting any joint but it's more elaborate. The neck must be grouped with the back because it is a continuation of the **spine,** which is really a series of interconnected joints, called **vertebrae.** Each vertebra is cushioned by a cartilagelike substance encased in a sac known as a **disk.**

Weak back muscles create a strain on the vertebrae when you bend over or lift something heavy. Certain sports can also injure the back and neck, particularly those that involve overarching for example, ballet dancing, figure skating, gymnastics, swimming, and weight training. Other sports, particularly those with a high number of head injuries such as horseback riding, can damage the neck.

The back also contains the most complex muscle group of the body. This complex muscle group is united by the **spinal cord,** which is a network of nerves stretching from the base of your neck all the way down your back to your **coccyx** (tailbone). The spinal cord is protected by the **spine,** which is affected by neck, upper back (e.g. rhomboids, trapezius), and lower back muscles. The lower back is also affected by your abdominal muscles and your front and back thigh muscles.

Back-strengthening exercises, therefore, include stretching and strengthening for the head and neck, shoulders, chest, stomach, lower back and upper legs, because these areas all affect the balance and alignment of the spinal cord. Low-impact aerobic exercises also keep the back strong and healthy by stimulating blood flow to the area and by involving moderate amounts of turning and bending of the spinal cord.

Spinal rehabilitation starts with bed rest for one to four days. Thereafter, the best exercises are initially done lying down. In 90% of chronic low back pain or injury, recovery takes place within one month.

SHOULDERS, ELBOWS, HANDS, AND WRISTS

The most common injuries in the upper body are **shoulder** dislocations, **elbow** tendinitis, and arthritis of the **hands** and **wrists.** Sports injuries and falling accidents are more of a threat to shoulders, elbows, hands, and wrists than the side effects of disease. Such sports that rely on the use of hand and arm movements as baseball, boxing, football, handball, squash, and racquetball, are especially dangerous. These types of injuries, even though they are painful, will not threaten your whole health system in the way that comparable lower body or back injuries might. You will still be able to exercise your heart and circulatory system using your legs by walking, arching, or walking in water. You may also be able to selectively use either your shoulder if your wrist or hand is injured, or your elbow and lower arm (by bending or extending it) if your shoulder is injured. If your foot, knee, or hip is also injured, however, it will prevent you from doing most, if not all, leg-based cardiovascular exercises. Additionally, it will take time and training to condition your arms, so that they can work by themselves continuously to raise your heart rate as much as your legs can. Rehabilitative exercises for shoulder, arm, wrist, and hand injuries are similar to preventive exercises, except they are done at a slower pace with a reduced amount of resistance.

KNEES

After the back, the **knees** are the second major musculoskeletal areas most subject to disease and injury; they are the most often injured of the group, probably because they bear more forces than any other joints. Men are more prone to suffer knee problems. However, before the age of recreational and competitive sports, both men and women experienced many fewer knee injuries. After being injured, the knee joint is more susceptible to becoming arthritic or reinjured.

The *ExRx* knee prevention exercises emphasize stretching and strengthening the front (quadriceps) and back (hamstrings) thigh muscles and avoiding high-risk movements that may injure the knee. Proper foot placement techniques (shown in Part Two), especially for walking and bicycling, can be applied to other such high-risk sports as jogging and football to help you avoid knee injuries.

HIPS

Hip joints are the third weakest area in the body, most often damaged by osteoporosis and rheumatoid arthritis (50% of patients have this disease in their hips). Such sports injuries as stress fractures (i.e. hairline cracks) among runners and impact injuries (i.e. hip pointers) among football players can also permanently damage this joint. In a young or middle-age person, it would take a very hard fall to break a hip, but in an older person with thinning bones, any fall could be quite harmful. Some doctors believe that with osteoporosis patients the hip bone can break spontaneously, thereby causing a fall. Such breaks can leave older victims of osteoporosis permanently disabled.

To strengthen the hip joint using bone strengthening and weight-bearing exercises, and to prevent hip diseases and injuries, you should also stretch and strengthen the muscles that surround the hip joint, buttocks, hip flexors and thigh muscles. To prevent falls, you should stand and move using wider foot placements. The runway model's narrow stance and foot placements and racewalker's overlapping foot placements, in addition to closed leg positions (e.g. crossing your legs when you sit) unnecessarily strain and tug at the hip joint. You can also lessen the degree that your leg and hip muscles pull at your hip joint by stretching and strengthening them in a balanced way.

After you have injured a hip, practice the same preventive exercises, only do so more carefully and slowly and when it's less painful. Hip pain can cause you to stop moving or even keep you from sitting up. For this reason alone, the hip joint is a body area that you must try to preserve and protect.

ANKLES, FEET, LOWER LEGS, AND TOES

Ankle and **lower leg** injuries are often associated with such youthful sports and activities as ballet dancing, gymnastics, soccer, running, and skiing. Sprains or breaks in the ankles are usually caused by wear and tear, but can be prevented by practicing lower leg posture exercises for foot placement and leg stance. Properly aligning your lower and upper leg before, during, and after any movement will put the least stress on the muscle joint. It is also important to stretch and strengthen the tendons and muscles that hold your leg in place—the **calf** and **shin.** At the same time that you work your ankle joint, you will be stretching and strengthening your **foot** and **toes.** Placing your feet down properly will help you work your ankle through its full range of motion with every step, slide, or pedal rotation you make.

Ankle, foot, and lower leg injuries can be fully rehabilitated, however, repeated injuries can weaken these areas. Diabetes and other joint and circulatory-related diseases, for example, rheumatoid arthritis, intermittent claudication, and Raynaud's disease often strike the lower leg most severely. The same exercises that can rehabilitate a sprained or broken ankle will help you manage the symptoms of these diseases, too

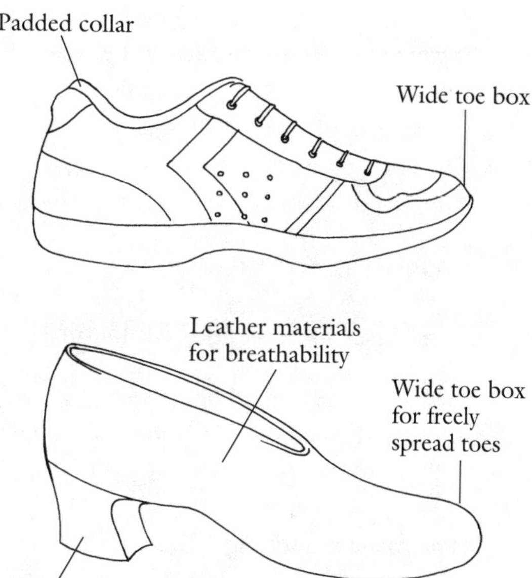

In addition to correct, low-impact, preventive or rehabilitative exercise, you should also wear proper shoes. Well-constructed exercise or walking shoes with arch supports, a roomy toe box, soft upper, firm heel counter, and, in some cases (i.e. for hiking and climbing), good ankle support, will help keep your lower leg, ankle, and foot properly aligned. Despite the claims, however, no shoe can cushion the impact caused by repeated running and jumping steps. You must switch to low-impact activities to avoid the shock effect.

YOUR MUSKEL PROFILE

To determine the amount of MuSkel exercise you should be doing, rate your MuSkel health and weaknesses using the MuSkel System Profile. If you rate I, II, or III, practice the MuSkel Preventive Exercises in Part Two. If you rate IV or V, practice the MuSkel Rehab program in Part Three.

Circle each of the major risk factors as they apply to you and multiply the number of these factors by the number of point values assigned in each category. Total up your points for the category before continuing on to the next category. You may also use this questionnaire to evaluate the medical risk factors of a child or adult under your care and supervision. The final score will ascertain which of the five health systems are the weakest and will determine where you should concentrate the *Exercise Rx* program.

MuSkel System Profile

Compute your MuSkel-risk factor by rating the severity of your diseases, symptoms, and physical weaknesses on a scale of 1 point (least severe) to 5 points (most severe). After finishing the entire MuSkel system profile questionnaire, add up all your point scores and divide by 10. Next, convert your scores and average scores to an overall rating that corresponds to the intensity or difficulty level for which you will begin your prevention or rehabilitation exercises. Please note: No answer equals a score of 0.

1. Rate your MuSkel age-risk factor
Score: ____

By comparing your subjective rating to your overall score at the end of this questionnaire, circle the score that best describes the condition of your MuSkel system or that of your child/patient.

Performance vs. Age Group	***Score***
Over 20 yrs. more fit than age group	1
10 to 20 yrs. more fit	2
Equal to age group	3
10 to 20 yrs. less fit	4
Less than 20 yrs. less fit	5

2. Rate your MuSkel gender-risk factors
Average Score: ____

Circle the gender-specific MuSkel diseases you already have (or have had), and then circle their corresponding point value using the point values listed below. The average onset age is shown in parentheses after each disease. Example: gout (30+). For those illnesses without an average onset age, score your level of disability from 1 (least severe) to 5 (most severe). If you haven't had any MuSkel disease, give yourself a 0.

Disease Onset	***Point Value***
Later than norm	1
Within the norm	2
Up to 5 yrs. before	3
5–10 yrs. before	4
10+ yrs. before	5

Common or Predominantly Male Diseases

gout (30+)	1	2	3	4	5
herniated disk (under 45)	1	2	3	4	5
larynx cancer (50–65)	1	2	3	4	5
malignant lymphomas	1	2	3	4	5
Paget's disease (40+)	1	2	3	4	5
retinal detachment	1	2	3	4	5

Common or Predominantly Female Diseases

carpal tunnel syndrome (30–60)	1	2	3	4	5
hammer toe	1	2	3	4	5
humpback, adolescent (12–16)	1	2	3	4	5
osteoporosis (50+)	1	2	3	4	5
scoliosis, adolescent (12–19)	1	2	3	4	5

Total Score ____ ÷ # of Items (that apply to you) ____ = Average Score ____

3. Rate your MuSkel genetic-risk factors
Average Score: ____

Circle and score the severity of any inherited MuSkel diseases that you already have (or have had) or that a close relative may have (or have had). (Only count grandparents, parents, their siblings, and your siblings related by blood.) Next, circle the corresponding point value. For those illnesses without an average onset age, score the level of disability from 1 (least severe) to 5 (most severe).

back problems	1	2	3	4	5
foot abnormalities	1	2	3	4	5
osteoarthritis	1	2	3	4	5
osteoporosis	1	2	3	4	5
rheumatoid arthritis (45)	1	2	3	4	5
joint problems	1	2	3	4	5

Total Score ____ ÷ # of Items (that apply to you) ____ = Average Score ____

4. Rate your MuSkel habits- and addictions-risk factors
Average Score: ____

Circle and score the severity of the MuSkel-related habits and addictions that apply to you from 1 (least severe) to 5 (most severe).

alcohol overconsumption	1	2	3	4	5
cigarette smoking	1	2	3	4	5
daredeviling	1	2	3	4	5
driving over speed limit	1	2	3	4	5
drug overconsumption	1	2	3	4	5

List and score any others

____________________	1	2	3	4	5
____________________	1	2	3	4	5
____________________	1	2	3	4	5

Total Score ____ ÷ # of Items (that apply to you)____ = Average Score ____

5. Rate your MuSkel personality traits-risk Factors
Average Score: ____

Circle and score your unhealthy MuSkel-related personality traits from 1 (least severe) to 5 (most severe).

accident-prone	1	2	3	4	5
careless	1	2	3	4	5
reckless	1	2	3	4	5
sloppy	1	2	3	4	5
violent	1	2	3	4	5

List and score any others

________________________	1	2	3	4	5
________________________	1	2	3	4	5
________________________	1	2	3	4	5

Total Score ____ ÷ # of Items (that apply to you) ____ = Average Score ____

6. Rate your MuSkel environmental risk factors
Average Score: ____

Circle and score the unhealthy environmental risk factors that apply to you from 1 (least severe) to 5 (most severe).

cluttered living space	1	2	3	4	5
strenuous job	1	2	3	4	5
workplace stress	1	2	3	4	5

List and rate any others

________________________	1	2	3	4	5
________________________	1	2	3	4	5
________________________	1	2	3	4	5

Total Score ____ ÷ # of Items (that apply to you) ____ = Average Score ____

7. Rate your existing MuSkel diseases- and injuries-risk factors
Average Score: ____

Circle any of the major aging diseases and injuries already sustained, and then circle the corresponding point value. For those illnesses without an average onset age, score the level of disability from 1 (least severe) to 5 (most severe).

Disease Onset	***Point Value***
None or later than norm	1
Within the norm	2
Up to 5 yrs. before	3
5–10 yrs. before	4
10+ yrs. before	5

arm fractures	1	2	3	4	5
back problems	1	2	3	4	5
bursitis	1	2	3	4	5
cancer surgeries (muscle and bone)	1	2	3	4	5
carpal tunnel syndrome (wrist)	1	2	3	4	5
dislocations and subluxations	1	2	3	4	5
eye muscle strain	1	2	3	4	5
fibromyalgia (chronic muscle pain)	1	2	3	4	5
foot abnormalities	1	2	3	4	5
joint problems or injuries (see injuries list pp. 39–40):					
ankle	1	2	3	4	5
elbow	1	2	3	4	5
fingers	1	2	3	4	5
hands	1	2	3	4	5
hip	1	2	3	4	5
knee	1	2	3	4	5
neck	1	2	3	4	5
shoulder	1	2	3	4	5
toes	1	2	3	4	5
wrist	1	2	3	4	5
joint replacement	1	2	3	4	5
leg fractures	1	2	3	4	5
muscular dystrophy	1	2	3	4	5
osteoarthritis	1	2	3	4	5
paralysis	1	2	3	4	5
puncture wounds	1	2	3	4	5

rheumatoid arthritis	1	2	3	4	5
sciatica	1	2	3	4	5
scoliosis	1	2	3	4	5
sexual problems (physical)	1	2	3	4	5
shin splints	1	2	3	4	5
spinal injuries	1	2	3	4	5
sports injuries	1	2	3	4	5
sprains	1	2	3	4	5
strains	1	2	3	4	5
stuttering (neck)	1	2	3	4	5
surgeries (muscle, bone, or joint)	1	2	3	4	5
tendinitis and bursitis	1	2	3	4	5
tennis elbow	1	2	3	4	5
whiplash	1	2	3	4	5

List and rate any others

____________________	1	2	3	4	5
____________________	1	2	3	4	5
____________________	1	2	3	4	5

Total Score ____ ÷ # of Items (that apply to you) ____ = Average Score ____

8. Rate your MuSkel symptoms-risk Factors
Average Score: ____

Circle and score the severity of the MuSkel symptoms that apply to you from 1 (least severe) to 5 (most severe).

bone pain	1	2	3	4	5
joint pain	1	2	3	4	5
muscle pain	1	2	3	4	5
joint or muscle stiffness	1	2	3	4	5

List and rate any others

____________________	1	2	3	4	5
____________________	1	2	3	4	5
____________________	1	2	3	4	5

Total Score ____ ÷ # of Items (that apply to you) ____ = Average Score ____

9. Rate your MuSkel physical condition- and fitness-risk factors
Average Score: ____

Add up and compute your average scores in the following seven categories. (a.–g.):

a. Rate your MuSkel functional weakness
Average Score: ____

Score your functionability from 1 (most able) to 5 (least able).

strength	1	2	3	4	5
stature	1	2	3	4	5
flexibility	1	2	3	4	5

Total Score ____ ÷ 3 = Average Score ____

b. Rate your body area weakness
Average Score: ____

Score your body areas from 1 (strongest) to 5 (weakest).

upper body	1	2	3	4	5
legs	1	2	3	4	5
trunk	1	2	3	4	5

Total Score ____ ÷ 3 = Average Score ____

c. Rate your joint stiffness or lack of joint mobility
Score: ____

Score flexibility in performing everyday activities:

Level of Stiffness	***Description***	***Point Value***
None	Can bend over and reach above head	1
Slightly	Can't bend over	2
Moderately	Can't reach above head	3
Very	Can't reach above shoulders	4
Extremely	Can't perform most reach-out or reach-over movements	5

d. Rate your bone strength
Average Score: ____

Your average score for bone strength is determined by two distinct subcategories: (1) body-frame type, and (2) bone-fracture rate. First, determine your scores for the two subcategories, and then add the two scores together and divide by 2 to determine your average bone-strength score.

(1) Rate your body frame
Score: ____

Determine your body-frame type by placing your index finger and thumb of one hand around the wrist of the other. (If you are measuring your child or patient, use only their hands and wrists to measure their body frame.) If your fingers don't meet at all, you are large-framed; if you can squeeze your fingers together to make them meet (or almost meet), you are medium- to large-framed; if your fingers meet easily (but do not overlap), you are medium-framed; if your fingers overlap slightly, you are small- to medium-framed; if your fingers overlap past the nail, you are small-framed.

Body Frame	***Score***
large	1
medium to large	2
medium	3
small to medium	4
small	5

(2) Rate your bone-fracture rate

Score: ____

# of Fractures	***Score***
0–1	1
1–2	2
2–3	3
3–4	4
5+	5

e. Rate your level of anatomical abnormalities

Score: ____

Total the number of anatomical abnormalities that you have to arrive at your anatomical abnormality rating. These include bow legs, flat feet, high arches, uneven leg lengths, heel inversion, knocked knees, duck feet, pigeon toes, and any other musculoskeletal abnormalities.

# of Abnormalities	***Score***
0	1
1	2
2	3
3	4
4+	5

f. Rate your muscle strength

Average Score: ____

Test muscle strength by doing sit-ups for trunk strength (i.e. stomach, hip, and lower back) and push-ups for upper body strength (i.e., arms, chest, shoulders, and back). Average the two scores (i.e. add the two scores together and divide by 2) to determine your overall muscle rating. Compare the scores to those of other age groups on Table 3.2, Sit-Ups, p. 60, and then convert the score to an age-group rating.

(1) Rate your trunk strength (sit-ups test)

Score: ____

Do as many sit-ups as you can in one minute. Lie down on your back with your feet flat on the floor, your knees bent at a 90 degree angle. If needed, you may anchor your feet under an object such as a bed or have a friend hold them in place. Fold your arms across your chest with your hands touching the opposite shoulder, keeping your arms flat against your chest. Sit up until your arms touch your knees. Then, lower yourself back down until your lower and middle back touch the floor again. Always sit up with your back straight, not arched or bowed. For a modified sit-up, curl the torso upward so that the shoulder blades lift off the floor, then curl down.

Number of sit-ups done in one minute: _____

Look up your age group on Table 3.2 and compare your number of sit-ups to the average. Convert your number of sit-ups into a performance rating of 1 (excellent) to 5 (poor) (the ratings are listed above the age groups on Table 3.2).

(2) Rate your upper body strength (push-ups test)
Score: ____

Do as many regular push-ups until you are unable to go on or until one minute has elapsed. (Females and children may do modified push-ups if they have less upper body strength.)

For regular push-ups, start by lying face down with your hands under your shoulders, palms on the floor, back straight, legs extended, and feet balanced on the balls of the feet. Raise your body up off the floor by pushing down on the ground and straightening arms while supporting your body with your arms and forefeet. Lower your body until your chest touches the ground, but do not rest your body on the ground. Keep your head in line with your back and do not bend at the waist. (For modified push-ups, rest your weight on your knees rather than the balls of the feet and raise your feet off the ground.)

Number of push-ups done in one minute: _____

Look up your age group on Table 3.3, Push-Ups, p. 60, and compare your number of push-ups to the average. Convert your number of push-ups into a performance rating of 1 (excellent) to 5 (poor) (the ratings are listed above the age groups on Table 3.3.

g. Rate your muscle flexibility
Average Score: ____

Muscle flexibility is the ability to move arms, legs, and trunk through a full range of motion without straining or injuring muscles and tendons. Your average score for muscle flexibility is determined by two tests: (1) prone test, and (2) seated test. First, determine your scores for the two tests, and then add the two scores together and divide by 2 to determine your average muscle flexibility score.

(1) Prone test

Score ____

Lie down, with your face up and your arms and legs spread out in a V. Knees should be slightly bent. Cross one leg over the other and try to touch the ground with the foot on the other side of the body from ankle level to hip level. Keep both shoulders flat on the ground. At what level can you touch the floor?

Level of Touch	***Score***
Ankle to hip	1
Ankle to thigh	2
Ankle to knee	3
Foot to ankle	4
Can't perform the exercise	5

(2) Seated test

Score ____

Sit on the floor, legs fully extended with your feet about one foot apart and a yardstick or measuring tape on the floor between the legs so that the "zero end" starts at the heels and extends away from the legs. Bend forward at the waist and stretch out your arms with your hands overlapped and palms facing down. How far can you touch the tape without bouncing? Also, be sure to keep your legs against the floor or have someone hold down the thighs to avoid bending knees.

Look up your age group on Table 3.4, Flexibility, p. 61, and compare your flexibility to that of the average for your age group. Convert your level of flexibility into a performance rating of 1 (excellent) to 5 (poor) (the ratings are listed above the age groups on Table 3.4).

10. Rate your MuSkel exercise- and activity-risk factor

Score: ____

Choose the rating that best fits your MuSkel exercise level:

Stretching/Strengthening exercises	
At least once a day	1 (excellent)
Five times a week	2

Two to three times a week	3
Once a week	4
Never/hardly at all	5 (poor)

Profile Summary

Compute your average score for each category, then convert it to a risk rating (which you will use later) as follows:

Average Score	*Risk Rating*
0.0–1.4	I
1.5–2.4	II
2.5–3.4	III
3.5–4.4	IV
4.5–5.0	V

Write in average scores and converted ratings for all ten risk-factor categories, then compute your overall average Muskel system score:

Risk Categories	*Average Score*	*Converted Rating*
1. Age	_____	_____
2. Gender	_____	_____
3. Genetic	_____	_____
4. Habits and addictions	_____	_____
5. Personality traits	_____	_____
6. Environment	_____	_____
7. Diseases and injuries	_____	_____
8. Symptoms	_____	_____
9. Physical condition and fitness	_____	_____
10. Exercise and activity	_____	_____

Total Score ____ ÷ 10 ____ = Average Muskel System Score ____

TABLE 3.2: SIT-UPS

Children's Sit-Ups[1]

	6 years		7 years		8 years		9 years		10 years	
	Boys	Girls	Boys	Girls	Boys	Girls	Boys	Girls	Boys	Girls
Excellent	20	20	24	24	26	26	30	28	34	30

	11 years		12 years		13 years		14 years		15 years	
	Boys	Girls	Boys	Girls	Boys	Girls	Boys	Girls	Boys	Girls
Excellent	36	33	38	33	40	33	40	35	42	35

	16 years		17 years		18 years	
	Boys	Girls	Boys	Girls	Boys	Girls
Excellent	44	35	44	35	44	35

Adult's Sit-Ups

	1	2	3	4	5	5	5	5
Age	19–29	30–39	40–49	50–59	60–69	70–79	80–89	90–99
Men	37–42	29–36	24–28	19–23	14–18	10–13	9–13	7–10
Women	33–38	25–33	19–24	15–18	10–14	7–9	6–8	0–5

TABLE 3.3: PUSH-UPS

Children's Push-Ups[2]

	6–9 years		10–13 years		14–18 years	
	Boys	Girls	Boys	Girls	Boys	Girls
Average	10–15	10–15	20–30	20–30	30–40	20–30
Excellent	16–30	16–30	31–40	31–40	41–50	31–40

Adult's Push-Ups

	1	2	3	4	5	5	5	5
Age	19–29	30–39	40–49	50–59	60–69	70–79	80–89	90–99
Men	35–44	25–34	20–24	15–19	10–14	7–9	5–8	0–4
Women	17–33	12–16	8–11	6–8	3–5	1–2	1–2	1

TABLE 3.4: FLEXIBILITY[3]

Children's Flexibility (in Inches)

	6 years		7 years		8 years		9 years		10 years	
Flexibility	Boys	Girls	Boys	Girls	Boys	Girls	Boys	Girls	Boys	Girls
Average	15	17	16	17	15	17	16	17	15	17
Excellent	17	19	18	20	18	20	18	21	18	21

	11 years		12 years		13 years		14 years		15 years	
Flexibility	Boys	Girls	Boys	Girls	Boys	Girls	Boys	Girls	Boys	Girls
Average	16	18	16	19	16	20	16	20	17	21
Excellent	18	21	18	21	18	23	19	23	20	23

	16 years		17 years		18 years	
Flexibility	Boys	Girls	Boys	Girls	Boys	Girls
Average	18	21	17	21	17	21
Excellent	20	23	20	24	20	24

Adult's Flexibility (in Inches)

	1	2	3	4	5	5	5	5
Age	19–29	30–39	40–49	50–59	60–69	70–79	80–89	90–99
Men	17–20	15–16	13–14	13–14	12–11	12–11	5–10	0–4
Women	21–24	19–20	17–18	17–18	13–16	13–16	9–12	0–8

[1]If your child scores above the "excellent" target on this table, his or her score is 1 point (most fit); if the number of sit-ups accomplished is at the "excellent" target or within 5 sit-ups of that target, his or her score is 2 points; 3 points should be awarded for 6 to 10 sit-ups below the "excellent" target; 4 points for between 11 and 15 sit-ups below the "excellent" target; and 5 points (least fit) for 16 or more sit-ups below the "excellent" target.

[2]If your child reaches the "average" range, he or she scores 3 points. If the "excellent" range is reached, score 2 points. If your child accomplishes more push-ups than the "excellent" range, score him or her at 1 (most fit). If, however, your child is 5 push-ups or below the "average" range, his or her score is 4. If your child is ten push-ups or below the "average" range, his or her score is 5 (least fit).

[3]If your child reaches the "average" flexibility, he or she scores 3 points. If the "excellent" target is reached, score 2 points. If your child accomplishes a flexibility that is higher than the "excellent" target, score him or her at 1 (most fit). If, however, your child is 2 inches below the "average" target, his or her score is 4. If your child is 4 inches or below the "average" target, his or her score is 5 (least fit).

CHAPTER 4

Fighting the Fat Gene

Saving Your Metabolic System

What is Metabolism?

Metabolism (Meta) refers to your body's ability to convert or metabolize food into energy, store it, and then burn off that stored energy. Whereas cardiovascular health (Chapter Five) is focused on improved blood and air flow, Meta health is focused on nutrient absorption and burning off fat and blood sugar.

The Meta System

The Meta system of your body includes three subsystems: nutritional, digestive, and excretory. These subsystems are located primarily in the lower torso—between the heart and the pubic bone—but they also work through the bloodstream. The Meta system body areas include the pelvic floor and perineal muscles and also include the muscles of the abdomen, lower back, hips, buttocks, groin, and inner thighs.

The Nutritional Subsystem

This is the subsystem that delivers the digested nutrients through the bloodstream to the internal organs and glands ending in the energy-conversion process. It also includes hormone-secreting glands.

The Digestive and Excretory Subsystems

The digestive subsystem includes such organs as the stomach, which digests food, and the liver, gallbladder, and kidneys, which process nutri-

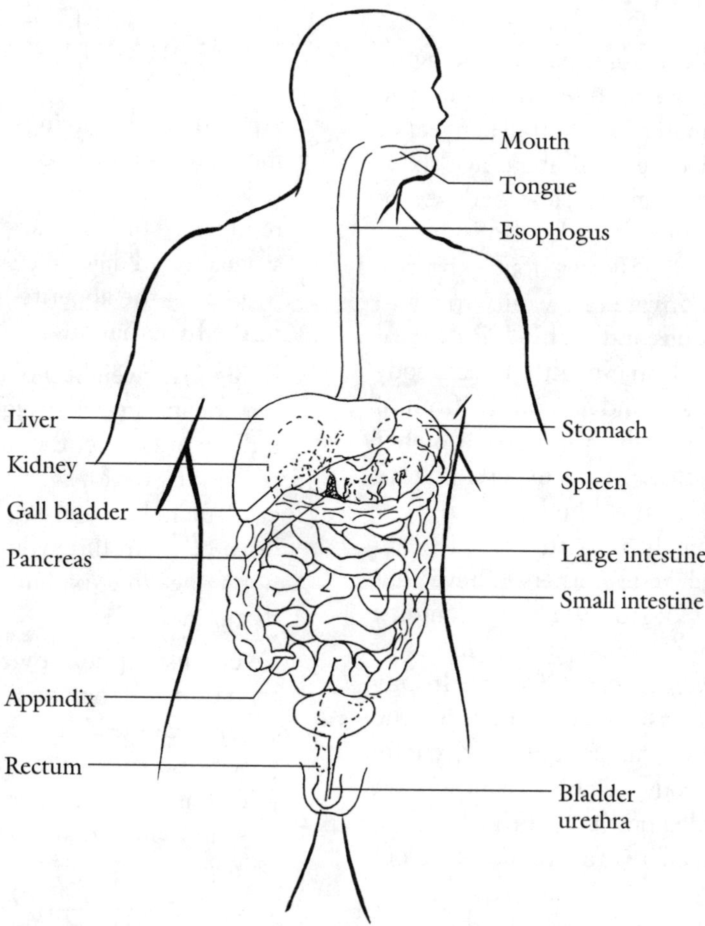

Digestive System

ents and chemicals that aid in digestion. The liver and kidneys also filter waste products from the blood as does the urinary system. Both the colon and intestines process waste products from the stomach to form the excretory subsystem.

THE KEY TO YOUR METABOLIC HEALTH

What thinning bones are to the MuSkel system, excess body fat is to the Meta system—the central health problem and the measuring stick for Meta system health. Yet, being overweight can significantly impair not only the health of your Meta system, but all the other four health systems as well. Fat determines the weight load or burden that we must bear daily—physically as well as emotionally. Excess fat can also be a sign of the prolonged decline of other such metabolic functions as nutrient and fluid flow. Being overweight will also affect the level and balance of your blood sugar.

MONITORING BODY FAT

Growing fatter is a natural part of the aging process. After age twenty-five, on average you will gain approximately one pound per year or ten pounds per decade until about age sixty-five. This process can be slowed down or reversed by increasing your level of physical activity and making better food choices. Many of us are motivated by vanity to try to take off extra pounds and inches but the real motivation should be our health. Excess body fat on the upper body and around the front of the stomach is believed to indicate a higher risk for heart disease. Many experts believe that fat on these areas of the body can work its way more quickly into the bloodstream thereby clogging arteries; others believe that arteries become clogged by a more complex process involving vascular injury, levels of cholesterol, as well as other factors. In any case, exercise experts still advocate using the percentage of body fat as a more accurate measure of ideal body weight. For most of us, the weight recorded on the bathroom scale is still the most reliable way to monitor our body fat.

MAJOR SYMPTOMS

The major symptoms (see Table 4.1) of the Meta health system include appetite stimulation (both above and below normal levels), blood sugar or insulin imbalance, body fat or muscle imbalance, cravings (e.g. for sugar, alcohol, and so on), constipation, incontinence, and thirst. All of these symptoms can be improved by exercise because exercise helps you control your Meta symptoms by evenly regulating the flow and absorption of nutrients throughout the body.

TABLE 4.1
MAJOR META SYMPTOMS

Appetite and Cravings Regular, moderate, whole-body exercise reduces your appetite for food by redirecting blood flow away from the stomach and digestive system and regulating the appetite mechanisms in the hypothalmus

Being Overweight Four out of five Americans are overweight and 34 million are obese; too much body fat is a risk factor for many major diseases including diabetes and heart disease; controlling your weight is not a one-time fix, but a continuous discipline

Overconsumption Ingesting more food or drink than your body requires can lead to stomach and pelvis discomfort and weight gain; overconsumption of alcohol, sugars, fats, and salt can also lead to organ damage

Loss of Pelvic Control Regular exercise, especially abdominal and pelvic floor exercises, will improve the regularity of metabolic functions and will help you avoid both chronic constipation, stress, and incontinence

Here is a list of Meta symptoms ranked from the least severe (1) to the most severe (33). Use this list to rate the severity of your symptoms and to gauge when they are becoming worse (and are therefore a warning to stop exercising and seek a doctor's attention).

Meta Symptoms List

1. Slightly overweight (5–10 lbs.) (least severe)
2. Moderate fatigue
3. Appetite
   a) poor (under)
   b) ravenous (over)
   c) abnormal thirst
4. Inactivity
5. Moderate weight gain
6. Moderate weight loss
7. Abdominal bloating
8. Moderately overweight (10–20 lbs.)
9. Food craving
10. Sugar craving
11. Frequent urination
12. Water retention
13. Constipation
14. Pelvic discomfort
15. Irritability, weakness
16. Overconsumption
17. Dry mouth
18. Diarrhea
19. Obesity (20–60 lbs.)
20. High blood sugar
21. Low blood sugar
22. Dehydration
23. Stomach pain
24. Incontinence
25. Rapid weight loss
26. Stomach and internal cramps
27. Menstrual cramps
28. Severe fatigue
29. Excessive weight (60+ lbs.)
30. Blurred vision
31. Dizziness
32. Faintness
33. Vomiting, nausea (most severe)

NUTRIENT BALANCE

In general, exercise promotes the absorption of **nutrients** that—as in the case of calcium into the bones—will not be properly absorbed unless you are physically active. Exercise has the greatest impact on the major diseases and disorders that are the result of imbalances between: (1) fat and muscle, (2) sugar and insulin, and (3) water and salt. Exercise also helps to restore and maintain other balances and to correct the deficiencies of almost all the body's nutrients.

To avoid certain metabolic and nutritional disorders, the long list of body nutrients that must be in balance includes: calcium, chloride, galactose, iodine, magnesium, phosphorus, potassium, protein, sodium, vitamins, and so forth. As exercise aids in the absorption of these nutrients, it not only helps maintain the balance, but, if the balance starts to tip in either direction, it also helps restore it to normality even faster.

FAT TO MUSCLE RATIO

Body fat is not only a store of fuel but also a layer of protection and insulation for all the organs that make up the metabolic system. (Body fat is also connected to the factor of blood sugar.) The Meta system's basic health is measured by a shortage or an excess of fat; body composition is measured by both your percentage of body fat and your lean body mass. Ideal body weight is an estimate of body composition. If you have to lose extra body fat you must increase your activity level and/or lower your calorie intake. If you are not at your ideal body weight, or within 5% of it (see Table 4.2 Ideal Body Weight, page 67), then the fat to muscle ratio portion of your metabolic system is out of balance and you will need to reduce your body fat. Reproductive organs can also be affected by the fat to muscle ratio.

BLOOD SUGAR TO INSULIN RATIO

Blood sugar is an important source of energy but an excess of sugar or insulin (the hormone that allows the processing of your sugar) can lead to organ damage.

Produced by the pancreas, **insulin** is a hormone that transports glucose into cells for use as energy and storage as glycogen. Insulin also stimulates protein synthesis and the storage of free fatty acids in fat deposits. When there is either an insulin deficiency or resistance, your body tissues have less access to essential nutrients for fuel and storage. You become energy-deprived and feel fatigued. Insulin-dependent diabetics (IDD or Type I) are deficient, whereas non-insulin-dependent diabetics (NIDD or Type II) are resistant and may also be deficient.

Insulin deficiency or resistance causes high levels of blood sugar or excessive glucose (sugar). High levels of blood sugar can be life threatening because it can lead to a metabolic crisis, such as ketoacidosis. It can also lead to fluid loss (i.e. frequent urination, dehydration, excessive thirsts, dry mucous membranes, dry skin). Excess sugar can also cause damage to the nervous system, kidneys, eyes, and blood vessels (i.e. it stimulates plaque buildup by causing lesions on artery walls). High blood sugar levels also encourage bacterial growth and reduce the body's resistance to infection.

Diabetes mellitus (DM), including Types I (insulin-dependent) and II (non-insulin-dependent), is a hormone disorder that affects the metabolic system (Type II accounts for 90 to 95% of these patients) and is a major risk factor for many other major diseases and disorders including heart disease, kidney disease, high blood pressure, nerve damage, loss of vision, impotence, tissue damage leading to amputation, and peripheral vascular disease. Diabetes is the ultimate metabolic disease, the prime example of how your Meta health can deteriorate when your body can't metabolize food in a balanced and efficient way. The most common symptom is fatigue caused by the abnormal processing of fats, carbohydrates, and proteins. But even nondiabetics can overtax their metabolism by burning sugar at the expense of other nutrients.

The goal of diabetes treatment is to control blood sugar levels. This is accomplished with diet, insulin injections, and exercise. Diabetics who exercise must monitor their insulin and blood sugar levels because too much exercise can cause low blood sugar. The balancing effect must be in the amount of exercise as well as the medication and food intake.

TABLE 4.2
IDEAL BODY WEIGHT (IN POUNDS)

HEIGHT	Age 25 S→M→L*	Age 35 S→M→L	Age 45 S→M→L	Age 55 S→M→L	Age 65+ S→M→L
4'10"	84 98 111	92 106 119	99 113 127	107 121 135	115 129 142
4'11"	87 101 115	95 109 123	103 117 131	111 125 139	119 133 147
5'	90 105 119	98 113 127	106 121 135	114 129 143	123 138 152
5'1"	93 108 123	101 116 131	110 125 140	118 133 148	127 142 157
5'2"	96 112 127	105 121 136	113 129 144	122 138 153	131 147 163
5'3"	99 113 131	108 124 140	117 133 149	126 142 158	135 152 168
5'4"	102 119 135	112 129 145	121 138 154	130 147 163	140 157 173
5'5"	106 123 140	115 132 149	125 142 159	134 151 168	144 162 179
5'6"	109 127 144	119 136 154	129 147 164	138 156 174	148 166 184
5'7"	112 130 148	122 141 159	133 151 169	143 161 179	153 172 190
5'8"	116 135 153	126 145 163	137 156 174	147 166 184	158 177 196
5'9"	119 138 157	130 149 168	141 160 179	151 171 190	162 182 201
5'10"	122 142 162	134 154 173	145 165 184	156 176 195	167 187 207
5'11"	126 147 167	137 156 178	149 170 190	160 181 201	172 193 213
6'	129 150 171	141 162 183	153 174 195	165 186 207	177 198 219
6'1"	133 155 176	145 167 188	157 179 200	169 191 213	182 204 225
6'2"	137 159 181	149 172 194	162 184 206	174 197 219	187 210 232
6'3"	141 164 186	153 176 199	166 189 212	179 202 225	192 215 238
6'4"	144 168 191	157 181 205	171 196 218	184 208 231	197 221 244

*S = Small frame, M = Medium frame, and L = Large frame. The weights correspond to each age/height range. Smaller frames will tend to fall toward the lower end of the range, medium frames in the middle, and large frames toward the high end of the range.

WATER TO SALT RATIO

As with blood flow, your body also needs sufficient water flow to move nutrients to organs and carry away waste products. Sodium helps the body to concentrate and balance those body fluids necessary for proper nerve and muscle function, glandular secretion, and water balance. A disruption in the potassium and sodium balance affects the way the body transports chemicals between cells and the fluid surrounding them.

Exercise promotes the flow of water through the body and creates a need for the body to ingest fresh water. Exercise also plays the role of a diuretic by making you urinate and defecate more frequently to remove waste products. The function of lower body organs is also improved through exercise by strengthening the muscles that surround these organs such as the pelvic, sphincter, and perineal muscles.

WHAT CAN GO WRONG?

BALANCING YOUR BODY COMPOSITION

For your body system to run efficiently, it must have the proper mix of fuels to fluids. An imbalance indicates that your body has either a deficiency or an excess of one or more nutrients. For example, being overweight is an indication that your body has stored too much fat. Imbalances can also appear as symptoms, for example internal muscle spasms and twitching, tingling sensations, fatigue, irregular heartbeat, frequent urination, or abdominal pain.

Meta exercise helps bring your body's system of internal organs into better balance. Untreated, metabolic imbalances can lead to serious diseases and disorders and permanent organ damage. The three most common disorders or diseases of the metabolic system are: alcoholism, diabetes, and obesity. Alcohol also causes excess fat to accumulate and can cause permanent liver damage.

BODY COMPOSITION

Body fat, by itself, is not a threat to your health. Indeed, fat is a valuable nutrient that helps the body regenerate itself. **Body composition** is a term referring to the balance of fat to muscle. Remember: It's not the absolute amount of fat your body holds, but rather the percentage of fat to your total body mass that is important. If fat comprises more than 30% of your total body composition, then you are medically at risk. Lower than 25% for women and lower than 20% for men is considered optimum. Men have a higher percentage of bone and muscle; women have a higher percentage of fat to maintain the reproductive system. Thus, the average twenty- to twenty-four-year-old man might be composed of 15% body fat, 44% muscle, 15% bone, and the remaining 26% would be blood, water, and softer tissues. The average twenty- to twenty-four-year-old woman might be composed of 27% fat, 36% muscle, 12% bone, and the remaining 25% would be blood, water, and softer tissues. As part of the aging process, the body-fat percentage goes up while muscle and bone density go down. But positive lifestyle changes can slow down or even reverse this process. Theoretically, if you work hard building up your muscles, you should be able to lower your body-fat percentage—depending on the amount and consistency of exercise.

WEIGHT CONTROL

Ninety percent of the U.S. population is overweight. A much smaller percentage, perhaps 2%, are underweight. The rest, maybe 5 to 8%, are at their normal weight when mea-

TABLE 4.3
WAIST-TO-HIP RATIOS AND RISK OF DISEASE

	Age	*Low Risk*	*Moderate Risk*	*High Risk*	*Very High Risk*
Women	20–29	0.6–0.72	0.72–0.78	0.78–0.83	0.83+
Men	20–29	0.6–0.83	0.83–0.88	0.88–0.95	0.95+
Women	30–39	0.6–0.73	0.73–0.79	0.79–0.85	0.85+
Men	30–39	0.6–0.84	0.84–0.92	0.92–0.97	0.97+
Women	40–49	0.6–0.74	0.74–0.80	0.80–0.88	0.88+
Men	40–49	0.6–0.88	0.88–0.95	0.95–1.10	1.10+
Women	50–59	0.6–0.75	0.75–0.83	0.83–0.89	0.89+
Men	50–59	0.6–0.90	0.90–0.96	0.96–1.20	1.20+
Women	60–69	0.6–0.78	0.78–0.85	0.85–0.92	0.92+
Men	60–69	0.6–0.91	0.91–0.98	0.98–1.30	1.30+

Use the hip-waist ratio measure to determine the percent of body fat on your body. The lower the percent of fat, the higher the percentage of muscle mass. Compare your ideal weight in pounds to your actual weight. For each point you scored on your hip-waist ratio test, you can add at least one pound to your ideal weight. Thus, if you score 5 points, you can add 5 pounds to your ideal weight. To compute your waist-to-hip ratio, see p. 85, Rate your body composition.

sured by the ideal weight tables issued by the Metropolitan Life Insurance Company. Now you know why these weight tables are called "ideal" and not "real."

The Bridge from Being Overweight to Being Obese

Being **overweight,** which is between 5 to 19% above the ideal or normal weight, is an unhealthy condition that is more a symptom than a disease. It is the central symptom affecting nearly all metabolic system diseases and disorders. Being overweight is an indication that you have not been physically active and that your body is consuming more calories than it burns off. Being overweight is a condition that can lead up to **obesity.** To qualify as being obese you have to remain at least thirty pounds overweight for a period of more than three years.

New guidelines have been issued for health professionals on measuring overweight and obesity by body mass index (BMI), which measures body weight relative to height. This method is designed primarily for use by health professionals. In practical terms, it means that the more muscular you are, the more you can weigh based on your ideal height and weight tables. Measuring BMI requires special testing equipment, such as a water tank or a body mass scanner. A quick way to find your ideal body weight is to adjust your waist-to-hip ratio score (Table 4.3) to your weight on the ideal weight table (Table 4.2).

How to compute body mass index:

1. Multiply weight by 703.
2. Multiply height in inches by height in inches.
3. Divide the answer in Step 1 by the answer in Step 2 for your body mass index.

BMI	*Points*
30 or more	1 Severely Obese
25–29.9	2 Obese
20–24.9	3 Very overweight
15–19.9	4 Moderately overweight
14.9 or less	5 Overweight

META GENETICS: BORN TO BE FAT

Being overweight is linked to genetic-inheritance factors. It is also a product of early childhood development. If your son or daughter is born into an overweight family he or she will probably inherit the genetic factor to grow more fat cells than a child born to a normal-weight family. This is also true if a child is allowed to overeat; she or he will grow more fat cells than a normal-weight child. Later on in life, those fat cells, which never completely disappear, will continue to influence body weight and percentage of body fat.

Each fat cell craves to be filled with fat and sends your brain signals to increase your appetite until you eat enough fat to fill them up. (This is one of the most important reasons to lead your child to a physically active life and to teach good eating habits.) The excess of unused energy is stored as body fat. Over weeks and months, this adds up to being overweight.

WHEN OVERWEIGHT GOES OUT OF CONTROL

Once upon a time, fat people kept their fat genes in check by remaining physically active. Perhaps the body's ability to slow down the basal metabolic rate and store fat was an evolutionary advantage. In the last eighty years, however, the percentage of obese people has grown probably because our health habits have changed. If you are obese, it can be very difficult to bring your weight into the ideal range, but you might be able to bring it down into a safer range. More important than this, however, is that you can create a fitter, more muscular body, which can more easily support the greater weight you are carrying. Regular exercise, when accompanied by a low-fat diet will help keep your body weight consistent. (See the exercise program in Part Three, Chapter Sixteen.)

ACHIEVING FAT BALANCES

The number of calories you burn to decrease or maintain your weight will depend on your daily activity level. Your average daily activity level will determine both your **BMR (basal metabolic rate)** and how many calories you burn at rest. Your BMR is expressed as hourly values of heat production per square meter of body surface area, which is estimated according to a person's height and weight. Your **active metabolic rate** is how many calories you burn when you are moving around, playing sports, exercising, and so forth. Both rates

TABLE 4.4
BODY MASS INDEX (BMI)

25 OVERWEIGHT LIMIT

WEIGHT HEIGHT	100	105	110	115	120	125	130	135	140	145	150	155	160	165	170	175	180	185	190	195	200	205
5' 0"	20	21	21	22	23	24	**25**	26	27	28	29	30	31	32	33	34	35	36	37	38	39	40
5' 1"	19	20	21	22	23	24	**25**	26	26	27	28	29	30	31	32	33	34	35	36	37	38	39
5' 2"	18	19	20	21	22	23	24	**25**	26	27	27	28	29	30	31	32	33	34	35	36	37	37
5' 3"	18	19	19	20	21	22	23	24	**25**	26	27	27	28	29	30	31	32	33	34	35	35	36
5' 4"	17	18	19	20	21	21	22	23	24	**25**	26	27	27	28	29	30	31	32	33	33	34	35
5' 5"	17	17	18	19	20	21	22	22	23	24	**25**	26	27	27	28	29	30	31	32	32	33	34
5' 6"	16	17	18	19	19	20	21	22	23	23	24	**25**	26	27	27	28	29	30	31	31	32	33
5' 7"	16	16	17	18	19	20	20	21	22	23	23	24	**25**	26	27	27	28	29	30	31	31	32
5' 8"	15	16	17	17	18	19	20	21	21	22	23	24	24	**25**	26	27	27	28	29	30	30	31
5' 9"	15	16	16	17	18	18	19	20	21	21	22	23	24	24	**25**	26	27	27	28	29	30	30
5' 10"	14	15	16	17	17	18	19	19	20	21	22	22	23	24	24	**25**	26	27	27	28	29	29
5' 11"	14	15	15	16	17	17	18	19	20	20	21	22	22	23	24	24	**25**	26	26	27	28	29
6' 0"	14	14	15	16	16	17	18	18	19	20	20	21	22	22	23	24	24	**25**	26	26	27	28
6' 1"	13	14	15	15	16	16	17	18	18	19	20	20	21	22	22	23	24	24	**25**	26	26	27
6' 2"	13	13	14	15	15	16	17	17	18	19	19	20	21	21	22	22	23	24	24	**25**	26	26
6' 3"	12	13	14	14	15	16	16	17	17	18	19	19	20	21	21	22	22	23	24	24	**25**	26
6' 4"	12	13	13	14	15	15	16	16	17	18	18	19	19	20	21	21	22	23	23	24	24	**25**

Sources: *Shape Up America; National Institutes of Health*

vary with each individual, with BMR's ranging between thirty and seventy calories per minute. If you are at the high end of the scale, you are probably naturally thinner; if you are at the low end, you are apt to be naturally fatter. Exercise increases your BMR, revving up your body's internal engine for many hours even after you finish your workout.

To bring your body composition into balance, you have to burn off as many calories as you take in each day. Over a long period of time (as much as a year or more), your body composition will reflect how active a person you have been.

METABOLIC EXERCISE

If you are overweight because you have been inactive temporarily, or if you only have a minor weight control problem (between five and twenty pounds), you can exercise regularly and return your body composition to normal without any special actions. Medical studies show that such continuous exercises as walking and stationary bicycling are the best types for weight reduction and control. Swimming and water exercise are not as effective for minor weight loss because movement in water does not burn calories as fast as walking and cycling do.

For more severely obese people, it becomes even more important to practice varied types of exercise. To lose weight, an obese person should stay active for a total of one to three hours each day, something that is very hard to do with one form of exercise alone. Therefore, on a daily basis, an obese person should supplement water exercise with land-based exercise practiced in short bouts. Moving continuously for more than five minutes is difficult for an obese person; therefore, shorter exercise bouts are more practical and safe.

Strength exercises performed with weights or resistance are the best way for building up the percentage of your muscle mass, but continuous muscle movement against resistance can also provide a substitute for weight training. Pumping hand weights while walking, and cycling against pedal resistance are two excellent options.

To raise your metabolic rate, you must increase your level of physical activity and involve your whole body by moving many parts simultaneously. Just as continuously working major muscles draws and pumps more blood to and from your heart, these same muscles work to move your arms, legs, torso, and so on, which, in turn, burns more more calories. Your leg muscles moving your legs in addition to your whole body contributes at least 60% of your total body calorie burn rate. When exercising in water, your arm muscles are moving your arms in addition to the rest of your body, and that can be the extra edge you need to keep your body composition in balance. And, if these muscles are bigger and stronger from strength training, they will burn calories at a higher rate. That's why a well-muscled body is like a V-8 engine rather than a 4-cylinder: It burns more fuel per mile. Remember: Even when they are at rest, muscles consume calories; fat doesn't.

With cardiovascular exercise, you concentrate on continuous motion; with metabolic exercise, it is cumulative. Therefore, you can start and stop as much as you need to, as long as your total activity, daily and weekly, reaches certain minimum levels. (See Meta Ex, pp. 200–215.)

METABOLIC BENEFITS OF EXERCISE

1. With exercise, you can concentrate your required daily body-system maintenance activities into a couple of hours.
2. Exercise can help you maintain the balance and flow of the various nutrients (e.g. vitamins, minerals, fats, proteins) in your body by stimulating their absorption and burning off the excess.
3. Exercise controls fat and sugar levels, the two central fuels for maintaining your energy balance.
4. Moderate exercise, in particular, regulates or suppresses your appetite for food and other nutrients. Vigorous exercise often sends the body into a state of imbalance, burning off too much sugar and causing feelings of hunger and weakness. Low blood sugar can also contribute to feelings of hunger.
5. Exercise speeds up the rate at which your body metabolizes stored fat by increasing both your **BMR** and your **active metabolic rate,** thereby raising the cumulative number of calories your body burns every day.
6. Exercise is the best way to effectively control your body composition (i.e. the balance between muscle and fat).
7. Exercise prevents water retention, which makes you feel and look fat, despite the fact that you will increase your consumption of water by two to four pints daily.
8. Exercise also increases the blood flow to internal organs, which balances out nutrient deficiencies while delivering white blood cells and antibodies to fight off infections.

METABOLIC EXERTION TRAINING STANDARD

Metabolic Exertion Training Standard (METS) is an additional technique for measuring the intensity of exercises or physical activity expressed as a multiple of your resting metabolic rate. One METS equals the resting metabolic rate, and therefore, 2–20 METS correspond to increasing levels of physical activity.

A METS rating lets you evaluate certain types of activities as to their ability to make your body work harder. Walking slowly is a "2 METS" activity. Playing tennis is a "6 METS" activity. Cross-country skiing at a racer's pace is a "20 METS" activity. A METS rating can also be correlated to the amount of oxygen your body needs to continue to perform the activities. For more information concerning METS, refer to Table 4.5, Clinically Significant Key Metabolic Equivalents for Maximum Exercise, and Table 4.6, Normal Values of Maximum Oxygen Uptake. Also see Table 4.7, Walking Speeds and Their METS Equivalents.

TABLE 4.5
CLINICALLY SIGNIFICANT KEY METABOLIC EQUIVALENTS FOR MAXIMUM EXERCISE

1 METS	= resting
2 METS	= level walking at 2 mph
4 METS	= level walking at 4 mph
<5 METS	= poor prognosis; usual limit immediately after MI; peak cost of basic activities of daily living
10 METS	= prognosis with medical therapy as good as coronary artery bypass surgery
13 METS	= excellent prognosis regardless of other exercise responses
18 METS	= elite endurance athletes
20 METS	= world class athletes

METS indicates metabolic equivalent or a unit of sitting, resting oxygen uptake; MI, myocardial infarction. 1 METS = 3.5 mL · kg^{-1} · min^{-1} oxygen uptake.

TABLE 4.6
NORMAL VALUES OF MAXIMUM OXYGEN UPTAKE

Age, y	*Men*	*Women*
20–29	43±7.2 12 METS	36±6.9 10 METS
30–39	42±7.0 12 METS	34±6.2 10 METS
40–49	40±7.2 11 METS	32±6.2 9 METS
50–59	36±7.1 10 METS	29±5.4 8 METS
60–69	33±7.3 9 METS	27±4.7 8 METS
70–79	29±7.3 6 METS	27±5.8 8 METS

METS indicates metabolic equivalent: 1 METS = 3.5 mL · kg 1 · min oxygen uptake. Values are expressed as milliliters per kilogram per minute.

Exercise and Dieting

Dieting and exercise can work together, provided you do not reduce the total calories you consume to anything less than 500 below your minimum daily requirement. (See Table 4.8, Matching Calorie Cuts to Weight-Loss Goals, (p. 000) for sensible calorie cutting for weight loss.) The key to keeping both your body fat and your metabolic system in balance is to maintain a level of daily physical activity commensurate with both your ideal body weight and your calorie intake. Your activity level will also determine the number of calories you need to consume to reduce or maintain your weight. Dieting alone tends to keep your body inactive and deprive it of the internal stimulation that exercise provides through increased metabolism and fluid and nutrient flow. In addition to these drawbacks, when you diet without exercise, your body fights off starvation by slowing down the metabolic system. At rest, carbohydrates supply 40% of your energy needs. With moderate exercise, the fuel mix is 50% fat and 50% carbohydrates. After twenty minutes, more fats than carbohydrates are being burned. After you become fatigued, carbohydrates again supply your energy needs. During short-duration,

TABLE 4.7
WALKING SPEEDS AND THEIR METS EQUIVALENTS

METS	*Walking Speed* (MI/M)	*Minute-Miles* (MM)
1	at rest	at rest
2	1.5	40
3	2	30
4	3	20
5	3.5	17
6	4	15
7	4.25	14
8	5	12
9	5.5	11
10	6	10
11	6.5	9.2
12	7	8.5
13	7.5	8
14	8	7.5
15	9	6.7
16	9.5	6.3
17	10	6

high-intensity cardiovascular exercise, carbohydrates provide 80% of the fuel, and fat only 20%. With strength training, the percentages increase to 95% and 5%, respectively.

The types of food you eat can also help you reduce your body fat and act as a type of exercise for your digestive system. For example, you should eat reduced amounts of processed and sugary foods and increase your intake of complex carbohydrates and fibrous foods. This will make your digestive system work harder and, consequently, it will burn more calories. Consuming food that is low in fat and high in fiber, complex carbohydrates, and protein increases the thermic effect of food (TEF), which makes up about 10% of the energy you expend each day. Your body expends more energy to metabolize carbohydrates and convert them into glycogen to store, burning 25% of the calories consumed. By contrast, your body only expends 4% of fat calories to convert, process, and store in fat cells. You should also keep in mind that your body only burns off these extra calories if it processes food regularly, so skipping meals or not eating to lose weight only keeps your metabolism from helping you expend energy.

If you are overweight or obese, you do not have to exercise as much as a thin person does to burn the same number of calories. If your ideal weight is 150 pounds and you weigh 200 pounds, your exercise effort will be that of an unfit 150-pound person walking or swimming while wearing a fifty-pound backpack. This clearly illustrates why an overweight or obese person must exercise more carefully and slowly, increasing speed and intensity gradually as the muscles and heart become fit enough to carry the extra load. The best way to become fit is through the MuSkel Ex of duration exercises and segmented activities (see pp. 180–199).

YOUR META PROFILE

To determine the amount of Meta exercise you should be doing, rate your Meta health and weaknesses using the Meta System Profile. If you rate I, II, or III, practice the Meta Preventive Exercises in Part Two. If you rate IV or V, practice the Meta Rehab program in Part Three.

Circle each of the major risk factors as

TABLE 4.8
MATCHING CALORIE CUTS TO WEIGHT-LOSS GOALS

Level	*Calories to Cut Per Day*	*Days Needed to Lose One Pound*	*Pound Loss Per Year*
I	50–200	70–18	5–20
II	200–300	18–11	20–34
III	300–500	11–7	34–50
IV	500–1000 (in two stages)	7–4	50–90
V	1000–1500 (in three stages)	4–2	90–150

To lose one pound of weight, you must burn 3,500 calories. Translate your weight-loss goal into calories and divide by 365 days. (That is, take the number of pounds that you are overweight and multiply that number by 3,500. Divide that number by 365. For example, if you are ten pounds overweight, you must burn an additional ninety-six calories per day for one year to lose that extra ten pounds—10 lbs. × 3,500 = 35,000 ÷ 365 = 95.89.) This will be your year-long activity schedule, exercising that extra amount per day to burn off your extra pounds.

they apply to you and multiply the number of these factors by the number of point values assigned in each category. Total up your points for the category before continuing on to the next category. You may also use this questionnaire to evaluate the medical risk factors of a child or adult under your care and supervision. The final score will ascertain which of the five health systems are the weakest and will determine where you should concentrate the *Exercise Rx* program.

Meta System Profile

Compute your Meta-risk factors by rating the severity of your diseases, symptoms, and physical weaknesses on a scale of 1 point (least severe) to 5 points (most severe). Average your points and convert your averages to an overall rating that corresponds to the intensity or difficulty level for which you will begin your prevention or rehabilitation exercises. Please note: No answer equals a score of 0.

1. Rate your Meta age-risk factor
Average Score: ____

Weigh yourself (or that of your child or patient) and compare your body weight to the norm for your age group according to Table 4.2, Ideal Body Weight, p. 67.

Weight	*Score*
Equal to or less than your age group	1
Up to 5 lbs. more	2
5–10 lbs. more	3
10–20 lbs. more	4
20+ lbs. more	5

2. Rate your Meta gender-risk factors
Average Score: ____

Circle the gender-specific Meta diseases you already have (or have had), and then circle the corresponding point value. The average onset age is shown in parentheses after each disease. Example: bladder cancer (50 +). For those illnesses without an average age, score your level of disability from 1 (least severe) to 5 (most severe). If you haven't had any Meta diseases, your score is 0.

Disease Onset	*Point Value*
Later than norm	1
Within the norm	2
Up to 5 yrs. before	3
5–10 yrs. before	4
10+ yrs. before	5

Common or Predominantly Male Diseases

alcoholism	1	2	3	4	5
bladder cancer (50+)1	1	2	3	4	5
cirrhosis of the liver	1	2	3	4	5
diverticulosis (40+)	1	2	3	4	5
enlarged prostate (50+)	1	2	3	4	5
groin hernia	1	2	3	4	5
kidney cancer	1	2	3	4	5
kidney stones	1	2	3	4	5
legionnaires' disease	1	2	3	4	5
leukemia, chronic lymphocytic (50+)	1	2	3	4	5
liver cancer (60+)	1	2	3	4	5
malignant lymphomas	1	2	3	4	5
pancreatic cancer (50+)	1	2	3	4	5
pilonidal disease (18–30)	1	2	3	4	5
prostate cancer (50+)	1	2	3	4	5
stomach cancer (40+)	1	2	3	4	5
testicular cancer (20–40)	1	2	3	4	5
urinary reflux (infants, inherited)	1	2	3	4	5

Common or Predominantly Female Diseases

acute pyelonephritis	1	2	3	4	5
amenorrhea (secondary)	1	2	3	4	5
aphthous stomatitis (up to adolescence)	1	2	3	4	5
cardiovascular disease (during pregnancy)	1	2	3	4	5
cervical cancer (30–50)	1	2	3	4	5
colitis (55–60)	1	2	3	4	5
colitis, juvenile (15–20)	1	2	3	4	5
cystitis	1	2	3	4	5
diabetes complications (during pregnancy)	1	2	3	4	5

gallstones (20–50)	1	2	3	4	5
inflammation of the thyroid	1	2	3	4	5
inflammation of vulva/vagina	1	2	3	4	5
lower urinary tract infections (1–12)	1	2	3	4	5
ovarian cancer	1	2	3	4	5
painful menstruation (adolescence)	1	2	3	4	5
rectal prolapse (45)	1	2	3	4	5
urethritis	1	2	3	4	5
urinary reflux (3–7, inherited)	1	2	3	4	5
uterine cancer (50–65)	1	2	3	4	5
vulvar cancer (mid-60s)	1	2	3	4	5

Total Score ____ ÷ # of Items (that apply to you) ____ = Average Score ____

3. Rate your Meta genetic-risk factors
Average Score: ____

Circle and score the severity of any inherited Meta diseases that you already have (or have had) or that a close relative may have (or have had). (Only count grrandparents, parents, their siblings, and your siblings related by blood.) Next, circle the corresponding point value. For those illnesses without an average onset age, score the level of disability from 1 (least severe) to 5 (most severe).

alcoholism	1	2	3	4	5
colon cancer	1	2	3	4	5
diabetes	1	2	3	4	5
drug addiction	1	2	3	4	5
hiatal hernia	1	2	3	4	5
obesity	1	2	3	4	5
pregnancy complications	1	2	3	4	5
prostate cancer	1	2	3	4	5

Total Score ____ ÷ # of Items (that apply to you) ____ = Average Score ____

4. Rate your Meta habits- and addictions-risk factors
Average Score:____

Circle and score the severity of unhealthy Meta-related habits and addictions that apply to you from 1 (least severe) to 5 (most severe).

fatty diet	1	2	3	4	5
overeating	1	2	3	4	5
sugary diet	1	2	3	4	5
undereating	1	2	3	4	5

List and rate any others

____________	1	2	3	4	5
____________	1	2	3	4	5
____________	1	2	3	4	5

Total Score ____ ÷ # of Items (that apply to you) ____ = Average Score ____

5. Rate your Meta personality traits-risk factors
Average Score: ____

Circle and score your unhealthy Meta-related personality traits from 1 (least severe) to 5 (most severe).

anxiety	1	2	3	4	5
boredom	1	2	3	4	5

List and rate any others

____________	1	2	3	4	5
____________	1	2	3	4	5
____________	1	2	3	4	5

Total Score ____ ÷ # of Items (that apply to you) ____ = Average Score ____

6. Rate your Meta environmental risk factors
Average Score: ____

Circle and score the unhealthy environmental risk factors that apply to you from 1 (least severe) to 5 (most severe).

overcrowded living	1	2	3	4	5
contaminated/spoiled food	1	2	3	4	5
workplace carcinogens	1	2	3	4	5
workplace stress	1	2	3	4	5

List and rate any others

______________________	1	2	3	4	5
______________________	1	2	3	4	5
______________________	1	2	3	4	5

Total Score ____ ÷ # of Items (that apply to you) ____ = Average Score ____

7. Rate your Meta diseases- and injuries-risk factors
Average Score: ____

Your Meta system disease and injury score is based on three distinct subcategories: (1) Nutritional, (2) Digestive and Excretory, and (3) Reproductive.

Score each of your three Meta subsystems by circling and scoring the severity of the diseases and injuries that apply to you from 1 (least severe) to 5 (most severe). Then, add the scores for the three subsystems and divide by 3 to compute your whole Meta system disease and injury average score.

a. Nutritional Subsytem
Score: ____

alcoholism	1	2	3	4	5
anemia	1	2	3	4	5
drug addiction	1	2	3	4	5
high cholesterol	1	2	3	4	5

hypoglycemia	1	2	3	4	5
obesity	1	2	3	4	5
overweight	1	2	3	4	5

List and rate any others

____________________	1	2	3	4	5
____________________	1	2	3	4	5
____________________	1	2	3	4	5

Total Score ____ ÷ # of Items (that apply to you) ____ = Average Score ____

b. Digestive and Excretory Subsystem
Score: ____

Addison's disease (adrenal insufficiency)	1	2	3	4	5
cirrhosis of the liver	1	2	3	4	5
colitis	1	2	3	4	5
colon cancer	1	2	3	4	5
constipation	1	2	3	4	5
Cushing's syndrome (adrenal excess)	1	2	3	4	5
diabetes	1	2	3	4	5
enlarged prostate	1	2	3	4	5
esophageal cancer	1	2	3	4	5
gallstones	1	2	3	4	5
gastroenteritis	1	2	3	4	5
hemorrhoids	1	2	3	4	5
hiatal hernia	1	2	3	4	5
incontinence	1	2	3	4	5
irritable bowel syndrome	1	2	3	4	5
kidney stones	1	2	3	4	5
neurologic bladder	1	2	3	4	5

List and rate any others

____________________	1	2	3	4	5
____________________	1	2	3	4	5
____________________	1	2	3	4	5

Total Score ____ ÷ # of Items (that apply to you) ____ = Average Score ____

c. Reproductive Subsystem
Score: ____

amenorrhea	1	2	3	4	5
cardiovascular disease (during pregnancy)	1	2	3	4	5
diabetic complications (during pregnancy)	1	2	3	4	5
dysmenorrhea	1	2	3	4	5
high blood pressure (pregnancy-induced)	1	2	3	4	5
impotence	1	2	3	4	5
menopause	1	2	3	4	5
postmenopausal bleeding	1	2	3	4	5
testicular cancer	1	2	3	4	5

List and rate any others

____________________	1	2	3	4	5
____________________	1	2	3	4	5
____________________	1	2	3	4	5

Total Score ____ ÷ # of Items (that apply to you) ____ = Average Score ____

8. Rate your Meta symptoms-risk factors

Average Score: ____

Circle and score the severity of the Meta symptoms that apply to you from 1 (least severe) to 5 (most severe).

constipation	1	2	3	4	5
fatigue	1	2	3	4	5
frequent urination	1	2	3	4	5
lightheadedness	1	2	3	4	5
menstrual cramps	1	2	3	4	5
overweight—5 lbs. (1), 10 lbs. (2), 15 lbs. (3), 20 lbs. (4), 30+ lbs. (5)	1	2	3	4	5
stomach cramps	1	2	3	4	5

List and rate any others

____________________	1	2	3	4	5
____________________	1	2	3	4	5
____________________	1	2	3	4	5

Total Score ____ ÷ # of Items (that apply to you) ____ = Average Score ____

9. Rate your Meta physical condition- and fitness-risk factors

Average Score: ____

Your Meta physical condition- and fitness-risk factor score is determined by two distinct subcategories: (a) body type and composition, and (b) Meta excesses and deficiencies. First, determine your body type by matching up your body to the types listed below (1). Then, determine your body composition by computing your waist to hip ratio (2). Next, compute your average score by adding these two scores together and dividing by 2. Finally, determine your Meta excesses and deficiencies score. Your average score for your Meta physical condition- and fitness-risk factors is computed by adding together your body composition score and your Meta excesses and deficiencies score and then dividing that number by 2.

a. Rate your body composition
Average Score: ____

Your body type is determined by the relative amount of muscle and fat you carry. Estimate and test your body type by using the following two methods.

(1) Rate your body type
Score: ____

Body Type	***Description***	***Score***
ectomorph	skinny (low fat, low muscle)	1
ecto/endo	between skinny and muscular	2
endomorph	muscular (high muscle, low fat)	3
endo/meso	between muscular and fat	4
mesomorph	fat (high fat, low muscle)	5

(2) Rate your body composition
Score: ____

(a) Use a tape measure to measure your buttocks at the widest part. The tape should be tight, but should not indent your flesh.

Hip measurement: _____.

(b) Next, measure your waist at the slimmest part, but, again, do not indent the flesh.

Waist measurement: _____.

(c) Divide your waist measurement in inches by your hip measurement in inches. This will give you a result expressed in decimal form. For example, if a twenty-eight-year-old man measures his waist at thirty-four inches and his hips at forty inches:

34 ÷ 40 = .85

According to Table 4.3, a .85 ratio places the man under "moderate risk" for disease.

(d) Compare your computed ratio to your age norm on Table 4.3, Waist-to-Hip Ratios and Risk of Disease, p. 69 to determine your body composition and your risk of disease.

b. Rate your Meta excesses and deficiencies
Average Score: ____

Circle and score only the items that you have had tested. Score 1 (least severe) to 5 (most severe).

calcium imbalance	1	2	3	4	5
chloride imbalance	1	2	3	4	5
insulin excess	1	2	3	4	5
iodine deficiency	1	2	3	4	5
lactose intolerance	1	2	3	4	5
magnesium imbalance	1	2	3	4	5
metabolic acidosis/alkalosis	1	2	3	4	5
phosphorous imbalance	1	2	3	4	5
potassium imbalance	1	2	3	4	5
protein–calorie malnutrition	1	2	3	4	5
sodium imbalance	1	2	3	4	5
vitamin deficiency:					
Vitamin A	1	2	3	4	5
B	1	2	3	4	5
C	1	2	3	4	5
D	1	2	3	4	5
E	1	2	3	4	5
K	1	2	3	4	5

List and rate any others

____________________	1	2	3	4	5
____________________	1	2	3	4	5
____________________	1	2	3	4	5

Total Score ____ ÷ # of Items (that apply to you) ____ = Average Score ____

10. Rate your Meta exercise- and activity-risk factors
Average Score: ____

Refer to your heart-training rate responses in your Cardio Profile (pp. 114–117) and convert these into metabolic (METS) rates (the capacity to burn calories) by using Table 4.5, Clinically Significant Key Metabolic Equivalents for Maximum Exercise on p. 74.

Next, circle and score the number of METS that apply to you from 1 (least severe) to 5 (most severe).

METS	*Score*
1–2	1
3–4	2
5–7	3
8–12	4
13–17	5

Profile Summary

Compute your average score for each category, then convert it to a risk rating (which you will use later) as follows:

Average Score	*Risk Rating*
0.0–1.4	I
1.5–2.4	II
2.5–3.4	III
3.5–4.4	IV
4.5–5.0	V

Write in your average scores and converted ratings for all ten risk factor categories, then compute your overall average Meta system score:

Risk Categories	*Average Score*	*Converted Rating*
1. Age	_____	______
2. Gender	_____	______
3. Genetic	_____	______
4. Habits and addictions	_____	______

5. Personality traits	_____	______
6. Environment	_____	______
7. Diseases and injuries	_____	______
8. Symptoms	_____	______
9. Physical condition and fitness	_____	______
10. Exercise and activity	_____	______

Total Score ____ ÷ 10 ____ = Average Meta System Score ____

CHAPTER 5

Buns of Steel, but a Heart of Mush

Saving Your Cardiovascular System

Heart Disease in America

The statistics on heart disease in the United States are themselves enough to cause a heart attack. Sixty million Americans have some form of heart disease or disability. Forty-two million of those have hypertension, and the balance suffer from severe heart disease. For the past fifteen years, the numbers have gradually gone from 200 thousand to 350 thousand heart bypass operations performed annually. Each year, one million Americans survive heart attacks and approximately five million Americans have symptomatic coronary artery disease.

A sedentary lifestyle, cigarette smoking, hypertension, and elevated cholesterol have been identified as major risk factors for developing heart disease. As the heart is central to the cardiovascular respiratory system, many heart patients also suffer respiratory or circulatory problems and diseases.

Cardiovascular Respiratory System Health

Your body needs a steady flow of oxygenated blood to the heart, brain, skeletal muscles, skin, and the rest of your body. Without it, your organs will suffocate and die. Cardiovascular system health depends on the health of the three major parts of the cardiovascular system: a strong heart, flexible and unobstructed blood vessels, and lungs with a deep-breathing capacity.

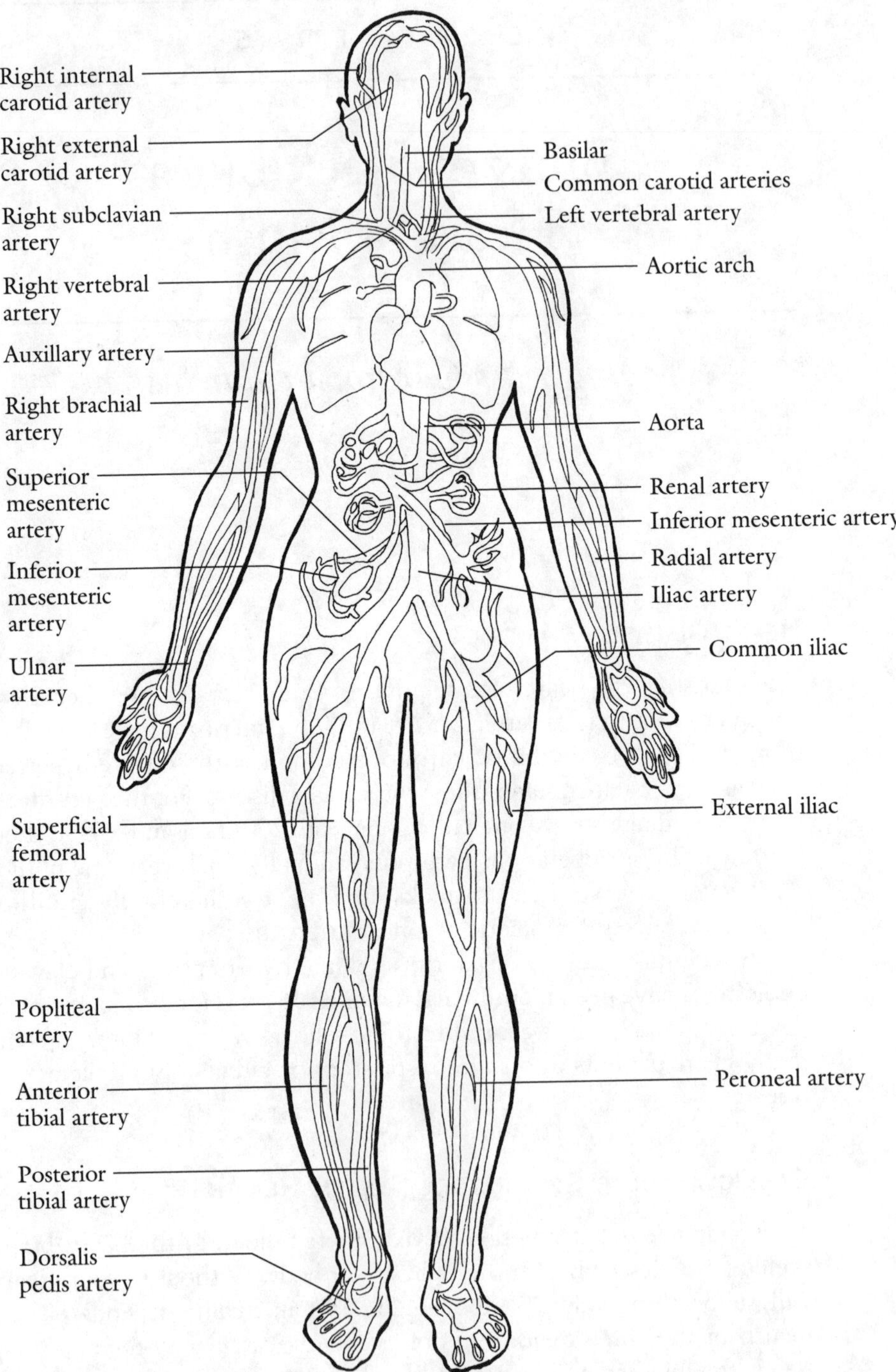

Circulatory System

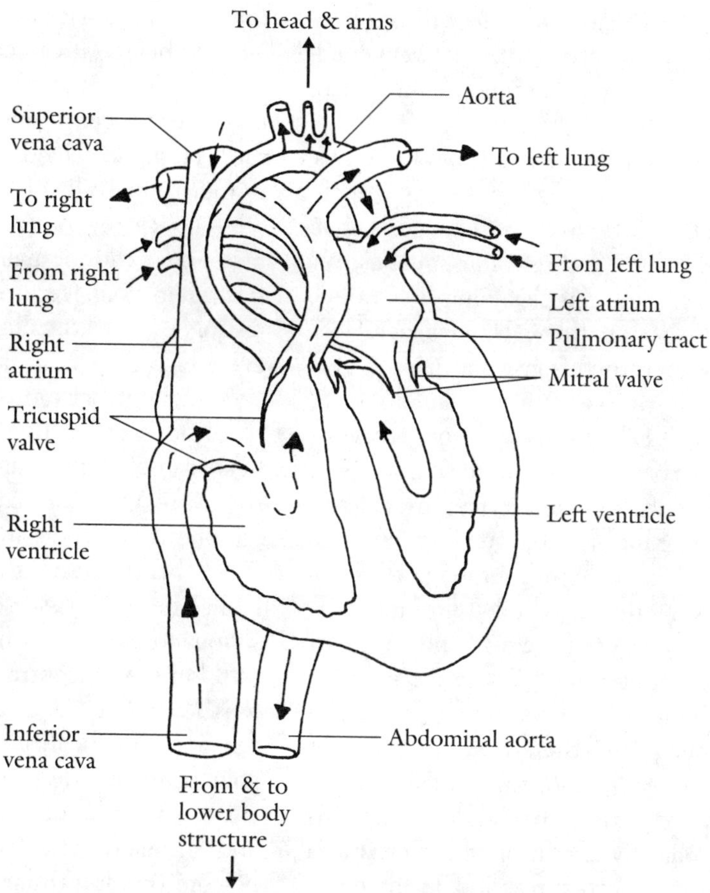

How Your Cardiovascular Respiratory System Works

Your cardiovascular respiratory system is the pump and air-delivery system of your body. It is really three subsystems working together, the heart, blood vessels, and lungs ("cardio"—heart; "vascular"—vessels; "respiratory"—lungs). At the center of this system is the heart muscle, the main pump. Various muscle groups strategically located in different parts of your body act as subsidiary pumps. The calf muscle is one: It pumps blood back to the heart from your lower legs. Other muscles also draw and pump deoxygenated blood from various areas of your body creating a greater demand on the heart muscle to pump fresh oxygenated blood back to them.

Your Heart Muscle: How It Works

Your heart is an eggplant-shaped muscle about the size of your fist (if you are a marathon runner, your heart can be the size of your biceps muscle). It is a super muscle that weighs approximately seven to twelve ounces. Long periods of physical inactivity, however, can shrink and weaken the heart muscle, just as a biceps muscle will weaken when it is not exercised. In this weakened state, your heart pumps less blood with each beat and becomes less efficient.

The inside of your heart is hollow and has four separate chambers: left and right **ventricles,** and left and right **atria.** The walls that contract (or "beat") and relax are muscles. As they contract, these muscles pump fresh oxygenated blood out through your **arteries.** Blood is then returned from your muscles and other organs to your heart via a smaller system of blood vessels called **veins.** As your left ventricle pumps oxygenated blood to your arteries, your right ventricle pumps oxygen-depleted blood into your lungs for oxygenation and ridding carbon dioxide. From your lungs, the oxygenated blood returns to the left atrium.

A healthy heart muscle is one that can keep a steady beat and a high stroke volume. **Stroke volume** is the amount of blood the heart can pump into the arteries in one beat or stroke. A well-conditioned heart pumps out more blood with each beat. This explains why an aerobically conditioned athlete has a lower heart rate, both at rest and during physical exertion. A sedentary person's heart must beat more often to accomplish the same level of blood flow. Starting out with a strong heart gives you the pumping power to maintain healthy blood flow and better efficiency.

A well-conditioned heart can do much more work than any other muscle in your body. At rest, it beats or contracts forty to seventy times per minute. During exercise, it may beat ninety to 200 beats per minute, or a total of sixty to 100 thousand times per day. A strong heart can pump nine pints of blood per minute at rest and fifty-four pints during work. Try to do as many continuous curls or contractions with your buttocks or biceps muscles! The only other muscle that can come close to the heart is your calf muscle, often called the "second heart." It can contract twenty to sixty times per minute during a slow walk and sixty to 120 times per minute during a fast walk or run. Though trained marathon walkers and runners can walk or run for extended periods—up to seventeen hours a day during a race—they cannot maintain that pace forever. But when your feet are up and your legs are resting, your heart still keeps beating, each and every second of your lifetime.

Your buttocks muscle, (your "buns"), on the other hand, is five times bigger than your heart muscle but it cannot do anywhere near the work of your heart. Imagine squeezing your buns 100 thousand times a day!

A heart muscle that is weak or that has had some of its tissue destroyed is a far more serious threat to your life and well-being than soft buns. Concentrating on your buttocks muscle and neglecting your heart is a folly. On a list of health and exercise priorities, your heart muscle should be at the top, your calves in the middle (right below your back and stomach), and your buttocks near the bottom (pardon the pun).

ARTERIES

A stronger flow of blood may also prevent the clogging and stiffening of your blood vessels throughout your body. As with your heart muscle, your blood vessels need physical activity by way of maintained blood flow throughout the system. Also, without a steady flow of blood, arteries can more quickly become clogged and less flexible. This condition, which can also be caused by elevated cholesterol levels, is called **atherosclerosis** (or hardening of the arteries). Hardened or constricted blood vessels, in turn, cause pain in the muscles fed by those arteries such as chest (or pectoral) muscles (see angina, p. 398) or calf muscles (see intermittent claudication, p. 408).

VEINS

Veins are smaller and less muscular blood vessels than the arteries. Their job is to bring blood back to the heart from the muscles and the organs. There are superficial veins, and larger, deep-seated veins within muscles. As with arteries, physical activity and exercise, particularly walking, promote vein growth and flexibility and improve circulation.

Circulation problems in veins, such as blood vessel narrowing, start at a less serious level and are expressed in such symptoms as increased cold sensitivity, blood pooling, varicose veins, and swelling of limbs. Symptoms can also escalate into vein blockages, called **blood clots,** and ruptured or leaking capillaries. These, in turn, can cause ulcers or sores on the surrounding skin.

Deep-seated blood clots can be life threatening. If a clot breaks away and enters the lungs, it is called a **pulmonary embolism** or blood clot of the lung. Clotting in deep veins requires serious medical attention, including blood-thinning medication, and a Cardiovascular Rehab Rx (see pp. 421–426). (Vein Rehab from vein clotting and phlebitis is covered in Part Three.)

LUNGS

The lungs work in concert with the heart by oxygenating oxygen-depleted blood, which then returns to the heart.

Air containing oxygen is inhaled into the lungs and exchanged for carbon dioxide that has been released from the oxygen-depleted blood. This process is called **gas exchange.** The fresher blood leaves the lungs via blood vessels and flows into the left atrium of the heart and from there to the left ventricle where it is pumped back into the arteries.

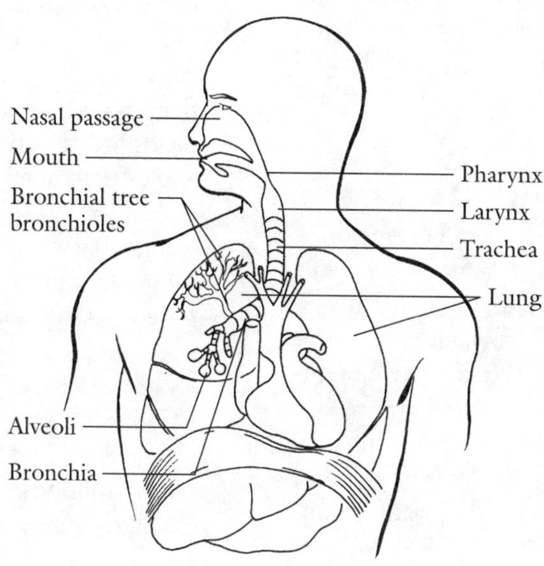

Respiratory System

WHAT CAN GO WRONG?

With the advent of fatty, processed foods and the growth of sedentary lifestyles in the last forty years, the environmental factors clearly overwhelm any inherited disposition to heart disease. For this reason, exercise medicine is central in the war against heart, artery, and lung disease—a human-made cure for human-made diseases. With the highest death rate of all the major diseases and the highest rate of occurrence (one in four people have some form of heart disease), you are at risk if you ignore your heart health.

Additionally, a disease in one part of the cardiovascular respiratory system can threaten all the other parts. Lung disease and breathing disorders can weaken the heart muscle and impair the circulation. Reduced circulation, in turn, may contribute to the formation of plaque on the inside arterial wall of the heart. Ironically, the weakest areas of the cardiovascular respiratory system are the blood vessels themselves. After they become diseased or blocked, they impede the flow of blood to the heart, lungs, and other such vital organs as the brain, stomach, and kidneys. The greatest and probably earliest sign of cardiovascular trouble will be in the blood vessels, which can cause high blood pressure.

High blood pressure or **hypertension** is both a condition and a risk factor for heart disease and is related to other such health system diseases as diabetes. If hypertension goes undetected and untreated, it can permanently damage the blood vessels and the rest of the cardiovascular system. Exercise can often favorably modify high blood pressure and may prevent further damage to other body organs and systems.

TABLE 5.1 CARDIOVASCULAR AND RESPIRATORY DISEASES AND DISORDERS

asthma Asthma is a highly treatable often reversible lung disease suffered by thirteen million Americans. One-third are under eighteen, but half of new cases are under ten; two-thirds are girls. Breathing passages become narrow and blocked and easily inflamed, overresponding to various types of stimulation including airborne irritants, emotional stress, fatigue, overexercise, and humidity and temperature changes. Wheezing, coughing, and chest tightness, as well as sweating are common symptoms. Even with treatment, asthma can be chronic, and in some instances can produce severe breathing problems.

atherosclerosis or coronary artery disease (CAD) is the blockage or hardening of arteries that supply blood to the heart muscle and can cause heart attack or stroke. Although most doctors believe there is an inherited tendency toward heart disease, a healthy lifestyle of diet and exercise may reduce many of the negative effects of heredity. More men than women have this disease, but the balance is rapidly shifting as high-fat diets, cigarette smoking, and stressful work conditions are becoming common for women, too. Most serious are blockages in the coronary artery and the renal (kidney) artery; heart and kidney failure are often fatal conditions. Brain artery occlusons can also cause strokes and various other arteries can also become clogged.

emphysema and **chronic bronchitis** Emphysema is a chronic lung disorder more common in men (probably because men smoke more than women do). Apart from smoking, both emphysema and chronic bronchitis are believed to have family- and hereditary-risk factors.

heart attack A heart attack chokes off or damages your heart muscle caused by a blockage of blood and/or oxygen. A serious heart attack can lead to the death of part of the heart muscle tissue and can inhibit the heart's capacity to function properly. **Myocardial infarction** (the medical term for heart attack) means "myo"—muscle, "cardium"—heart, "infarcation"—death, that is "death of the heart muscle."

high blood pressure or **hypertension** Half of all Americans have high blood pressure; one-quarter of all deaths are related to heart disease. Hypertension is a condition that can lead to heart attack, stroke, and other lethal diseases. As with other forms of heart disease, there are strong hereditary and familial components, but in many people, it can be controlled with diet and exercise.

high cholesterol This is a condition of too much fat in the blood. It is usually related to diet, but is also found in families with heart disease.

lung cancer As with emphysema, lung cancer can severely and permanently reduce your breathing capacity and cause excruciating chest and shoulder pain. Even though the prognosis is poor (i.e. a five-year survival rate—it's the most common cause of cancer death in men and is quickly becoming the most common for women), the disease is largely preventable by either avoiding or quitting cigarette smoking. Regular exercise, especially aerobic exercise, can help you break the cigarette habit. Polluted air and air containing industrial carcinogens have also been associated with certain types of lung cancer.

Stroke Stroke is the third major cause of death in the United States (of the 500 thousand sufferers per year, only half survive). It is classified officially as a cerebrovascular accident and is caused by impaired blood circulation in one or more of the blood vessels supplying the brain. It most often occurs in middle-age and elderly persons, but currently younger people can also have cocaine-induced strokes.

Strokes are caused by three types of blockages: (1) **thrombus** (blood clot), (2) **embolism** (pieces of fragmented clot usually originating in the heart), and (3) **hemorrhage** (rupture and bleeding). The major risk factors associated with strokes are: hardening of the arteries, high blood pressure, irregular heartbeat, rheumatic heart disease, diabetes, abnormal blood pressure when standing, an enlarged heart, high serum triglyceride levels, lack of exercise, use of oral contraceptives, and cigarette smoking. By quitting smoking, getting more exercise, and medical treatment, you can seriously reduce your chances of stroke or **transient ischemic attacks** (deficiency of blood in a part, usually caused by a constriction or an actual obstruction of a blood vessel).

varicose veins These blue, spidery veins

often appear in the backs of thighs and legs. Although they are not considered life threatening, the condition is inherited and two-thirds of patients are women. This condition can be favorably modified but not eliminated or reversed. Exercise improves leg circulation and reduces the risk of varicose veins, which contribute to more serious health problems such as phlebitis.

vascular disease This disease of the arteries causes impaired circulation in those blood vessels that supply the body's major organs, including the brain, kidneys, and stomach. It may be caused by such risk factors as high blood pressure, high cholesterol, obesity, and cigarette smoking.

HEART DISEASE, VASCULAR DISEASE, AND HEART ATTACKS

The single greatest threat to your cardiovascular system is heart disease itself. **Heart disease** is an umbrella term for hundreds of heart-related diseases that strike the heart and blood vessels. Heart disease accounts for half of the deaths in America. In one form or another, 25% of Americans suffer from heart disease.

Heart disease does not start with a weak heart muscle nor does it start with a heart attack. Heart disease begins with either a diseased blood vessel system (vascular system) or one that is prone to the accumulation of cholesterol-laden plaque along its inner walls.

Also called **coronary artery disease (CAD),** the most life-threatening form of heart disease is blockage of the arteries that feed blood directly to the heart muscle. When this happens, the heart can't receive enough oxygen. If a blood vessel (i.e. coronary artery) feeding the heart muscle becomes completely blocked or occluded, a **heart attack** (or **myocardial infarction**) results, in which your heart muscle literally suffocates.

A heart attack is the most traumatic disorder that can disable your cardiovascular system. "My kingdom for a heart!" could be the battle cry of many people in their forties, fifties, and sixties, who have been stricken by a heart attack. Heart attacks are usually the culmination of heart disease. Each heart attack can damage more living heart tissue, leaving the heart less and less able to function as the body's primary pump. Although traditionally regarded as a man's disease, many women (particularly those who are executives, smokers, postmenopausal, and diabetic) are having more and more heart attacks. Their risk factors are age, sex, heredity, obesity, diabetes, high blood pressure, high cholesterol, physical inactivity, smoking, birth control pills, and a frenetic or stressful lifestyle.

Despite cancer and AIDS, heart attacks still remain the number-one killer of men and women throughout the industrialized world. Exercise, along with a proper diet, can help save your cardiovascular system from this totally modern, largely environmental disease, which is almost entirely a product of an unhealthy lifestyle.

LUNG DISEASE

Even though lung diseases contribute to the weakening of your heart and vascular system, they are generally not caused by weaknesses in the system but by unhealthy habits and environmental factors, most particularly smoking cigarettes, and polluted, carcinogenic air and infections. Keeping your lungs healthy is important because they are the only mechanism for bringing oxygen into your blood stream. Severely damaged lungs cannot do the job and can ultimately play a role in heart attack and heart failure. Exercise can keep your lungs strong and healthy by increasing their breathing capacity. Exercise, however, can also improve your lungs after disease has damaged them—depending of course on the degree of damage. Because those risk factors that affect your heart and blood vessels may also affect your lungs, an effective exercise program must be aimed at all three diseases—heart disease, lung disease, and vascular disease.

Cardiovascular Risk Factors

The cardiovascular system requires lifelong physical activity to maintain its health, to counteract its natural aging, and to slow down the onset of heart, lung, and blood vessel diseases. It is important to monitor your body for such early signs of heart disease as high cholesterol and high blood pressure. Even if you do not have a single predisposing risk, an unconditioned heart muscle can cause you unnecessary fatigue. High blood pressure, in turn, has its own special risk factors. This is because it is a disorder that can also exist without any underlying heart disease or symptoms.

Cardiovascular risk factors generally come in multiple combinations. This is bad news if you are a nonexerciser, but very good news if you exercise to renew your health. Controlling one risk factor—such as weight or diabetes—with exercise often helps control the other risk factors at the same time.

Cardiovascular Exercise

Cardiovascular exercise is an important component of any health program. The amount of exercise is more important than the intensity of exercise. Indeed, most exercise should be done at moderate intensity. Those at lower risk can do at least thirty minutes or more of moderate intensity exercise every day of the week, (preferably) as suggested by the American College of Sports Medicine and the Centers for Disease Control. Those with a higher risk of cardiovascular disease should build up to a daily exercise regimen from every other day, but overall, people at high risk need to practice a greater amount of cardiovascular exercise than those at low risk. Whether you are in the high or low cardio risk category, healthy or diseased, you should make it a high priority to practice at least a minimum amount of cardiovascular exercise every day.

The Big City Factor: Bad Diet and High Stress

The pattern is familiar, predictable, and sad. Many people from farms and rural areas who lived into their nineties have offspring who moved to the city and succumbed to the rich food, stressful life, and lack of physical activity; they became smokers, became overweight, and never adopted counteracting health and exercise habits. They developed high cholesterol, high blood pressure, and, eventually, heart disease, and had their first heart attack while still in their forties. Meanwhile, back on the farm, the physical activity is not what it used to be, and instead of fresh farm products, rural folks began to eat processed foods. Thus, those who stayed on the farm or in the countryside have nearly equal the risk as their stressed-out city siblings.

Heart disease is one of the few diseases in which healthy living and exercise can help to keep the disease in check, perhaps for a lifetime. Sometimes exercise is not the only solution, however. If you already have heart disease or a familial component for it, and you also have high blood pressure, blood pressure medication and a strict diet are often required. The shocking early death of running guru Jim Fixx is a dramatic example of how severe heart disease cannot entirely be treated by exercise alone. Sadly, Fixx's health profile showed a family history of heart disease and high blood pressure, a prior smoking habit, and a diet of high-fat foods. As a result, despite many years of running and exercise, Fixx succumbed to a heart attack.

Many experts say diet is half the battle. To reduce body fat, you should reduce both the fat in the foods you eat as well as the total amount of calories you ingest. But your concern about body fat should be heightened even further if your familial predisposition is toward obesity, high cholesterol, high blood pressure, or heart disease.

AGE AND GENDER

If you are a male over age forty, you have a greater chance of having heart disease than females under the ages of fifty to fifty-five. If you are female and over the age of fifty to fifty-five, your chances of contracting heart disease are equal to males after the age of forty. After menopause, the loss of your natural production of estrogen causes you to lose a gender-related immunity to heart disease.

Thus, while age and gender do contribute to the risk of disease, one or more of the other risk factors (e.g. poor diet, stress, high blood pressure or familial tendency) must also be present to cause concern. Preventing disease is a matter of controlling the risk factors that you can change (e.g. diet and stress) so you can make the most of the factors you inherit and cannot control (e.g. age, race, genetics).

The risk factors that follow include ones you can control (such as diet) and those you can't control (such as age and race). Wherever possible, we have rated the factors on a scale of 1 (least severe) to 5 (most severe), to indicate the weight you should place on each risk in relation to others.

HIGH BLOOD PRESSURE: FACTOR OF 3 TO 4

High blood pressure or hypertension is a condition in which your blood pressure is above normal when your body is at rest. It is a major risk factor for heart disease deaths, especially heart attacks and strokes (i.e. 90% of stroke victims have high blood pressure). Unfortunately, you can't feel it. It must be measured with a blood pressure meter.

Blood pressure control is as central to the health of your cardiovascular system as bone strengthening is to your musculoskeletal system. When your blood pressure is too high, the probability of incurring severe damage to your arteries and of having a heart attack or stroke may be increased by a factor of three to four times that of a person with normal blood pressure levels. Table 5.2 shows the levels of blood pressure from low to severely high. This table serves to assist you in evaluating your own blood pressure level.

HIGH BLOOD PRESSURE RISK FACTORS

1. **Familial tendency:** 50% of hypertensives have other immediate blood relations with high blood pressure or such related diseases as diabetes, kidney disease, and thyroid conditions.
2. **Age:** The tendency of blood pressure to rise with age. Over half of men and women over the age of sixty have high blood pressure.
3. **Gender:** Hypertension is more prevalent in men than women over the age of fifty.
4. **Race:** Blacks are twice as likely as whites to be hypertensive at any age.
5. **Being overweight:** Each extra pound of body weight above the ideal puts an increased burden on the circulatory system.
6. **Salt and salty foods:** If you are genetically predisposed to hypertension, too much salt intake can be a risk factor. Foods that contain 40% or more of the recommended daily allowance (RDA) of salt cause water retention and increase blood volume. This puts increased pressure on artery walls. Although exercise can have a diuretic effect, you should also consider reducing your sodium intake to below five grams per day especially if you have a genetic factor for high blood pressure.
7. **Stress:** For people with moderate to severe hypertension, stress can further increase blood pressure levels.
8. **Cigarette smoking:** This addiction can double the risks associated with high blood pressure. Smoking also causes blood vessel constriction and contributes to plaque buildup in the arteries.
9. **Saturated fats:** A diet high in saturated fats can lead to a buildup of cholesterol in the bloodstream, which, in turn, can cause arteriosclerosis.

TABLE 5.2
BLOOD PRESSURE SCALE

1	2	3	4	5
Low	Normal	Mildly High	Moderately High	Severely High
under 120/80	120/80 to 140/90	140/90 to 159/104	160/105 to 180/115	over 180/115

Your blood pressure varies throughout the day and rises when you exercise or are anxious; doctors try to gauge your blood pressure at rest. Normal blood pressure is in the range of 120/80 up to 140/90. The first number represents **systolic** pressure, which is the pressure on your artery walls when blood is pumped out of your heart. A high systolic blood pressure increases your probability of having a stroke by several fold. The second number is the **diastolic** pressure, which is the pressure on your arteries when your heart is between heartbeats.

For each ten-point reduction of your systolic pressure, your chances of heart attack decrease by one-third. Low to moderately high blood pressure may be controlled with a daily cardiovascular exercise program, proper diet, and stress reduction. Severely high blood pressure may also be favorably modified with regular cardiovascular exercise, in addition to some level of blood pressure medicine. After you have been diagnosed as hypertensive, cardiovascular exercise should become a priority not only for a stronger heart, but also to enhance blood circulation throughout the seventy thousand miles of your vascular network.

CHOLESTEROL: FACTOR OF 2 TO 3

Cholesterol is a fatlike substance found in such animal by-products we eat as meat and dairy products. Because saturated fats (i.e. fats that are solid at room temperature, such as butter and lard) can increase your cholesterol level, it makes good health sense to reduce your intake of butter, marbled meats, and other foods that are high in saturated fats. Your body also manufactures its own cholesterol for the healthy functioning of hormones and cell membranes. The buildup of too much cholesterol in your bloodstream, however, can clog your arteries by forming a type of plaque that sticks to your artery walls, narrowing them and causing the passage of blood to slow down. Although high cholesterol is often associated with being overweight, people who are at normal or even below normal weight can also have high cholesterol. Indeed, experts believe that atherosclerotic plaque does not always start as circulating bodies that stick to vessel walls, but instead they begin as microscopic injuries to blood vessel walls that consequently protrude as they collect cholesterol and other products.

Two components of your cholesterol count that are important in determining your risk for heart disease are **high-density lipoprotein (HDL,** so-called "good cholesterol") and **low-density lipoprotein (LDL,** so-called "bad cholesterol"). Low-density lipoprotein forms the plaque that collects in the arteries; HDL helps remove LDL from your bloodstream. Studies show that exercise may decrease levels of LDL and increase HDL levels, which can help reduce the potential for plaque buildup. Cardiovascular exercise also reduces body weight and the stores of fat, which helps decrease your total cholesterol count—especially if it is elevated. Also, controlling your insulin levels by eating smaller meals more often is another important protective measure. Ideally, your LDL levels should be 130 or lower and less than 100 if you already have heart disease, while your ideal HDL levels should be 35 or higher. Indeed, an HDL level that is higher than 60 is considered a negative risk factor for heart disease. For every 1% decrease in total cholesterol, there is a 2 to 3% drop in the risk of heart disease. Your ratio of total cholesterol to HDL is one of the most important health indicators. A ratio of 4.5 or less puts you in the low-risk category for heart disease; 4.6 or more indicates a higher risk.

Your cholesterol count must be judged safe based on your age and gender. An adult's cholesterol level ideally should be under 200. If you are a young adult between the ages of twenty and thirty-three your ideal total cholesterol should be under 180 if you are male; and your cholesterol count should be under 177, if you are female. Children (age 0 to 19) who fall within the moderate to high range of cholesterol levels are at risk of eventually getting heart disease. Recent studies show that one-third of all American children have moderate to high cholesterol (see Table 5.3, Safe Cholesterol Counts).

CIGARETTE SMOKING: FACTOR OF 2 TO 3

Smoking cigarettes increases your heart attack risk by two to three times that of a nonsmoker. Smoke damages your cardiovascular system and it artificially stimulates your heart to beat faster and often irregularly as well. Smoking replaces oxygen in your blood with **carbon monoxide** while damaging the lining of the arteries and thus enhancing plaque buildup. The nicotine found in cigarettes also constricts your arteries and raises your blood pressure. This also possibly contributes to more cholesterol plaque buildup. Cigarettes also damage your lungs and deprive your organs of needed oxygen, which increases your risk of heart attack and stroke by thirteen times that of a nonsmoker. This is especially true for women who smoke and also take birth control pills.

By smoking, you can also become addicted to the artificial stimulation of your mental activity. Additionally, it is difficult to smoke only one or two cigarettes: The longer you smoke, the more your body becomes addicted to the repetitive activity of craving and then inhaling greater amounts of smoke or nicotine. Cardiovascular exercise may help you to kick the smoking habit by weaning you off of this artificial stimulation. Vigorous exercise may be even more effective as a prescription for smoking addiction than moderate exercise because it does a better job of increasing your natural breathing capacity and introducing more fresh oxygen into your blood and lungs. Exercise provides a new, positive habit to take the place of the dangerous habit of smoking while teaching you self-control and self-confidence—two vital weapons needed to fight cigarette smoking addiction.

BEING OVERWEIGHT: FACTOR OF 3 TO 5

Although weight and fat gain are a natural part of the aging process after age twenty-five, inactivity and processed foods contribute to even greater weight gains than is ideal for your age, gender, and body build (i.e. more than ten pounds per decade). This extra weight and fat stresses your heart, arteries, and lungs. An overweight person (i.e. more than ten pounds over the ideal weight) has three times more heart attack risk than a normal weight person; this risk increases to five times if a person is thirty pounds overweight.

With or without dieting, a weight-loss program that includes moderate cardiovascular exercise is the best way to lose weight and maintain an ideal weight. Moderate-intensity exercise has the best track record for both long-term results and appetite suppression. If you are more than thirty pounds overweight you should begin your comeback with a Meta Rehab Rx exercise program (see pp. 350–395).

TABLE 5.3: SAFE CHOLESTEROL COUNTS

AGES 20–39

Total Cholesterol	*Ideal*	*Moderate Risk*	*High Risk*
Male	under 180	180–202	over 202
Female	under 177	177–197	over 197
LDL			
Male	under 118	118–137	over 137
Female	under 109	109–127	over 127
HDL			
Male	over 51	37–51	under 37
Female	over 63	45–63	under 45

AGES 40–59

Total Cholesterol	*Ideal*	*Moderate Risk*	*High Risk*
Male	under 210	210–233	over 233
Female	under 210	210–235	over 235
LDL			
Male	under 141	141–162	over 162
Female	under 129	129–155	over 155
HDL			
Male	over 52	37–52	under 37
Female	over 69	49–69	under 49

Stressful Living—Type A Personality Plus Chronic Hostility: Factor of 5

Heart attacks can be brought on by or at least coincide with a physically and mentally or emotionally stressful event. However, remaining in a constant or recurring state of stress or hostility is probably an even more significant cause (see Chapter Six, The Mind/Body Connection, for more details about personality traits and stressful reactions). People who

SAFE CHOLESTEROL COUNTS *(continued)*
AGES 60+

Total Cholesterol	*Ideal*	*Moderate Risk*	*High Risk*
Male	under 214	214–240	over 240
Female	under 228	228–252	over 252
LDL			
Male	under 144	144–165	over 165
Female	under 150	150–175	over 175
HDL			
Male	over 60	40–60	under 40
Female	over 74	50–74	under 50

are regularly in this state are considered to have **Type A personalities**—especially if they are also angry and hostile.

Many experts believe that being under stress or having continuous stressful reactions makes the body secrete too many stress hormones, for example, cortisol and adrenaline. These, in turn, release fat into the bloodstream, which increases cholesterol and blood pressure, which can eventually damage arteries. Type A, chronically hostile personalities, have five times the risk factor for having a heart attack than a person who is not stressed-out or hostile.

Many Type As have learned to limit the number and duration of their stressful reactions through exercise. By reducing the physical effects (muscle tension) of your stressful reactions, exercise decreases the flow of hormones that can cause organ damage. At the same time, exercise releases such hormones as endorphines, which have mood-elevating effects that counteract the results of stress-related hormones.

Recent studies also indicate that socially isolated people who shun interaction with other people (the same as with chronically hostile people) are also at a higher risk for heart disease and other chronic diseases.

DIABETES: FACTOR OF 2

Diabetics (both Types I and II) have twice the risk of a nondiabetic person for having a heart attack or stroke. This is because diabetics are usually overweight and also have high blood pressure. Diabetes also carries a greater risk for having atherosclerosis, therefore causing more heart attacks and strokes. Moderate cardiovascular exercise may help control these complications and reduce the risk of a potential heart attack or stroke.

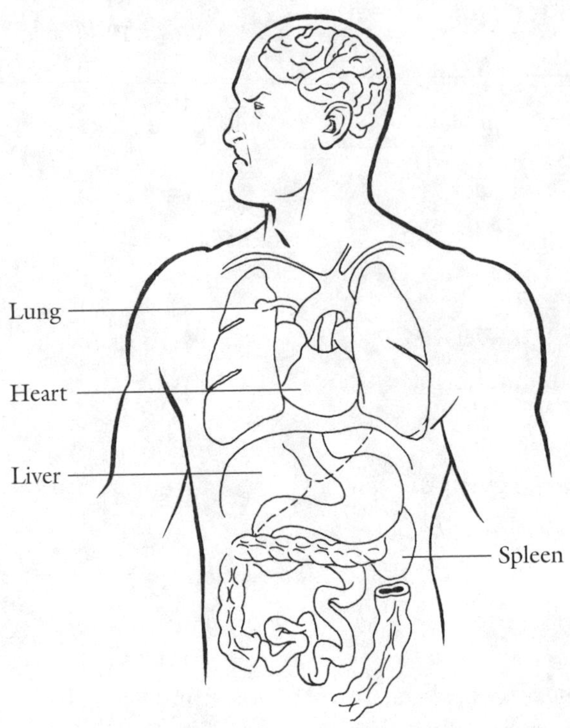

Effects of Stressful Reactions and Type A Personality

A SEDENTARY LIFESTYLE: FACTOR OF 4

Lifelong physical inactivity (also known as living a sedentary lifestyle) may increase your risk of not surviving a heart attack by a factor of four. But how much does it increase your risk of having the heart attack in the first place? We are just beginning to find out. We do know that your risk of developing the conditions that cause most heart attacks (i.e. high blood pressure, high cholesterol, being overweight) are reduced with being moderately active your whole life. Some doctors believe that a sedentary lifestyle may turn out to be as dangerous as high blood pressure, high cholesterol, and cigarette smoking. Perhaps it is an even greater risk factor, because your activity level is both part of the problem and the solution.

CARDIOVASCULAR RESPIRATORY EXERCISE RISKS AND BENEFITS

When you are at rest, your lungs take in about twelve pints of air per minute. When you are fully conditioned and are exercising at peak capacity, your lungs can take in more than 200 pints per minute, an almost twenty-fold increase. Greater air flow, as with better blood flow, increases the amount of oxygen that your working muscles receive and allows you to work harder without tiring.

Lung disease reduces your breathing capacity. However, mild symptoms such as occasional breathlessness, coughing, and wheezing can still be helped with Cardiovascular Rehab exercises (see pp. 216–220).

The major risk factors for lung disease are cigarette smoking and air pollution. These can cause **chronic bronchitis** (an inflammation of the lungs that causes a three-month-per-year cough for two years in a row), and which can lead to **emphysema,** which causes a loss of elasticity and actual damage to the lungs.

Diseased lung tissue, the same as with diseased heart tissue, cannot be restored. The body compensates, instead, by shifting the some of the lung's work load to the heart. If severe lung deterioration takes place, the right ventricle of the heart cannot pump the used blood out of the heart and into the lungs fast enough and the right side of the heart fills with the extra blood. This is **right-sided heart failure** caused by lung disease. A heart attack usually causes **congestive heart failure** or **left-sided heart failure,** which is fluid buildup in the lungs resulting from damage to the left ventricle. **Asthma,** another lung disorder, and **allergies** can also inhibit your breathing as a result of muscle spasms and the accumulation of mucus in your breathing tubes.

Strengthening the good lung tissue that you have often compensates for the weakness of or damage to other tissue. Cardio exercise not only strengthens the breathing muscles but also helps clean the outflow of mucus from the tubes, which makes your breathing easier and more vigorous. For asthmatics, moderate cardiovascular exercise is best because it increases breathing gradually, so it will not cause muscles to go into spasm.

WHAT KIND OF EXERCISE IS MOST EFFECTIVE?

An effective cardiovascular exercise program promotes the smooth, continuous flow of oxygen and blood to your body's organs and muscles. Cardiovascular exercise—defined as continuous rhythmic movement of arms and legs—is the best prevention exercise for heart, blood vessel, and lung health.

Traditional aerobic exercise is a part of a cardiovascular exercise program, but is not all of it. The definition of aerobic exercise refers to any exercise that consumes a great deal of oxygen. Aerobic exercise intensity is achieved in two basic ways: a heart rate at least 60 to 80% of the maximum heart-training rate and a breathing rate of over twenty breaths per minute. You can estimate your maximum heart-training rate by subtracting your age from 220. Cardiovascular exercise should also include circulatory exercise as well, which is any exercise that generates blood flow to all or most major muscle groups.

As you will see if you follow the Cardiovascular Prevention Ex on pp. 216–230, the best overall exercises for the cardiovascular system are such moderate-paced exercises as walking, stationary bicycling, and swimming. These three exercises are easily accessible, produce the lowest injury rates, and simultaneously work three or more of the major muscle groups. Walking and cycling exercise the leg muscle group (i.e. thighs, buttocks, calves, and shins); swimming (and rowing, too) exercises the arm muscle group.

The Cardiovascular Prevention Ex (see pp. 216–230) can also be practiced even if you have mild to moderate heart, blood vessel, and/or lung disease including high blood pressure, arterial blockage, varicose veins, intermittent claudication, and angina pectoris. **Angina pectoris** is a symptom of coronary artery disease characterized by chest pain that occurs when your heart muscle temporarily does not receive enough oxygen and blood because one or more of the coronary arteries feeding the heart has been narrowed by arteriosclerosis. If you have had a heart attack, heart surgery, or have moderate or severe angina or intermittent claudication, you should start with the Cardiovascular Rehab Program (see pp. 421–426) and work your way up to the Preventive Program.

IT'S NEVER TOO LATE

Studies show that the signs and symptoms of heart disease (i.e. high blood pressure, circulatory blockage, chest pain) can be controlled, relieved, and sometimes even reversed, with an exercise and diet program. In other words, a cardiovascular exercise program may

CARDIOVASCULAR AND RESPIRATORY EXERCISE BENEFITS

1. Exercise increases your energy capacity or stamina. You can do more physical work daily without getting as fatigued.
2. Exercise improves your circulation or blood flow, which means your muscles and organs get the oxygen and nutrients they need. It also reduces the pain associated with poor circulation and blockage in chest and calf muscles.
3. Exercise helps you breath easier and deeper by making your lungs stronger and more flexible. You also feel more relaxed.
4. Exercise improves the flow of all fluid and may help to prevent infections by flushing mucus buildup in lungs and nasal passages.
5. Exercise lowers blood pressure, which helps prevent plaque formation on artery walls and also reduces the impact of high blood pressure as a risk factor for various forms of heart disease.
6. Exercise increases HDL, which helps protect against heart disease.
7. Exercise lowers your heart rate while at rest, thereby allowing your heart to beat more efficiently.
8. Exercise increases your maximum heart-training rate by letting you work out at a higher intensity without becoming breathless and fatigued.
9. Exercise also reduces the risk of having a second heart attack or stroke, after the first one has occurred.
10. Most important, exercise may reduce the risk of getting heart, lung, and circulatory diseases and can slow down the progress of symptoms associated with these diseases (e.g. being overweight, irregular heartbeat, and so on).

improve the health of your heart to some degree no matter how weak it has become.

YOUR CARDIO PROFILE

To determine the amount of cardiovascular respiratory exercise you should be doing, rate your cardio health and weaknesses using the Cardio System Profile. If you rate I, II, or III, practice the Cardio Preventive Exercises in Part Two. If you rate IV or V, practice the Cardio Rehab program in Part Three.

Circle each of the major risk factors as they apply to you and multiply the number of these factors by the number of point values assigned in each category. Total up your points for the category before continuing on to the next category. You may also use this questionnaire to evaluate the medical risk factors of a child or adult under your care and supervision. The final score will ascertain which of the five health systems are the weakest and will determine where you should concentrate the *Exercise Rx* program.

Cardio System Profile

Compute your Cardio-risk factors by rating the severity of your diseases, symptoms, and physical weaknesses on a scale of 1 point (least severe) to 5 points (most severe). Average your points and convert your averages to an overall rating that corresponds to the intensity or difficulty level for which you will begin your prevention or rehabilitation exercises. Please note: No answer equals a score of 0.

1. Rate your Cardio age-risk factor
Score: ____

Average your scores for question 9, items a, b, c, and d and circle the rating that best describes the condition of your Cardio system (or that of your child or patient).

Performance vs. Age Group	*Score*
Over 20 yrs. more fit than age group	1
10 to 20 yrs. more fit	2
Equal to your age group	3
10 to 20 yrs. less fit	4
Less than 20 yrs. less fit	5

2. Rate your Cardio gender-risk factors
Average Score: ____

Circle the gender-specific Cardio diseases you already have (or have had), then circle their corresponding point value. The average onset age is shown in parentheses after each disease. For those illnesses without an average onset age, score your level of disability from 1 (least severe) to 5 (most severe). If you haven't had any Cardio diseases, your score is 0.

Disease Onset	*Point Value*
Later than norm	1
Within the norm	2
Up to 5 yrs. before	3
5–10 yrs. before	4
10+ yrs. before	5

Common or Predominantly Male Diseases

aneurysm (65)	1	2	3	4	5
arterial occlusive disease	1	2	3	4	5
Buerger's disease	1	2	3	4	5
chronic bronchitis/emphysema	1	2	3	4	5
coronary artery disease	1	2	3	4	5
heart attack (60)	1	2	3	4	5
high blood pressure (50)	1	2	3	4	5
legionnaires' disease	1	2	3	4	5
lung cancer	1	2	3	4	5

Common or Predominantly Female Diseases

migraine	1	2	3	4	5
Raynaud's disease	1	2	3	4	5
sarcoidosis (30)	1	2	3	4	5
varicose veins	1	2	3	4	5

Total Score ____ ÷ # of Items (that apply to you) ____ = Average Score ____

3. Rate your Cardio genetic-risk factors
Average Score: ____

Circle and score the severity of any inherited Cardio diseases that you already have (or have had) or that a close relative may have (or have had). (Only count grandparents, parents, their siblings, and your siblings related by blood.) Next, circle the corresponding point value. For those illnesses without an average onset age, score the level of disability from 1 (least severe) to 5 (most severe).

arteriosclerosis	1	2	3	4	5
emphysema	1	2	3	4	5
high blood pressure	1	2	3	4	5
high cholesterol	1	2	3	4	5
varicose veins	1	2	3	4	5

Total Score ____ ÷ # of Items (that apply to you) ____ = Average Score ____

4. Rate your Cardio habits- and addictions-risk factors
Average Score: ____

Circle and score the severity of the unhealthy Cardio-related habits and addictions that apply to you from 1 (least severe) to 5 (most severe).

alcohol consumption	1	2	3	4	5
cigarette smoking	1	2	3	4	5
compulsive gambling	1	2	3	4	5
driving over the speed limit	1	2	3	4	5
drug addiction	1	2	3	4	5
fatty diet	1	2	3	4	5
hygiene neglect	1	2	3	4	5
overeating	1	2	3	4	5
skipping meals	1	2	3	4	5
stressful living	1	2	3	4	5
sugary diet	1	2	3	4	5
undereating	1	2	3	4	5

List and rate any others

____________________	1	2	3	4	5
____________________	1	2	3	4	5
____________________	1	2	3	4	5

Total Score ____ ÷ # of Items (that apply to you) ____ = Average Score ____

5. Rate your Cardio personality traits-risk factors
Average Score: ____

Circle and score the unhealthy Cardio-related personality traits that apply to you from 1 (least severe) to 5 (most severe).

Chronic

anger	1	2	3	4	5

anxiety	1	2	3	4	5
compulsiveness	1	2	3	4	5
depression	1	2	3	4	5
hostility	1	2	3	4	5
type A behavior	1	2	3	4	5

List and rate any others

____________________	1	2	3	4	5
____________________	1	2	3	4	5
____________________	1	2	3	4	5

Total Score ____ ÷ # of Items (that apply to you) ____ = Average Score ____

6. Rate your Cardio environmental risk factors
Average Score: ____

Circle and score the unhealthy environmental risk factors that apply to you from 1 (least severe) to 5 (most severe).

air pollution	1	2	3	4	5
city living	1	2	3	4	5
second-hand smoke	1	2	3	4	5
workplace stress	1	2	3	4	5

List and rate any others

____________________	1	2	3	4	5
____________________	1	2	3	4	5
____________________	1	2	3	4	5

Total Score ____ ÷ # of Items (that apply to you) ____ = Average Score ____

7. Rate your Cardio diseases- and injuries-risk factors

Average Score: ____

Identify any of the major Cardio diseases and injuries that you have already sustained, then circle and score the severity of those diseases and injuries that apply to you from 1 (least severe) to 5 (most severe).

Heart and Vessels

arteriosclerosis	1	2	3	4	5
coronary artery disease	1	2	3	4	5
glaucoma	1	2	3	4	5
high cholesterol	1	2	3	4	5
intermittent claudication	1	2	3	4	5
orthostatic hypotension	1	2	3	4	5
phlebitis	1	2	3	4	5
renal hypertension	1	2	3	4	5
renal infarcation	1	2	3	4	5
renal vein clot	1	2	3	4	5
stroke	1	2	3	4	5

Lungs and Breathing

allergies	1	2	3	4	5
asthma	1	2	3	4	5
bronchitis	1	2	3	4	5
colds and flu	1	2	3	4	5
emphysema	1	2	3	4	5
lung cancer	1	2	3	4	5
pneumonia	1	2	3	4	5
sinus infection	1	2	3	4	5
sinusitis	1	2	3	4	5
tuberculosis	1	2	3	4	5

List and rate any others

________________	1	2	3	4	5
________________	1	2	3	4	5
________________	1	2	3	4	5

Total Score ____ ÷ # of Items (that apply to you) ____ = Average Score ____

8. Rate your Cardio symptoms-risk factors
Average Score: ____

Circle and score the severity of the Cardio symptoms that apply to you from 1 (least severe) to 5 (most severe).

angina pectoris	1	2	3	4	5
chronic breathlessness	1	2	3	4	5
chronic fatigue	1	2	3	4	5
palpitation	1	2	3	4	5

List and rate any others

________________	1	2	3	4	5
________________	1	2	3	4	5
________________	1	2	3	4	5

Total Score ____ ÷ # of Items (that apply to you) ____ = Average Score ____

9. Rate your Cardio physical fitness- and condition-risk factors
Average Score: ____

Your Cardio physical condition- and fitness-risk factor score is determined by four distinct subcategories: (a) heart and lung strength, (b) oxygen processing uptake capacity, (c) safe cholesterol count, and (d) vascular health. After performing all the tests (a.–d.), add all these scores together and divide by 4 to determine your heart and lung strength average score. If you skip any section or sections of these tests, divide by the number of tests that you actually perform.

a. Rate your heart and lung strength
Average Score: ____

After performing the following two tests of your heart and lungs, add your scores together and divide by 2 to determine your heart and lung strength average score.

1) Circle and rate the strength of your heart and lungs when doing any kind of strenuous activity (e.g. climbing stairs, brisk walking, jogging).

Breathless	*Score*
After 15+ min.	1
In 10–15 min.	2
In 5–10 min.	3
In 1–5 min.	4
In less than 1 min.	5

(2) Measure your heart- and lung-training rate by measuring your heart rate at different levels of exertion to determine the strength of your heart muscle. If you do not have access to a heart monitor you should take your pulse rate at the wrist or carotid artery, both of which are a good indicators of your actual heart beat.

Take the following two measurements:

(a) Maximum heart rate
Subtract your age from 220: _____.

(b) Resting heart rate
Measure your heart rate (or feel your pulse) while seated or lying down: _____

Resting Heart Rate (in beats per minute)	***Score***
60+	1
50–60	2
40–50	3
30–40	4
less than 30	5

b. Rate your oxygen processing uptake capacity
Average Score: ____

Oxygen uptake is the ability of your heart and lungs to efficiently work together and deliver oxygenated blood to your muscles. It is measured by your body's ability to complete a vigorous task in a limited amount of time. In terms of exercise, it is the ability to walk one mile, bicycle two miles, or swim one-quarter of a mile. In everyday terms, it is whether you become breathless whenever you climb a flight of stairs or rush to catch a bus. If you are in condition to exercise continuously for twelve to thirty minutes, you can take an exercise test. To score your VO_2 Max, have a test done at a doctor's office or at a lab. If you cannot have a lab test done, estimate your VO_2 Max based on your rate of breathlessness. See Table 4.6, Normal Values of Maximum Oxygen Uptake, p. 74.

c. Test your heartbeat response to different intensity levels
Average Score: ____

% of Maximum Heart-training Rate	***Exercise Pace***	***Score***
20–39%	Static	1
40–49%	Slow	2
50–59%	Moderate	3
60–69%	Vigorous	4
70–85%	Fast	5

If your heart-training rate is higher than the rate for that level, your rating is at that level. For example, if you can do moderate-paced exercise (Level 3), but your heart-training rate falls into Level 4, your health rating would fall into the level below your exercise level, in this case, Level 2.

d. Rate your safe cholesterol count
Average Score: ____

Rate your safe cholesterol count based on the laboratory measurement listed in Table 5.3, Safe Cholesterol Counts, p. 102.

e. Rate your vascular health

Average Score: ____

Blood pressure is the best indication of blood vessel health. Refer to Table 5.2, Blood Pressure Scale (p. 99) to match your actual blood pressure to the scores listed below. (You will either have to have a medical person measure your blood pressure or you will have to use a home blood pressure kit to obtain your actual blood pressure.)

Blood Pressure	*Score*
Normal	1
Slightly high or low	2
Mildly high or low	3
Moderately high or low	4
Severely high or low	5

10. Rate your Cardio exercise- and activity-risk factors

Average Score:____

The heart-training rate is the highest heart rate at which you can perform any Cardio exercise without breathing too hard. The heart-training rate is expressed as a percentage of the maximum heart rate. If your heart-training rate is above the standard for any type of exercise (see list below), it mans that you are less fit than the norm because your heart has to work harder than what is considered normal for that exercise. If your heart-training rate is below the standard, you are more fit than the norm for that exercise or activity.

To find your heart-training rate, first take your "exercise" pulse. To do this, stop exercising and count your pulse rate for six seconds immediately after you stop exercising. Convert your six-second pulse rate to the one-minute rate by multiplying that number by ten. Now, convert your one-minute pulse rate to your heart-training rate by dividing that number (your one-minute pulse) by your maximum heart rate. For example, let's say that you are forty years old. Your personal maximum heart rate is the maximum heart rate (220 beats per minute (bpm) minus your age (40), which equals 180 (220 – 40 = 180) bpm. This is your personal maximum heart rate (for this example, if you are forty years old). Your heart-training rate should be below your maximum heart rate; that is, within 70 to 85% of your personal maximum heart rate. For this example, this forty-year-old's heart-training rate is 126 to 153 beats per minute, or twelve to fifteen beats every six seconds. If you are above your heart-training range, you are exercising too hard and should exercise at a lower level or lower intensity.

You should be able to exercise continuously and stay within your heart-training range or you are not fit enough to exercise at that level of intensity. Ideally, you should be able to exercise continuously for twenty minutes or more in the moderate-to-brisk paced level.

To measure your Cardio fitness, pick one of the exercise levels that follow (see list below) and try to exercise at that level with that activity (i.e. walking, cycling, swimming) for twenty minutes or more. If you can accomplish this, you earn that score for that level. If you are unable to complete a twenty-minute session, give yourself a score of one point higher for every five minutes less than the twenty-minute goal. For example, if you chose to walk at the brisk-paced level (2) and you could not complete walking for twenty minutes at that level, but could only walk for five minutes, your score would be 5 instead of 2.

Because your heart-training rate is used later on to determine your level of exercise, do not overestimate your capacity; it is better in this case to be conservative and to rate yourself a little lower if you have any doubts about your score.

Exercise Levels	***Score***
Static exercise:	5
Standing up, posture, or balancing exercises	
Slow-paced exercise:	4
Walking (20–40 steps per minute)	
Cycling (20–40 revolutions per minute)	
Swimming (10–20 strokes per minute)	
Moderate-paced:	3
Walking (40–60 spm)	
Cycling (40–60 rpm)	
Swimming (20–30 spm)	
Brisk-paced:	2
Walking (60–90 spm)	
Cycling (60–90 rpm)	
Swimming (30–40 spm)	
Fast-paced:	1
Walking (90–120 spm)	
Cycling (60–90 rpm)	
Swimming (40–60 spm)	

Profile Summary

Compute your average score for each category, then convert it to a risk rating (which you will use later) as follows:

Average Score	***Risk Rating***
0.0–1.4	I
1.5–2.4	II
2.5–3.4	III
3.5–4.4	IV
4.5–5.0	V

Write in your average scores and converted ratings for all ten risk factor categories, then compute your overall average Cardio system score:

Risk Categories	***Average Score***	***Converted Rating***
1. Age	_____	_____
2. Gender	_____	_____
3. Genetic	_____	_____
4. Habits and addictions	_____	_____
5. Personality traits	_____	_____
6. Environment	_____	_____
7. Diseases and injuries	_____	_____
8. Symptoms	_____	_____
9. Physical condition and fitness	_____	_____
10. Exercise and activity	_____	_____

Total Score ____ ÷ 10 ____ = Average Cardio System Score ____

CHAPTER 6

The Mind/Body Connection

Saving Your Psyche-Immune System

What Is the Psyche-Immune System?

The psyche-immune system is actually composed of two systems in one: 1) the psyche, which includes the brain, hormones, nervous system, the mental processes, and emotions; and 2) the immune system, which is the system of white blood cells and antibodies.

Psychological fitness is similar to physical fitness, in that the damaging effects of negative thoughts and emotions accumulate just as those of inactivity do. These effects, in turn, lower your ability to cope with and overcome everyday challenges. As you weaken, both mentally and emotionally, not only is your psychological health threatened but so is the physical health of your four other health systems. For example, chronic anxiety, avoidance, compulsiveness, and fear can mount and become personality traits and habits that lead to overconsumption of food, alcohol, or cigarettes. Repeated overeating and excessive alcohol consumption can lead to such chronic disorders as alcoholism or obesity. These addictions then become risk factors for heart and liver disease and cancer among other diseases and disorders.

Exercise can help you take control of your life, that is, it can help you to limit stressful reactions and curtail bad habits, in addition to raising your spirits, building your psychological well-being, and boosting your immune response. When you are under chronic emotional distress, often your immune system shuts down, or if not, you may be driven to alcohol, drugs, and other addictive or dangerous behaviors—such as over- or undereating—which will weaken your immunity even further.

Your body fights off disease by delivering nutrients and antibodies to an infected area via **white blood cells** that attack disease-causing

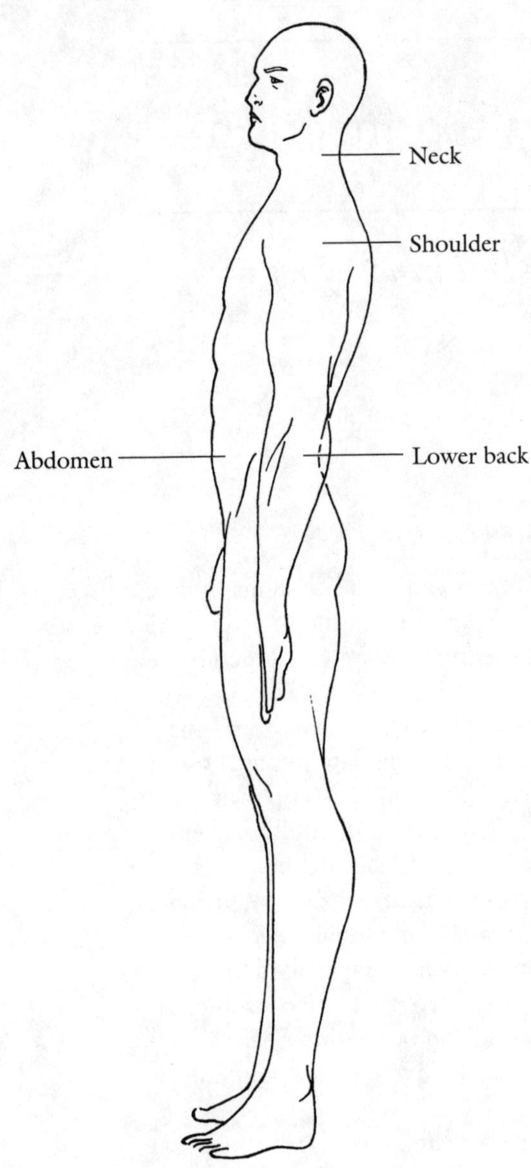

Major Areas of Tension

microorganisms. When your immune system is overworked, its ability to replace used up or dead white blood cells becomes impaired. Exercise—especially moderate exercise—fortifies your five body systems against diseases and their side effects, strengthens the various organs that help provide immunity, and reduces the impact of stressful events on the immune system by minimizing your stressful reactions.

STRESSFUL LIVING

Stressful living is a chronic condition involving repeated stressful reactions on a daily basis. Reactions to stress, for example chronic muscle tension and insomnia, can develop into patterns, conditions, or syndromes. These conditions alone may not be harmful to your health, but can become dominant medical risk factors for many such serious diseases as heart disease, alcoholism, autoimmune diseases, and diabetes. Additionally, the symptoms of any major disease you already have may be further complicated by stress.

One way to cope with stressful events is to ignore or avoid them. You can delegate responsibilities, avoid people who annoy you, leave potentially threatening letters unopened, or live in a plastic bubble. Some other ways to cope are to mask your feelings or sedate yourself with medications, food, or drink. Artificial ways of coping with stress offer only short-term results and leave you with side effects. In the end, we cannot escape life's trials and tribulations and we would be better off learning to face them. Like grieving, communicating, and coping, exercise is the one of the most natural and honest ways to deal with the stress of life.

STRESS-RELATED ILLNESSES

Stressful reactions and stressful living are not diseases themselves, but can increase the chances of developing such diseases and disorders as alcoholism, anorexia nervosa, bulimia, chronic fatigue syndrome, depression, heart attack, hypochondria, obsessive/compulsive disorder, and stroke. Stress-related diseases are not caused by stressful reactions alone but are worsened because of them.

Stress alone is not harmful. Indeed, many people are not affected by it. Your physical reaction to stress, however, can do harm. A stressful reaction is one in which your body gets ready to fight or flee: your heart races, your adrenaline flows, you sweat, and your muscles grow tense. Although this would be a healthy reaction to a *real* threat like a grizzly bear attack, it is overkill when the grizzly bear is just your boss checking on your work progress. You can learn to manage your stressful reactions by making yourself stress-hardy through exercise.

Well-Being

Well-being has to do with your basic attitude toward your current health and the future. A sense of well-being can be positive, negative, or, over a period of time, changeable. Usually, you start out in life with a feeling of positive well-being. Central to your feeling of well-being is your assumption of good health. Exercise promotes a positive outlook on life by giving you a sense of control over your body. Becoming stronger and more flexible, faster, quicker, and more coordinated provides a secure basis of self-confidence. Fitter people feel less threatened. Exercise also stimulates your body to secrete hormones, called endorphins, which are mood-elevators.

Exercise also promotes personal hygiene both externally and internally, which is another key to well-being. Because you sweat more when you exercise, you feel more compelled to shower and bathe. The increased exertion level and water loss also causes you to drink more fluids. Increased fluid flow washes away more bacteria and germs, leaving less work for your immune system to do.

What Can Go Wrong?

Your psyche-immune system can be impaired by major immune or stress-related diseases and disorders such as alcohol and drug addiction, heart disease, eating disorders, cancer, AIDS, chronic fatigue syndrome, and depression. Psyche-immune diseases carry with them stress-related symptoms such as anxiety, insomnia, chronic hostility, moodiness, low self-esteem, overconsumption, in addition to such psychosomatic responses as head, neck, and back aches. Your psyche system has its own unhealthy defenses—stressful reactions, bad habits, addictions, and personality changes. Exercise provides both short-term and long-term techniques for attacking the underlying disorders as well as your unhealthy defenses.

Major Risk Factors

Habits and Addictions

Addictions and habits start out as shortcuts and temporary solutions to everyday problems—a cup of coffee to wake you up, a cigarette to focus your mind, a shot of scotch or a tranquilizer to calm you down, a chocolate bar to boost your energy—but end up being repeated as often as problems arise. Such repetitive activities as gambling, being a workaholic, and even overexercising can also play similar unhealthy roles by letting you avoid everyday problems or traumatic crises. The problem with these coping shortcuts is

THE PSYCHE-IMMUNE BENEFITS OF EXERCISE

Exercise helps you:

1. Become stress-hardy.
2. Manage your stressful reactions by releasing muscular tension on a regular basis.
3. Overcome anxiety, depression, fear, and worry.
4. Cope with everyday problems, keeping small crises from becoming bigger.
5. Take positive control of your body functions and build self-confidence and self-esteem for life.
6. Improve your emotional balance and outlook.
7. Become more sociable.
8. Improve various mental functions such as memory, alertness, creative thinking, perception, concentration, and awareness by increasing the flow of oxygen and nutrients to your brain.
9. Break bad habits or addictions or keep them from forming.
10. Reduce muscular tension as it occurs.
11. Become more prepared to handle life's major traumas including such major psyche-immune diseases as depression and chronic fatigue.
12. By providing a substitute for various medications that stimulate, tranquilize, or provide pain relief.
13. Intervene with physical therapy for anxiety, panic attacks, overconsumption, appetite, and cravings.
14. Calm such emotional reactions as anxiety, fear, depression, anger, or hostility.

that artificial stimulants and depressants eventually cause permanent damage to your mind and body—even if used in moderation.

MUSCULAR TENSION

Muscular tension is probably the primary symptom of the psyche-immune system under stress. It overshadows the central emotional symptom of anxiety and the central cognitive symptom of loss of concentration. Eventually, if an emotional or mental symptom gets serious enough, it will be accompanied by muscular tension. If left untreated, muscular tension can become a prolonged condition, weakening and inflaming surrounding tissue.

Muscular tension occurs in a half-contracted muscle that is being deprived of blood flow and nourishment. The prolonged contraction causes the muscle to pull at surrounding tissues and joints, putting them out of alignment, and possibly pinching the surrounding nerves.

Unlike an exercise or exertive (lifting something) muscle contraction, muscular tension grows not out of physical work, but the muscle's reaction to a threat. By tensing itself, it is getting ready for action—for fight or flight. Muscular tension also rises out of keeping your body in the same position (i.e. seated or standing) for long periods. Postural muscles in the back, shoulders, arms, or legs contract to hold your body in a specific position.

If you are neglecting to exercise or are experiencing severe stress, regular exercise may not be enough to relieve muscle tension. If tension is not relieved daily it can become a chronic condition and can spread to other muscle groups causing overall fatigue. Tense muscles also pull on tendons and ligaments, which, in turn, pull at joints. Prolonged pressure can cause joint inflammation and can lead to chronic back, neck, and shoulder aches.

Similarly, when skeletal muscles are tense, your internal organs—heart, arteries, stomach, intestines, colon, bowel, lungs—are kept from functioning properly. Stomach cramps, heart palpitations, colitis, and irritable bowel syndrome are all symptoms similar to muscle tension. When your body is in a constant state of readiness, it can also prevent you from getting enough sleep. Repeated or alternating sleepless nights can wear down your immunity to diseases and can cause body areas to become fatigued and more subject to easy injury.

Finally, when muscles are constantly tense, they drain off energy that could be used in more productive activities. As a result, you can feel as tired at the end of a stressful day as if you had run a marathon.

Personality Traits

Psychologists use two basic personality poles to measure degrees of optimism and pessimism. Where you lie between these two extremes indicates how motivated you are to solve problems. According to this breakdown, human personalities can range from (1) the supercharged, aggressive, and extremely competitive Type A, to (2) the balanced and assertive Type B, to (3) the slow-moving and phlegmatic Type C. Each type has a specific set of emotional and mental reactions to stress. However, Type A behavior is the only personality type specifically noted as a substantial risk factor for disease—specifically heart disease and high blood pressure.

As children, we learn personality traits and mental skills from our parents, though some experts believe these traits have a genetic basis. Regardless, they can have a profound effect on our lives. Awareness, assertiveness, creativity, friendliness, motivation, optimism, and self-control are traits that positively affect our overall psychological health. Addictive behavior, anger, boredom, compulsiveness, hostility, phobias, and self-centeredness, on the other hand, adversely affect our psychological health.

Psyche-Immune Symptoms

Psyche-immune symptoms are physical, emotional, and mental reactions to differing levels of stress you experience every day over a lifetime. They may be reactions to changes in your social life, in your career, and to the threat or onset of disease. The symptoms often start in your mind and your patterns of thought, spreading to your nervous system. Yet each of these three groups of symptoms become intertwined with and impact each other. Mental symptoms stimulate emotional symptoms that produce physical symptoms, but the process also flows in other directions. For example, your negative emotions can feed your negative thoughts, and both can cause a physical reaction that in turn can worsen your mental and emotional symptoms.

Therefore, finding ways to manage a stressful mental or emotional reaction can often head off a physical symptom. Similarly, physical exercise also helps calm down emotional or mental reactions, by diverting the mind's attention away from your symptoms.

MENTAL SYMPTOMS

Mental symptoms are the thoughts or patterns of thinking, like memory lapse or absentmindedness, that can change over time or become connected with your illness.

From least to most severe, common mental symptoms are:

1. Memory lapse
2. Absentmindedness
3. Creativity blocks
4. Poor perception
5. Indecision
6. Insomnia
7. Attention deficiency
8. Obsessive/compulsive disorder
9. Irrationality
10. Amnesia
11. Dementia

EMOTIONAL SYMPTOMS

Like mental symptoms, emotional symptoms are linked to your thought processes, but also to the sum total of your personality, attitudes, behaviors, and life skills. Some emotional symptoms are (from least to most severe):

1. Boredom
2. Dieting
3. Moodiness
4. Egocentricity
5. Fears
6. Phobias
7. Depression
8. Family conflicts
9. Intimacy problems
10. Emotional fatigue
11. Low self-confidence
12. Low self-esteem
13. Chronic sleep problems
14. Addictive behavior
15. Panic
16. Manic depression
17. Sexual dissatisfaction
18. Suicidal tendencies

PHYSICAL SYMPTOMS

The physical symptoms on this list can overlap with those caused by injury and disease, but they may be substantially aggravated by stress and other disorders in the psyche-immune system. Furthermore, physical symptoms often seem to be the culmination of aggravated mental and emotional symptoms.

From least severe to most severe, some common physical symptoms are:

1. Appetite loss
2. Caffeine dependency

3. Muscle tension
4. Headaches (mild)
5. Mild fatigue
6. Muscle aches
7. Back aches
8. Weight loss
9. Colitis
10. Activity addiction
11. Overexercise
12. Workaholism
13. Compulsive gambling
14. Sexual addiction
15. Chronic fatigue syndrome
16. Drug addiction
17. Ulcers
18. Migraines

PSYCHE-IMMUNE EXERCISES

Psyche-immune exercises are aimed at reducing muscle tension. Although a regular exercise program provides much relief from stressful reactions, special relaxation exercises may also be necessary when stress levels are abnormally elevated. Reducing muscle tension means stretching and strengthening muscles so that they will spring back faster from bouts of tension.

The intensity and duration of the psyche-immune exercise you undertake should vary according to the degree of muscle tension or stress in your life. If you are merely bored, the degree of tension is light, and thus the amount of exercising you need may also be light, for example slow-paced range-of-motion exercises. If you are experiencing a high level of anxiety, a more intense level or longer-lasting exercise period may be necessary. In Psyche-Immune Ex (pp. 231–248) the exercise intensity and duration is measured and graded. For certain symptoms, such as depression and fear, the choice of where you exercise is as important as how much you exercise—a claustrophobic exercise room can add to your emotional tension.

FIGHT STRESS WITH EXERCISE

By either increasing the total amount, or in some cases, the level of intensity of exercise, you can counteract psyche-immune symptoms. Level 1–5 psyche symptoms (top of Table 6.1, Addictive Consumption p. 126) can be counteracted by an equivalent quantity of points gained through regular exercise (bottom of Table 6.1).

EXERCISE FOR COGNITIVE AND EMOTIONAL STRESS

When your stressful reaction does not include muscular tension (e.g. moodiness, light depression, or boredom), it requires light exercise prevention: a cool-down walk, light stretching, or a slow, full-body, range-of-motion exercise. This exercise therapy may only last for seconds and minutes, but it offers much longer-lasting effects.

EXERCISE FOR PSYCHOSOMATIC SYMPTOMS

Psychosomatic symptoms mimic those of real physical diseases and disorders without an actual physical cause being present. Some common

TABLE 6.1
ADDICTIVE CONSUMPTION AND SAMPLE WALKING EXERCISE SOLUTION

Examples of Addictive Consumption					
Level	1	2	3	4	5
Amount of sugar per day(in teaspoons)	0–10	11–20	21–25	26–35	35+
Cups of coffee per day	0–2	3–4	5–6	7–10	10+
Cigarettes per day	0–5	6–10	11–20	21–40	40+
Alcoholic drinks per day*	0–1	1–2	2–3	3–5	5+
Alcoholic drinks per week*	0–5	5–9	10–14	15–21	21+
Example of Walking Exercise Solution					
Length of walks (in minutes)	5	10	10	10	15
Approximate number of walks per day	1–2	2–4	3–4	4–6	4–6
Walking speed (mph)	3–5.5	3–5.5	3–5.5	3–5.5	3–5.5
METS level of exercise:	4–15	4–15	4–15	4–15	4–15
Level at which to begin maintenance program	1	2	3	4	5

*One drink equals two ounces of hard liquor, four ounces of wine, or eight ounces of beer.

psychosomatic symptoms include headaches, back aches, insomnia, and such physical symptoms of heart and lung disease as asthma attacks, breathlessness, and chest pain. Some stressful reactions stem from anxiety or depression about disease, thus causing a snowball effect. *ExRx* treats both psychosomatic and physical symptoms the same way by having you exercise the body areas that are affected.

Exercising for Breaking Bad Habits and Addictions

Exercise works on a bad habit or addiction by substituting itself for repetitive behaviors and by rebuilding body systems that have been weakened by those habits or addictions. Intermittent exercise, such as taking a walk, a bicycle ride, stretching, or calisthenics, works well as a warm-up to take the place of the bad behavior or craving, to stimulate or relax your body.

EXERCISE FOR PERSONALITY CHANGES

Exercise can also have a long-term impact on your personality. While controlling your reaction to stress, you can begin to reshape your emotional and mental health, regaining calm much more quickly and easily. In addition to those benefits, during exercise your mind is freed up for reflection, giving you an opportunity to take a step back and collect your thoughts and plan your actions in a more deliberate and controlled manner. Type A behaviors can be transformed into Type B. However, exercise therapy can take many months and probably even years but eventually you will develop a more balanced, noncompetitive outlook on life.

YOUR PSYCHE-IMMUNE PROFILE

To determine the amount of psyche-immune exercise you should be doing, rate your psyche-immune health and weaknesses using the Psyche-Immune System Profile. If you rate I, II, or III, practice the Psyche-Immune Preventive Exercises in Part Two. If you rate IV or V, practice the Psyche-Immune Rehab program in Part Three.

Circle each of the major risk factors as they apply to you and multiply the number of these factors by the number of point values assigned in each category. Total up your points for the category before continuing on to the next category. You may also use this questionnaire to evaluate the medical risk factors of a child or adult under your care and supervision. The final score will ascertain which of the five health systems are the weakest and will determine where you should concentrate the *Exercise Rx* program.

Psyche-Immune Profile

Compute your Psyche-Immune-risk factor by rating the severity of your diseases, symptoms, and physical weaknesses on a scale of 1 point (least severe) to 5 points (most severe). Average your points and convert your averages to an overall rating that corresponds to the intensity or difficulty level for which you will begin your prevention or rehabilitation exercises. Please note: no answer equals a score of 0.

1. **Rate your Psyche-Immune age-risk factor**
   Average Score: ___

Circle and score the following age-related Psyche-Immune conditions that apply to you and rate your level of severity from 1 (least severe) to 5 (most severe).

absentmindedness	1	2	3	4	5
disorientation	1	2	3	4	5
frequent illnesses	1	2	3	4	5

List and rate any others

____________________	1	2	3	4	5
____________________	1	2	3	4	5
____________________	1	2	3	4	5

Total Score ___÷ # of Items (that apply to you) ___ = Average Score ___

2. **Rate your Psyche-Immune gender-risk factors**
   Average Score: ___

Circle the gender-specific Psyche-Immune diseases you already have (or have had), and then circle their corresponding point value. The average onset age is shown in parentheses after each disease. For those illnesses without an average onset age, score your level of disability from 1 (least severe) to 5 (most severe).

Disease Onset	***Point Value***
Later than norm	1
Within the norm	2

Up to 5 yrs. before				3	
5–10 yrs. before				4	
10+ yrs. before				5	

Common or Predominantly Male Diseases

impotence	1	2	3	4	5
Reiter's syndrome (20–40)	1	2	3	4	5
tic disorder (begins at 18)	1	2	3	4	5

Common or Predominantly Female Diseases

agoraphobia	1	2	3	4	5
arthritis	1	2	3	4	5
chronic fatigue syndrome (under 45)	1	2	3	4	5
major depression	1	2	3	4	5
pain disorder (30–50)	1	2	3	4	5
rheumatoid arthritis (30–60)	1	2	3	4	5
rheumatoid arthritis, juvenile	1	2	3	4	5
scleroderma	1	2	3	4	5
systemic lupus	1	2	3	4	5
vaginal spasms	1	2	3	4	5

Total Score ____ ÷ # of Items (that apply to you) ____ = Average Score ____

4. Rate your Psyche-Immune genetic-risk factors
Average Score: ___

Circle and score the severity of any inherited Psyche-Immune diseases that you already have (or have had) or that a close relative may have (or have had). (Only count grandparents, parents, their siblings, and your siblings related by blood.) Next, circle the corresponding point value. For those illnesses without an average onset age, score the level of disability from 1 (least severe) to 5 (most severe).

Addictions to:

alcohol	1	2	3	4	5
drugs	1	2	3	4	5

food	1	2	3	4	5
breast cancer	1	2	3	4	5
depression	1	2	3	4	5

Total Score____ ÷ # of Items (that apply to you) ____ = Average Score ____

4. Rate your Psyche-Immune habits- and addictions-risk factors
Average Score: ___

Your Psyche-Immune habits- and addictions-risk factors average score is determined by three distinct subcategories: (a) your substance and activities habits and addictions level, (b) your drug dependencies and addictions level, and (c) your withdrawal symptioms. After finding your level for both of these subcategories, add your scores together and divide by 3 to determine your average score.

a. Rate your substance and activity habits and addictions
Average Score: ___

Circle and score your level of consumption of each of the following habits or activities. Circle the categories that apply to you, and rate the severity of consumption or overactivity for each one. To determine your individual level of consumption, refer to Table 6.2, Habits and Activities Levels, p. 144. After you have completed determining your level of consumption for any of the items that apply to you on the following list, total your points and divide that total by the number of items that you have circled. This represents your substance and activity habits rating.

alcohol consumption	1	2	3	4	5
cigarette smoking	1	2	3	4	5
compulsive gambling	1	2	3	4	5
driving over the speed limit	1	2	3	4	5
fatty diet	1	2	3	4	5
hygiene neglect	1	2	3	4	5
overeating	1	2	3	4	5
overexercising	1	2	3	4	5
reckless driving	1	2	3	4	5
sugary diet	1	2	3	4	5
skipping meals	1	2	3	4	5
stressful living	1	2	3	4	5

undereating	1	2	3	4	5
workaholism	1	2	3	4	5

List and rate any others

________________________	1	2	3	4	5
________________________	1	2	3	4	5
________________________	1	2	3	4	5

Total Score ____ ÷ # of Items (that apply to you) ____ = Average Score ____

b. Rate your drug dependencies and addictions
Average Score ___

Score your dependencies and addictions by circling any drugs taken and multiply by a point value based on use and level of addiction. Circle only those items that you have consumed or engaged in an at least once.

Number of times taken	***Score***
Up to once a year	1
Once a month	2
Up to 3 times a month	3
Once a week	4
Once a day or more	5

Soft Drugs

tranquilizers/sleeping pills	1	2	3	4	5
diet pills	1	2	3	4	5
marijuana	1	2	3	4	5

Hard Drugs

speed or amphetamines	1	2	3	4	5
cocaine	1	2	3	4	5
heroin	1	2	3	4	5

List and rate any others

____________________	1	2	3	4	5
____________________	1	2	3	4	5
____________________	1	2	3	4	5

Total Score ____ ÷ # of Items (that apply to you) ____ = Average Score ____

c. Rate your withdrawal symptoms
Average Score: ____

The length that you experience withdrawal symptoms can serve as a guide to the severity of your addiction and the level of therapy needed to break your dependency. Circle and rate your withdrawal symptoms, if applicable. For ratings, refer to Table 6.3, Withdrawal Times, p. 146.

5. Rate your Psyche-Immune personality traits
Average Score: ____

a. Overall traits
Average Score: ____

Circle your unhealthy personality traits and rate their severity, on a scale of 1 (least severe) to 5 (most severe).

aggressiveness	1	2	3	4	5
anxiety	1	2	3	4	5
attention deficiency	1	2	3	4	5
boredom	1	2	3	4	5
chronic hostility	1	2	3	4	5
compulsiveness	1	2	3	4	5
egocentricity	1	2	3	4	5
family conflicts	1	2	3	4	5
fear	1	2	3	4	5
hygiene neglect	1	2	3	4	5
indecisiveness	1	2	3	4	5

intimacy problems	1	2	3	4	5
irrationality	1	2	3	4	5
low confidence	1	2	3	4	5
moodiness	1	2	3	4	5
obsessiveness	1	2	3	4	5
phobias	1	2	3	4	5
poor communicativeness	1	2	3	4	5
sexual dissatisfaction	1	2	3	4	5
short temper	1	2	3	4	5
suicidal thoughts	1	2	3	4	5
Type A behavior	1	2	3	4	5
unclear or illogical thinking	1	2	3	4	5
violent outbursts	1	2	3	4	5

List and rate any others

______________________	1	2	3	4	5
______________________	1	2	3	4	5
______________________	1	2	3	4	5

Total Score ____ ÷ # of Items (that apply to you) ____ = Average Score ____

b. Rate type A–E behavior: _____
Average Score: ____

Personality is a mix of emotional, mental, and physical reactions presented in a behavior pattern. Personality is relevant to health and exercise purposes because it predicts the ability to take control of one's health and to control how one's body copes with physical and psychological trauma. Negative personality traits are similar to disease symptoms; they can cause pain, discomfort, and damage to the body and nervous system.

Circle the numbers that best represent your behavior for the list of fifteen questions found in Table 6.4, What Personality Type Are You?, p. 147. After answering all the questions, add up your points. Your score will range from fifteen to 105 points. Select your personality type from the following answer key.

Answer Key

Type C	Midpoint	Type B	Midpoint	Type A
1 point	2	3	4	5 points
0–21	21–40	41–60	60–89	90–105

Now add up your points by referring to the point scale after each question. If you could not answer all the questions, total your points and divide them by the number of questions you did answer. Example: 30 points divided by 10 questions yields an average score of 3. A score of 3 (or 41–60, if you answered all the questions) would indicate both that you are a Type B. If you scored 1, you are a Type C, the personality that is considered too lethargic. If you scored a 5, you are a Type A, and therefore prone to stress-related illnesses such as heart disease. The high score also indicates a need for a greater amount of physical exercise to help you diffuse the stress of the day. If you scored 2 or 4, you are considered a combination of either Type B or C (2) or Type B or A (4). These "midpoint" measures are also good for measuring your progress in transforming yourself from a Type C to a Type B or a Type A to a Type B.

6. Rate your Psyche-Immune environmental risk factors
Average Score: ____

Circle and score the unhealthy environmental risk factors that apply to you from 1 (least severe) to 5 (most severe).

carcinogen exposure	1	2	3	4	5
germ exposure	1	2	3	4	5
noise pollution	1	2	3	4	5
overcrowded living	1	2	3	4	5
workplace stress	1	2	3	4	5

List and rate any others

____________________	1	2	3	4	5
____________________	1	2	3	4	5
____________________	1	2	3	4	5

Total Score ____ ÷ # of Items (that apply to you) _____ = Average Score: _____

7. Rate your Psyche-Immune diseases- and injuries-risk factors

Average Score: ____

Your Psyche-Immune diseases- and injuries-risk factor is determined by three distinct subcategories: (a) emotional disorders, (b) mental disorders, and (c) physical disorders. Score and rate each of the following three subcategories by circling and scoring the severity of the diseases you have (or have had). To find your average score for your Psyche-Immune diseases- and injuries-risk factor, add together your scores for these subcategories and then divide by 3.

a. Emotional Disorders

Average Score: ___

alcoholism	1	2	3	4	5
anorexia nervosa	1	2	3	4	5
bulimia	1	2	3	4	5
fatigue	1	2	3	4	5
general anxiety disorder	1	2	3	4	5
hypochondriosis	1	2	3	4	5
low self-esteem	1	2	3	4	5
major depression	1	2	3	4	5
obsessive/compulsive disorder	1	2	3	4	5
panic disorder	1	2	3	4	5
personality disorder	1	2	3	4	5
phobias	1	2	3	4	5
posttraumatic stress disorder	1	2	3	4	5
schizophrenia	1	2	3	4	5

List and rate any others

____________________	1	2	3	4	5
____________________	1	2	3	4	5
____________________	1	2	3	4	5

Total Score _____ ÷ # of Items (that apply to you) _____ = Average Score _____

b. Mental Disorders
Average Score: ____

amnesia	1	2	3	4	5
attention deficit	1	2	3	4	5
creative blocks	1	2	3	4	5
memory loss	1	2	3	4	5

List and rate any others

____________________	1	2	3	4	5
____________________	1	2	3	4	5
____________________	1	2	3	4	5

Total Score _____ ÷ # of Items _____ = Average Score ____

c. Physical Disorders
Average Score: ___

acquired immune deficiency syndrome (AIDS)	1	2	3	4	5
chronic steroid use	1	2	3	4	5
colitis	1	2	3	4	5
chronic fatigue syndrome	1	2	3	4	5
fibromyalgia	1	2	3	4	5
gastroenteritis	1	2	3	4	5
insomnia	1	2	3	4	5
irritable bowel syndrome	1	2	3	4	5
pain disorder	1	2	3	4	5
psoriasis	1	2	3	4	5
psychoactive drug abuse	1	2	3	4	5
sexual dysfunction:					
arousal and orgasm disorders	1	2	3	4	5

impotence	1	2	3	4	5
painful intercourse	1	2	3	4	5
premature ejaculation	1	2	3	4	5
somatization disorder	1	2	3	4	5
stuttering	1	2	3	4	5
TMD, TMJ, and bruxism	1	2	3	4	5
trench mouth	1	2	3	4	5

List and rate any others

______________________	1	2	3	4	5
______________________	1	2	3	4	5
______________________	1	2	3	4	5

Total Score _____ ÷ # of Items (that apply to you) _____ = Average Score ____

8. Rate your Psyche-Immune symptoms-risk factors
Average Score: ____

Circle and score any of the Psyche-Immune symptoms that apply to you from 1 (least severe) to 5 (most severe).

muscle tension	1	2	3	4	5
sweating	1	2	3	4	5
rapid heart beat	1	2	3	4	5
itching	1	2	3	4	5

List and rate any others

______________________	1	2	3	4	5
______________________	1	2	3	4	5
______________________	1	2	3	4	5

Total Score _____ ÷ # of Items (that apply to you) _____ = Average Score ____

9. Rate your Psyche-Immune fitness- and condition-risk factors

Average Score: ____

Your Psyche-Immune fitness- and condition-risk factor is determined by two distinct subcategories: (a) stress-hardiness, and (b) immune-hardiness. Score and rate each of the subcategories. To find your average score for your Psyche-Immune fitness and condition-risk factors, add your two scores together and then divide by 2.

a. Rate your stress-hardiness

Average Score: ____

Stress-hardiness is how a person reacts to stressful events and the average time it takes to go through a stressful reaction. It is also influenced by the number of stressful events that a person experiences on a daily, weekly, monthly, or yearly basis. The following four tests of your stress-hardiness should serve to ascertain your level. When you complete all four areas, add all the scores together and divide by 4 to determine your overall stress-hardiness level.

1) Rate your stressful events

Score: ____

The following is a list of stressful events that can occur within a person's lifetime. Next to each event is a corresponding mean value number. Identify those events that you may have experienced recently and circle them and their mean value. Then record the total number of events and the total mean values. Next, add these numbers together to find a total point value. Last, select the rating from the list below that best corresponds to your total number of points.

Level V

Event	Mean value
1. Death of spouse	100
2. Diagnosis of cancer, AIDS, or other fatal disease	95
3. Unwed pregnancy (for women)	92
4. Divorce	73
5. Marital separation	65
6. Detention in jail or other institution	63
7. Death of close family member	63
8. Stroke or heart attack	53
9. Diagnosis of rheumatoid arthritis	53
10. Diagnosis of multiple sclerosis	53
11. Diagnosis of angina pectoris	53

Level IV

12. Getting married	50
13. Being fired from a job	47
14. Marital reconciliation with mate	45
15. Retirement	45
16. Major change in health or behavior of family member	44
17. Pregnancy	40
18. Quitting an addiction to cigarettes, drugs, or alcohol	40
19. Changing from "Type A" to "Type B" behavior	40
20. Sexual difficulties	39
21. Gaining a new family member (e.g., through birth, adoption, relative moving in, etc.)	39
22. Major business readjustment (e.g., merger, bankruptcy, etc.)	39
23. Major change in financial state (e.g., a lot better off or worse off)	38
24. Death of a close friend	37
25. Changing to a different line of work	36

Level III

26. Major change in the number of arguments with spouse (either more or less)	35
27. Taking on a mortgage greater than $100,000	31
28. Foreclosure on a mortgage or loan	30
29. Major change in responsibilities at work (either promotion, demotion, or a lateral move)	29
30. Son or daughter leaving home	29
31. In-law troubles	28
32. Outstanding personal achievement	28
33. Spouse beginning or ceasing work	26
34. Beginning or ceasing formal schooling	26
35. Major change in living conditions (building a home, remodeling, deterioration of home or neighborhood)	25

36. Revision of personal habits (e.g., dress, manners, association)	24
37. Troubles with the boss	23
38. Major change in working hours or conditions	20
39. Change in residence	20
40. Changing to a new school	20
41. Major change in usual type/amount of recreation	19
42. Major change in church activities (more or less)	19
43. Major change in social activities (clubs, dancing, movies, etc.)	18
44. Taking on a mortgage or loan of less than $100,000 (purchasing a car, TV, etc.)	17
45. Major change in sleeping habits (insomnia, sleeping more, or change in part of day you are asleep)	16
46. Major change in number of family get-togethers (more or less)	15
47. Major change in eating habits (dieting, eating more, or very different meal hours or surroundings)	15

Level I

48. Business travel	13
49. Vacation	13
50. Christmas	12
51. Minor violations of the law (traffic tickets, jaywalking, etc.)	11
52. Car trouble	11
53. Commuting	11

Total events: _____.

Total points: _____.

Total events and points _____.

1	2	3	4	5
0–49	50–99	100–199	200–299	300+

2) Rate your everyday stress
Score: ____

Circle one (refer to the list of stress events above for examples of stressful events).

Stressful Events Per Week	*Score*
0–7	1
8–15	2
16–28	3
29–35	4
36+	5

3) Rate your stressful reactions
Score: ____

Stressful Reactions	*Points*
Rare (monthly)	1
Infrequent (weekly)	2
Moderate (every work day)	3
Frequent (daily)	4
Constant (hourly)	5

4) Rate your average emotional, physical, and mental reaction time to an everyday stress event.
Score: ____

Circle one of the following:

	Score
0–1 minute	1
1–2 minutes	2

2–3 minutes	3
4–5 minutes	4
5+ minutes	5

b. Rate your immune-hardiness (frequency of respiratory illnesses and infections such as colds, flu, viruses)
Average Score: ___

	Score
Never sick	1
Sick once a year	2
Sick twice a year	3
Sick three times a year	4
Sick more than four times a year	5

10. Rate your Psyche-Immune activity level
Average Score: ____

Circle the rating that best describes the amount of time you spend relaxing. This includes time spent practicing hobbies, going on vacations, doing yoga, or just putting your feet up and laying back.

	Score
Some relaxation time (daily)	1
Moderate relaxation time (weekly)	2
Low relaxation time (monthly)	3
Little relaxation time (yearly)	4
No relaxation time	5

Profile Summary

Compute your average score for each category, then convert it to a risk rating (which you will use later) as follows:

Average Score	***Risk Rating***
0.0–1.4	I
1.5–2.4	II
2.5–3.4	III
3.5–4.4	IV
4.5–5.0	V

Write in your average scores and converted ratings for all ten risk-factor categories, then compute your overall average Psyche-Immune system Score:

Risk Categories	***Average Score***	***Converted Rating***
1. Age	_____	_____
2. Gender	_____	_____
3. Genetics	_____	_____
4. Habits and addictions	_____	_____
5. Personality traits	_____	_____
6. Environment	_____	_____
7. Diseases and injuries	_____	_____
8. Symptoms	_____	_____
9. Physical condition and fitness	_____	_____
10. Exercise and activity	_____	_____

Total Score ____ ÷ 10 ____ = Average Psyche-Immune System Score ____

TABLE 6.2
HABITS AND ACTIVITIES LEVELS

Alcohol:

Don't drink alcohol—0

1–7 drinks per week—1

8–15 drinks per week—2

16–25 drinks per week—3

26–33 drinks per week—4

35+ drinks per week—5

Cigarettes:

Don't smoke cigarettes—0

Less than 1 pack per day—1

1 pack per day—2

2 packs per day—3

3 packs per day—4

4+ packs per day—5

Compulsive gambling:

Don't gamble—0

1 time a month—1

2–3 times a month—2

1 time a week—3

2–3 times a week—4

4+ times a week—5

Driving over the speed limit:

Don't drive over speed limit ever—0

1 time a week—1

2–3 times a week—2

3–4 times a week—3

5–7 times a week—4

Every time I drive a car—5

Overeating:

Don't overeat—0

1 time a week—1

2–3 times a week—2

3–4 times a week—3

5–7 times a week—4

Every time I eat—5

Undereating:

Don't undereat—0

1 time a week—1

2–3 times a week—2

3–4 times a week—3

5–7 times a week—4

Every time I eat—5

Overexercising:

0–5 hours per week—1

6–8 hours per week—2

9–12 hours per week—3

13–18 hours per week—4

19+ hours per week—5

Fatty diet:

Don't eat fatty foods—0

1–2 meals per week—1

3–4 meals per week—2

5–7 meals per week—3

8–10 meals per week—4

11+ meals per week—5

Hygiene neglect:

Bathe/groom/brush teeth every day—0

Bathe/groom/brush teeth every other day—1

Bathe/groom/brush teeth every three days—2

Bathe/groom/brush teeth twice a week—3

Bathe/groom/brush teeth once a week—4

Bathe/groom/brush teeth less than 3 times a month—5

Reckless driving:

Don't ever drive recklessly—0

1 time a week—1

2–3 times a week—2

3–4 times a week—3

5–7 times a week—4

Every time I drive a car—5

Sugary diet:

Don't eat any sugar—0

1–2 meals per week—1

3–4 meals per week—2

5–7 meals per week—3

8–10 meals per week—4

11+ meals per week—5

Skipping meals (based on 3 meals per day):

Never skip a meal—0

Skip 1–3 meals per week—1

Skip 4–5 meals per week—2

Skip 6–7 meals per week—3

Skip 8–10 meals per week—4

Skip 11+ meals per week—5

Stressful living:

1–2 stressful events per week—1

2–3 stressful events per week—2

3–4 stressful events per week—3

5–6 stressful events per week—4

7+ stressful events per week—5

Workaholism:

0–40 hours worked per week—1

41–50 hours worked per week—2

51–70 hours worked per week—3

71–80 hours worked per week—4

80+ hours worked per week—5

TABLE 6.3
WITHDRAWAL TIMES

Sugar:

Withdrawal time:

1 day—1

2–3 days—2

3–4 days—3

5–6 days—4

7+ days—5

Caffeine:

Withdrawal time:

1 day—1

2–3 days—2

3–4 days—3

5–6 days—4

7+ days—5

Cigarettes:

Withdrawal time:

1 week—1

2–3 weeks—2

1–2 months—3

3–4 months—4

5+ months—5

Alcohol:

Withdrawal time:

3–4 days—1

5–6 days—2

1–2 weeks—3

3–4 weeks—4

5+ weeks—5

Marijuana:

Withdrawal time:

1–2 days—1

3–5 days—2

6–8 days—3

9–12 days—4

13+ days—5

Tranquilizers/sleeping pills:

Withdrawal time:

1–5 days—1

5–10 days—2

11–13 days—3

2–3 weeks—4

4+ weeks—5

Speed or amphetamines:

Withdrawal time:

1–5 days—1

5–10 days—2

11–13 days—3

2–3 weeks—4

4+ weeks—5

Cocaine:

Withdrawal time:

1–5 days—1

5–10 days—2

11–13 days—3

2–3 weeks—4

4+ weeks—5

TABLE 6.4
WHAT PERSONALITY TYPE ARE YOU?

The following test will help you to ascertain where you fall within the Type A to C personality spectrum. Circle the number that you feel most closely represents your own behavior.

1. Never late	7	6	5	4	3	2	1	Frequently don't keep appointments
2. Avoids competition	1	2	3	4	5	6	7	Very competitive
3. Finishes other people's sentences (interrupts others, etc.)	7	6	5	4	3	2	1	Doesn't pay attention when others speak
4. Always rushed	7	6	5	4	3	2	1	Never rushed
5. Does not mind waiting	1	2	3	4	5	6	7	Impatient
6. Always feel can give more	7	6	5	4	3	2	1	Everything is too much effort
7. Takes things one at a time	1	2	3	4	5	6	7	Tries to do many things at once
8. Emphatic and loud in speech	7	6	5	4	3	2	1	Speaks slowly and quietly
9. Gets no satisfaction from work	1	2	3	4	5	6	7	Needs work recognized by others
10. Fast (eating, walking)	7	6	5	4	3	2	1	Slow doing things
11. No motivation	1	2	3	4	5	6	7	Hard driving
12. Dwells on feelings	7	6	5	4	3	2	1	Hides feelings
13. Follower	1	2	3	4	5	6	7	Leader
14. Dominates social situations	7	6	5	4	3	2	1	Disappears in the crowd in social situations
15. Submissive	1	2	3	4	5	6	7	Inflexible to changes and suggestions

Now add up your points. Scores range from 15 to 105. The higher the score, the more Type A characteristics you have, and the closer the score is to 15, the more you are a Type C personality. A score of 60 would make you the quintessential Type B. Undoubtedly if you are a Type B, in some instances you will fall closer to Type A and in others closer to Type C. A high score (over 90) indicates that you may be at risk for stress-related illnesses, including heart disease, and should use ten-minute walks throughout the day to diffuse stress. If you scored below 90, you are not in any "danger," but walking can certainly help you recover from stressful times in your life. If your score was below 50, you may not have enough stress in your life. Remember, change is essential for a fulfilling life.

PART TWO

PREVENTION EX

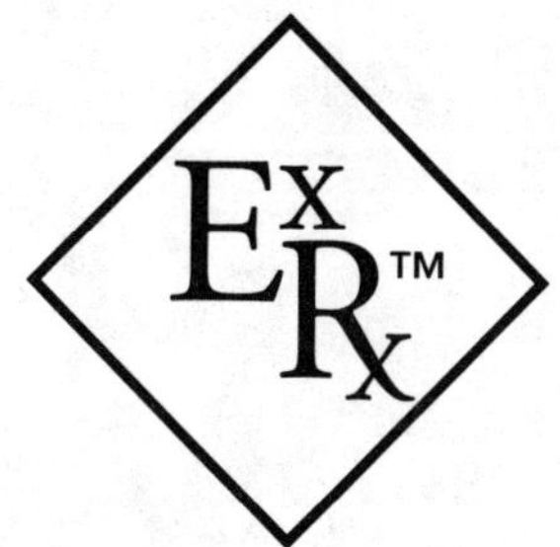

Introduction to Prevention Ex

Use Part Two as a basic preventive program and for a exercise program to get back in shape. The Part Two preventive exercises are designed to benefit the healthy parts of your body.

If you have any body area weaknesses or injuries, first use the Part Three exercises to rehabilitate those areas. Use the Part Two exercises only after you have rehabilitated any weak or injured body system.

If you are really out of shape and have not exercised for more than six months, be sure to evaluate both your body condition and medical conditions with your doctor before starting the Part Two or Part Three exercises.

How to Use Part Two

Practice the six prevention exercise routines in Part Two in the chapter order they are presented to you, as follows:

Health System	*Exercise Routine*
Chapter 7, Basic Techniques	Posture, Balance, and Breathing
Chapter 8, Ageing	Range of Motion and Warm-ups
Chapter 9, MuSkel	Stretching and strengthening
Chapter 10, Meta	Duration and resistance
Chapter 11, Cardio	Aerobic and circulatory
Chapter 12, Psyche-Immune	Cool down and relaxation

If you have no medical weaknesses, begin by doing the full exercise program at the minimum maintenance levels for your fitness level. If you are healthy, but just out of shape, start at Level I and build up to Level III.

If you have determined through the five questionnaires in Part I that you are weak in one of your five health systems, do more of those exercise routines that correspond to that weak health system. Start out at the Level I practice level and build up to a practice level that corresponds to your weakness level.

If you have also determined that you are weak in specific body areas or functions (e.g. posture function) do more of those specific exercises to improve those functions.

If your health system is very weak (i.e. Level IV or V), you should start with the rehabilitation exercise program in Part Three. If your weakness level is I, II, or III, you should start at that corresponding prevention exercise level as shown in the following:

Health Weakness	*Exercise Level*
I (Very Strong)	III (Advanced Prevention)
II (Strong)	II (Intermediate Prevention)
III (Moderately Strong)	I (Beginner Prevention)

In other words, a weaker health rating requires starting at an easier or lower exercise level.

If some of your health systems are weak, but others are strong, you may practice a split-level exercise program. In other words, if you have determined that your Cardio system is at Level V but your MuSkel system is at Level I, you will be doing rehabilitation exercises for your Cardio system and prevention exercises for your MuSkel system.

Your overall health rating for each system will determine how much time you spend doing each routine or which practice level you build up to.

Practicing Sports as Exercise

Traditional sports and exercise programs can be classified according to their risk of injury or disability: low risk, moderate risk, or high risk. Avoid high-risk sports and practice moderate-risk sports only one to two days a week. Low-risk sports and exercise can be played or practiced every day of the week, but you should avoid overdoing even these. The following list rates each sport or exercise as either high-risk (H), moderate-risk (M), or low-risk (L) activities. High-risk represents sports or exercise that can incur a large number of injuries (i.e. ten or more), moderate-risk represents sports or exercise that can incur a smaller number of injuries (i.e. five to nine), and low-risk represents those in which there are only a few number of injuries associated with that sport or exercise. If the rating for a particular sport also has an asterisk (*), this denotes that there is risk of head, neck, or back injury/pain associated with this sport or exercise.

Sports and Exercise Injuries List

- Aerobics, dance—M
- Aerobics, high-impact—H
- Aerobics, low-impact—L
- Aerobics, step—L
- Archery—L*
- Backpacking—L
- Badminton—Competition—H
- Badminton—Recreational—L
- Ballistic batting—M
- Baseball—H
- Basketball—H

- Biking, outdoor—M
- Billiards/pool—L
- Boating—L
- Bowling—M*
- Boxing—H*
- Calisthenics—L
- Canoeing—M*
- Climbing, artificial wall—M
- Climbing, rock—H*
- Croquet—L
- Curling—L
- Cycling, stationary—L
- Dance, ballet—H
- Dance, ballroom—L
- Dance, exercise—H
- Darts—L
- Diving—H*
- Equestrian sports—H*
- Exercise machines—L
- Fencing—H
- Fishing—L
- Football, contact—H*
- Football, touch—M
- Gardening—L
- Golf—M
- Gymnastics—H*
- Handball—H*
- Hang gliding—H*
- "Health riding" machines—M
- Hiking—L
- Hockey—H*
- Horse riding machines—H*
- Hunting—H
- Jogging—L
- Jumping, broad—H*
- Jumping, high—H*
- Jumping rope—M
- Karate—H*
- Kayaking—L
- Lacrosse—M
- Pole vaulting—H
- Racquetball—H*
- Resistance training—M
- Rowing machines—L
- Rowing sports—M
- Rugby—H*
- Running—H
- Sailing—L
- Scuba diving—M
- Skateboarding—H*
- Skating, figure—M
- Skating, ice—M
- Skating, inline—M
- Skating, roller—M
- Skiing, cross-country—L
- Skiing, downhill—H*

- Skiing, water—H*
- Sledding—H
- Snorkeling—L
- Snowboarding—H*
- Snowmobiling—H*
- Soccer—H*
- Softball—M*
- Squash—M
- Stretching—L
- Swimming—L
- Trampoline—H*
- Tennis, court—H
- Tennis, table—L
- Tobogganing—H
- Volleyball—M*
- Walking—L*
- Walking, treadmill—L
- Water exercise—L*
- Weight-bearing exercise—L
- Weight-lifting exercise—M*
- Wind surfing—L
- Wrestling—H*

CHAPTER 7

Basic Techniques

Posture, Balance, and Breathing Exercises

THE THREE BASIC TECHNIQUES

Body alignment has a direct effect on your medical health. Learning to breathe deeply, move properly, and maintain your physical balance will help you avoid many aches and pains and speed your recovery from accidents, injuries, and surgery. The posture and balance exercises can help you prevent or control musculoskeletal and neuromotor pains and disorders, while the breathing exercises may benefit those with cardiovascular respiratory diseases and disorders, while also offering relief from nervous and muscular tension.

After you have mastered the basic techniques—posture, balance, and breathing—you will know how to align your body and to make the necessary postural adjustments to manage various symptoms. For example, if you feel a tingling or numbness in your hand, adjusting the position of your neck may relieve these symptoms by unpinching and straightening out your nerve channel. If your foot has "gone to sleep," flexing your knee and straightening the alignment of your lower back may increase the blood flow to your foot.

You should practice the basic techniques before and after your warm-up routines or whenever you catch yourself slouching or breathing irregularly or incorrectly. By doing so, you'll learn to breathe more deeply as you warm up your body.

POSTURE GUIDELINES AND EXERCISES

Your body has a natural resting position where the least pressure is put on your spine and other joints, bones, and muscles. This position is called

proper body alignment. When you move around or exercise, you should maintain this proper alignment to avoid injury and to promote balanced body development. There are three basic body positions: lying, seated, and standing.

The three basic body positions are also the "starting positions" for doing the exercises that follow, and also serve as the "holding positions" that you maintain while practicing the exercises. Proper alignment is the standard by which we judge whether any exercise is safe or injurious to the musculoskeletal system.

Our bodies come equipped with two types of joints: (1) hinged, and (2) ball-and-socket. Hinged joints let us move in only two directions, in a back and forth motion. Ball-and-socket joints allow a circular range of motion. Our elbows, knees, fingers, and toes are hinged. Our shoulders, hips, wrists, and ankles are ball-and-sockets.

Poor posture increases your injury rate. Some exercises can also cause injury because they violate proper posture standards. When your posture is out of whack, extra stress is placed on your body parts. This can lead to muscle cramping, joint inflammation, and even the early onset of musculoskeletal diseases. After being injured, backs, knees, hips, ankles, or elbows are prone to further injury.

In this chapter, you will learn specific posture exercises and corrections that you can do daily to prevent injury and promote balanced body development. Practicing the simple act of straightening up will give you renewed alertness, vitality, and self-confidence, and reduce your chances of injuring yourself.

Our posture exercises are divided into three types:

1. **Basic posture exercises** help maintain body stature and strength for everyday activity and exercise.

2. **Therapeutic posture exercises** relieve pressure and eliminate pain in joints and muscles resulting from poor body alignment.

3. **Rehabilitative posture exercises,** are the basic strengthening techniques for surviving a convalescence in bed and getting back on your feet.

Benefits of Proper Posture and Alignment

When your posture muscles weaken, your body's weight presses down on the bones (called facets or vertebrae) in your spine. This can lead to a squeeze or herniation of the disks, which are the sac cushions between your vertebrae. When the facets are squeezed, they shift and become bony projections that pinch your nerves and can throw your neck and back muscles into spasm.

Our posture exercises teach you how to properly align your body parts and maintain their alignment by correcting common postural defects. Our techniques prevent injury and promote the healing of weakened or damaged body areas. Almost anyone can use posture training to improve overall mental and physical health, appearance, and exercise or athletic performance. Some of the specific benefits you may receive are:

- Better appearance, a slimmer look
- Better self-image, more confidence
- Less upper body tension

- Less head, neck, shoulder, back, and hip pain
- Less fatigue
- Lower accident and injury rate
- Quicker healing rate
- Balanced muscle and bone strength
- Easier breathing

POSTURE PRACTICE

Similar to any other exercise, good posture takes practice. You must develop strong, flexible, and balanced muscles to support your body from the front, back, and sides. As your first exercise, it is best to practice aligning your body in a series of integrated steps. As your alignment improves, you will begin to notice and correct postural flaws while you exercise and as you conduct your daily activities. You'll practice such exercises as the chin tuck, shoulder brace, stomach tuck, buttocks squeeze, elbow tuck, and parallel foot placement whenever you catch yourself slumping forward or overarching. Over a longer period of time, your body will learn to hold the proper posture on its own with less corrective action.

POSTURE POSITION GUIDE

To simplify the presentation of all the exercises in this book, simple exercise commands will be used to describe individual movements and specific and precise ways you should hold and move your body. To help you understand how to do the exercises, you should learn the following shorthand expressions:

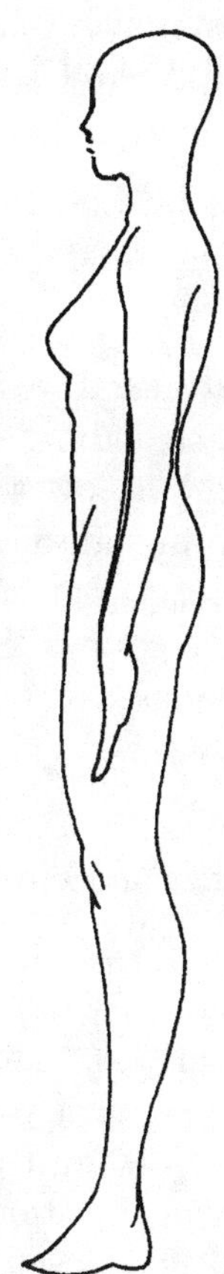

Neutral Spine Position

- **Head up** means hold your head so that your chin line is parallel to the floor. Your head should be centered over your shoulders and aligned with your shoulder joints to form an imaginary perpendicular line with the floor. Your eyes look straight ahead, not focusing any closer than fifteen feet in front of you.
- **Back straight** means holding your upper body erect and perpendicular to the ground so that your joints are properly

aligned—eyes straight, head up, shoulders back and down, back flat (see illustration, p. 157).

- **Palms down, in, out,** or **up** means the direction your palms face during any particular exercise.
- **Back flat,** also called "neutral spine position," means smoothing out an exaggerated curve in your lower back by pulling your stomach in and squeezing your buttocks. Now, relax your muscles until you feel your spine go into the neutral spine position (see illustration, p. 157).
- **Toes pointed straight** means your feet should be pointed straight ahead, parallel to one another and either hip-width or shoulder-width apart.
- **Heels flat** means your heels should be pressed or kept flat against the ground, bearing the weight of your body equally with your forefeet until you are ready to move and change positions. This position corrects the tendency to stand on your forefeet and put yourself off balance.
- **Heels pressed down** means to shift your weight from your forefeet to your heels.
- **Knees bent slightly (160 degrees—the angle at the back of leg), one-quarter bent (120 degrees), one-half bent (90 degrees),** or **full bent** are all positions of the knees that will be used in certain exercises in which you should not lock the knee joints. One-quarter bent allows you to stretch and strengthen your leg muscles. One-half bent means knees bent at 90 degrees. Full bent, which is a rare exercise position, means knees bent within 15 degrees of your body or when your calves touch your buttocks.
- **Do repetitions** means to repeat the exercise the same way for a specified number of times.
- **Hold** means to hold the position for a specified number of seconds.
- **Recumbent position** is a sitting-back posture that you can do on a bed or floor mat by resting your legs on the surface and bracing your upper body on your hands or elbows.
- **Building up to number of times or seconds** means to start at a lower number and gradually do additional repetitions or add seconds (i.e. time) over days and weeks of practice, making sure not to dramatically increase (no more than 10% increase) the movement at any one time.

Now that you know the exercise jargon, let's move on to the exercises.

STANDING POSTURE EXERCISES

HEAD TO TOE ALIGNMENT

Stand with your feet hip-width apart (shoulder-width if you want more stability). Your feet should be parallel to one another, toes pointed in front of you, your knees slightly bent, lower back slightly arched, your arms hanging down loosely by your sides, and your shoulders back.

In your mind's eye, you should see yourself properly aligned from the side. An imaginary straight line, perpendicular to the ground, should connect your ear with the joints in your shoulders, hips, knees, and ankles.

From the front view, your head should be in the center of your shoulders. Four imaginary lines running separately through your

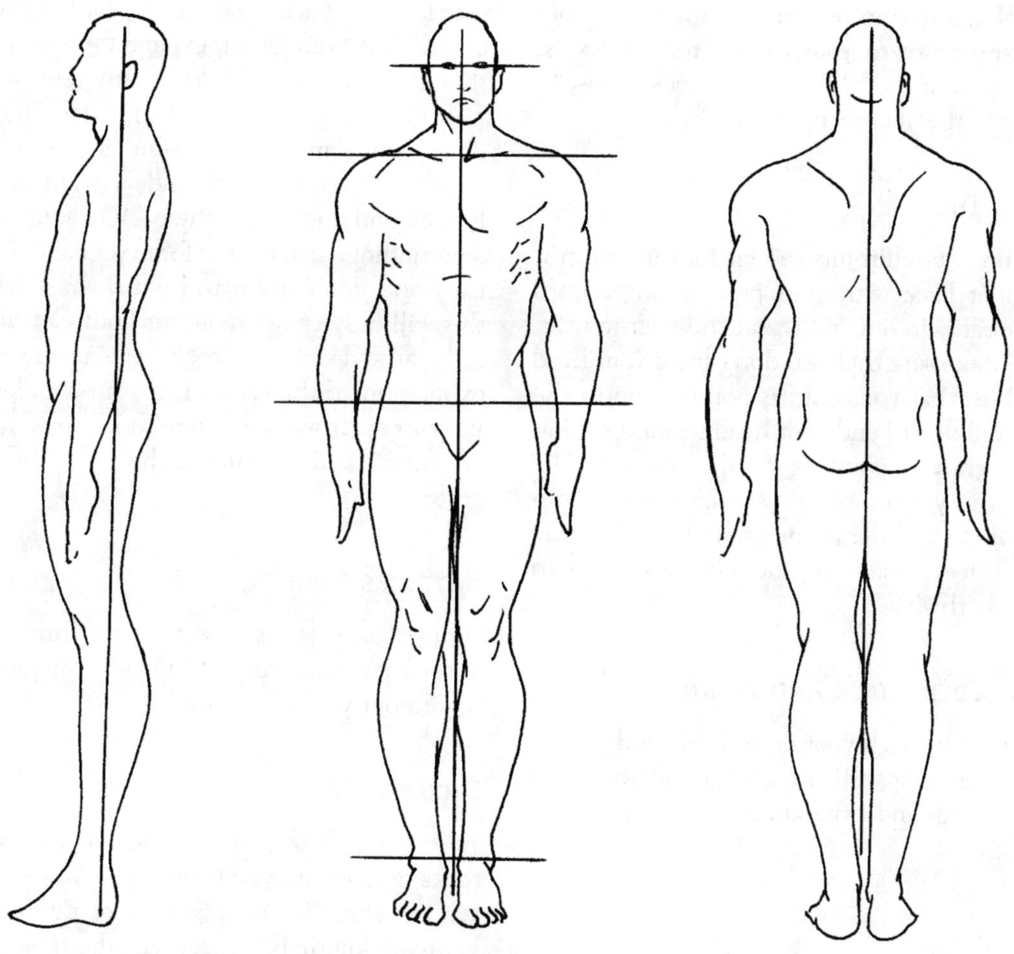

Proper Posture Alignment

eyes, shoulders, hips, and ankle joints should be parallel to the ground. Another line should extend perpendicularly from the top of your head, through your nose and belly button, down to the ground.

From the back, an imaginary line should run equidistant between your ears down through your spinal cord and between your legs.

HEAD CENTERING

Your head should be centered over your shoulders. Your eyes should focus on a point about five yards in front of you, so that you don't drop your head forward to look at the ground close to you. If you want to look down, cast your eyes down without moving your head. This move will also be useful when your are walking, jogging, or biking.

The position of your head controls your posture down to your waist. From the waist down, your stomach and buttocks muscles control the alignment of your hips.

Chin Tuck

When your chin juts too far forward, push it straight back with your pointer finger until your ear is in line with your shoulder joint.

Make sure that you don't bend your head back so that your chin is pointing up in the air, and don't bend your head forward so that your chin is pointing to the ground. The imaginary line running under your chin should be parallel to the ground. At first, you might feel tension in your neck muscles when you do this.

Shoulders Back And Down

Breathe through your nose slowly and deeply. Let your lungs fill up, beginning from your diaphragm and expanding through your buttocks, lower back, and rib cage up to your chest. Feel your chest expanding and your shoulders widening. Visualize any tension in your neck, upper back, and shoulders sliding down your arms, and out your fingertips. As you do this, allow your shoulders to fall slightly back and down. Feel the back of your neck lengthening. Don't try to force your shoulders back and don't strain to hold them there—this will only create more tension! Continue to breathe deeply. Let each exhalation be an exhalation of the tension in your shoulders. Be patient. It will take time to let go of years of tension and to unlearn the habits of bad posture.

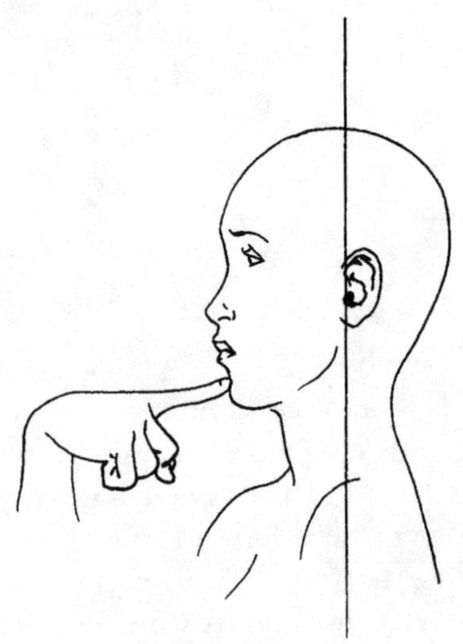

Head Alignment

Buttocks Squeeze

When you catch yourself overarching your lower back, squeeze your buttocks muscles to flatten out your lower back.

Stomach Tuck

At the same time as you squeeze your buttocks muscles in, you should pull your stomach in, which is called **bracing or tightening your abdominals.** Together, these adjustments strengthen and support your torso and lower back, and allow for steady forward, backward, and side-to-side movements. Bracing or tightening your abdominals is very important for any posture transition, for example, getting in and out of a car or a bed or changing exercise positions.

Elbow Tuck

To minimize the tension in your shoulders caused by holding your arms away from your body, pull your elbows into your sides.

Joint Bend

Bend your elbow and knee joints slightly to avoid pinching nerves and to allow blood to flow through them more easily. Bent elbows enable your arm muscles to relax. Bent knees provide greater stability by lowering your center of gravity.

Parallel Foot Placement

Place feet hip- to shoulder-width apart, so that your hips or shoulders are directly over your ankle joints. Avoid narrowing your foot placement or crossing your legs; such positions tug at your hip joints.

Seated Posture Exercises

Seated postures are necessary for those who exercise while sitting down, for example bicyclists, rowers, and wheelchair or other disabled exercisers. From your head to your hip, your correct seated posture is the same as your correct upright posture.

Head to Hip Alignment

This body alignment position (see illustration below) is the same as the standing head to toe alignment and is used with chairs that have backs. Sit with your lower back pressed against the chair back for extra support.

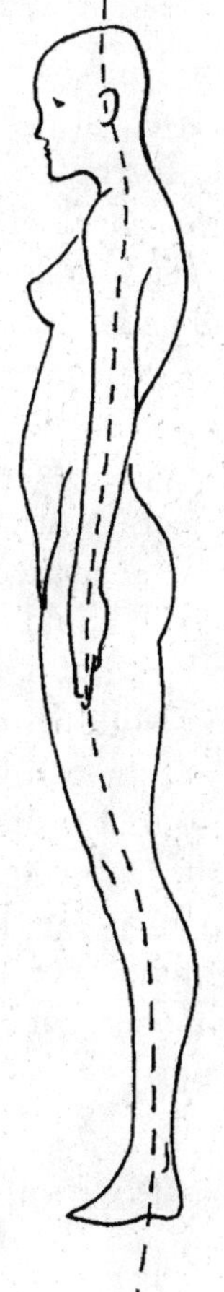

Incorrect Standing Posture

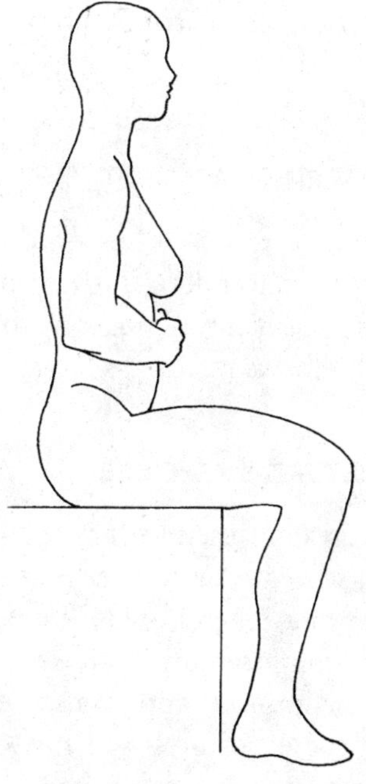

Starting Seated Position

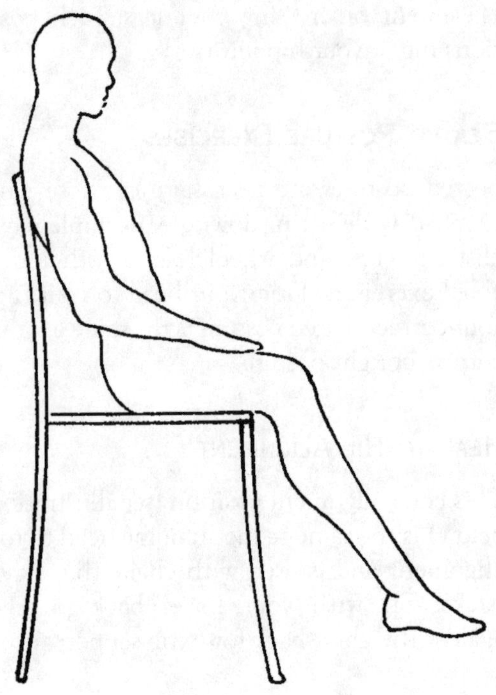

Incorrect Seated Position

Foot and Arm Placement

Foot placement: rest your feet on the ground, hip-width to shoulder-width apart. Arm placement: rest your hands on your upper thighs with elbows bent.

Lying Posture Exercises

Lying postures are useful for those who cannot sit up, who are bed bound, or who practice such prone exercises as floor and mat stretching, strengthening exercises and activities, or swimming and water exercises. Mastering these postures will not only help you to exercise more effectively, but allow you to rest and sleep better, too.

Chin Ups

Your chin should point up, so that your chin-line is perpendicular to the ground. Your head should be supported so that your ears and your shoulder joints are in proper alignment with hip joints.

Flattening Your Shoulders

Extend your arms out from your body, with elbows bent, until you feel your shoulder blades touching the ground or bed.

Flat Back (Lying)

Make sure you are lying on a firm surface, so that your body is equally supported on all sides and parallel to the ground. Bend your knees and bring your heels closer to your buttocks until you feel your lower back flatten out and make full and even contact with the bed or surface. Next, let your back and buttock muscles relax to achieve the neutral spine position. The neutral spine position is when your back feels most comfortable; it is midway between the arched and flat back positions. Your arms should be by your sides, elbows down, and palms up.

When resting while lying on your back, support your head or neck with a pillow or rolled up towel, so that your chin line makes a right angle with the bed or floor. Your eyes should look straight up at the ceiling. From both sides, your mind's eye should see a line running through your ears, shoulders, and ankle joints.

Alternative Leg Position

Your legs can be spread out again with knees bent at right angles. If you stretch out your

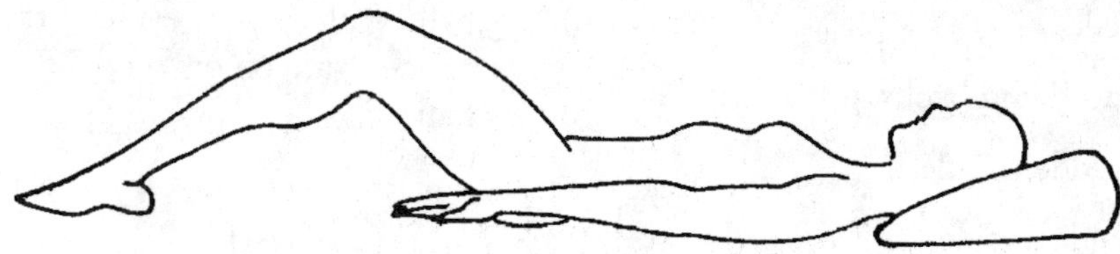

Position for Lower Back Pain

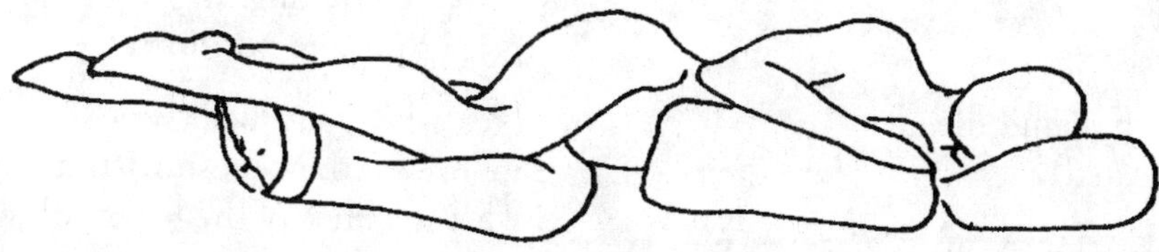

Alternative Position for Lower Back Pain

legs from this position, be sure to keep your knees slightly bent.

BALANCING EXERCISES

Our balancing exercises will enhance your muscle coordination (e.g. loosen up the neck and shoulder muscles) and enable you to overcome protective muscle spasms and the tendency to move stiffly. By training your eyes to move independently of your head, you will improve your everyday balance and overcome symptoms of giddiness or dizziness.

LEVEL I

Balancing #1: Eye and Head Movements (Lying)

Start by lying on your back, knees slightly bent, eyes facing the ceiling (see Lying Posture Exercises, p. 162).

Eyes

Move your eyes (do not move your head)—slowly at first, then more quickly:

- Up and down
- Side to side
- Diagonally, upper right to lower left and back again, then upper left to lower right and back again
- Follow your finger as you move it three feet away to one foot away

Head

- Move your head, keeping your eyes looking forward, first moving slowly, then more quickly, and then last with your eyes closed:

- bend forward and backward
- turn from side to side
- tilt from side to side
- Repeat with eyes and head moving in the same direction
- Repeat the eye and head movements in the seated and standing positions

LEVEL II

Balancing #2 : Eye and Head Movements (Seated)

- Repeat Balancing #1 in the seated position with eyes open and closed
- Shrug and circle shoulders
- Bend forward by flexing at the hips rather than rounding your back and pick up objects from the floor
- Be sure to maintain the "neutral" spine position when doing this exercise

Balancing #3: Stand Up Exercise

- Change your position from sitting to standing
- Repeat Balancing #1 in the standing position first with eyes open and then closed. Stand on a stable surface and keep a stable support nearby
- Throw a tennis (or similar-sized) ball from hand to hand above your eye level
- Throw the ball from hand to hand under knee
- As you throw, try to look away from the ball or close your eyes, so that you must concentrate on or "sense" the path of the ball

Balancing #4: Wide-Based Balancing

- First, practice stepping in place
- Start by placing your feet hip- to shoulder-width apart (approximately 8–12 inches or 20–35 centimeters apart); stand up straight, aligning your body in the proper posture position
- Next, lift your foot (your heel should be in line with your shin) until it is level with the knee of the leg on which you are still standing; balance yourself on one foot holding for as many counts as you can up to a maximum of sixty seconds
- Now, return to your starting position and repeat by lifting up your other foot
- Next, put your foot down, placing the heel down first and rolling onto the ball of your foot
- Now, try the same sequence with your eyes closed; again, try to balance yourself on one foot for as long as you can up to sixty seconds
- If balancing is difficult with your eyes closed, then hold onto a support (e.g. a chair) while you are doing this exercise

Balancing #5: Walking

- Perform first with your eyes open (practice as many times as you want), then once with your eyes closed:

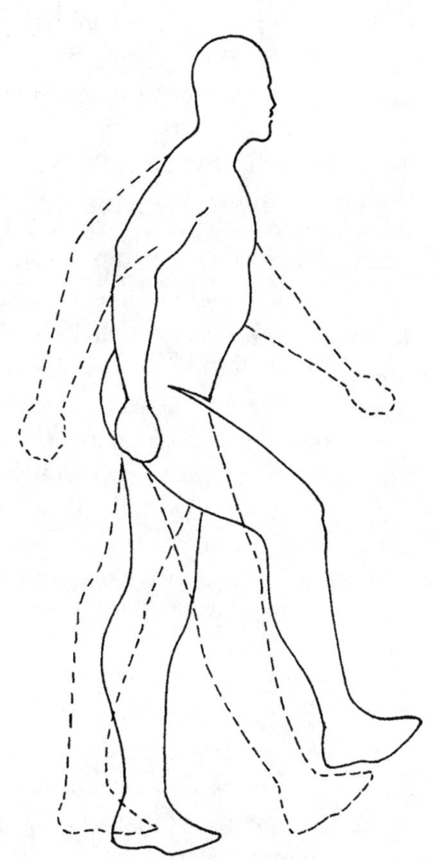

Step Balancing

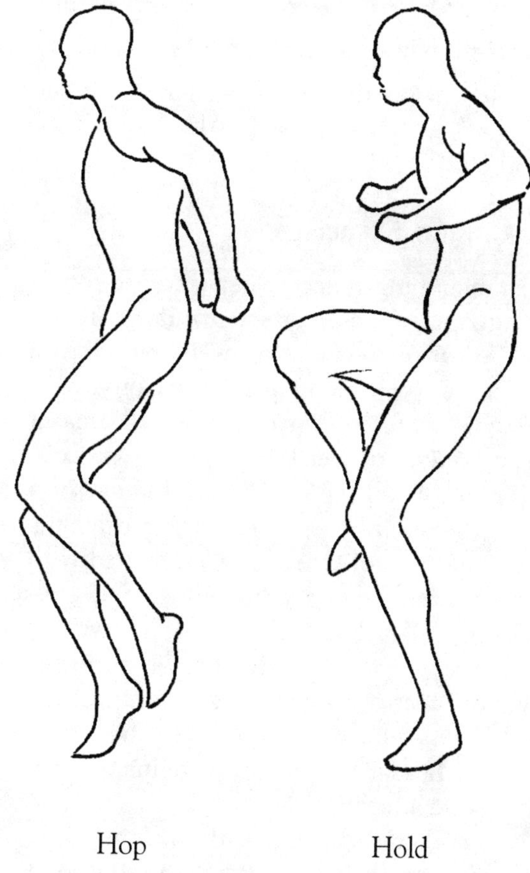

Hop Hold

LEVEL III

Balancing Exercise #6: Jumping (Hop and Hold)

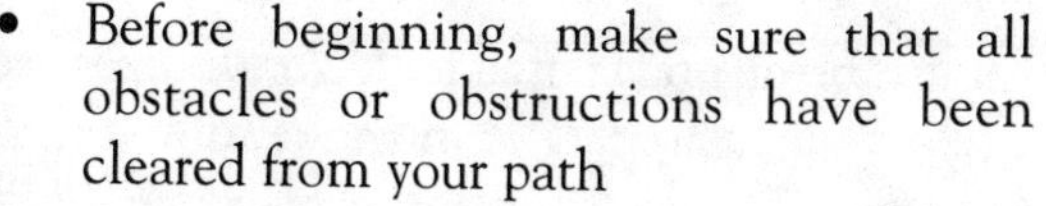

- Before beginning, make sure that all obstacles or obstructions have been cleared from your path
- Practice walking across the room
- Walk up and down a slope, staircase, or incline
- Walk up and down steps

- Try this exercise only after you can sink down until your knees are bent at approximately a 70-degree angle
- Start with a wide stance
- Raise one foot up, and place it on the side of your standing foot but don't let it touch the floor

- Bend the knee of the standing leg and then jump up, landing on your standing foot; hold for five seconds
- Repeat on the other leg; repeat all the steps with your eyes closed

BREATHING EXERCISES

Your breathing reflects your state of conditioning, as well as your state of mind. If you hold your breath when you exert yourself, you can raise your blood pressure. Conversely, bringing more oxygen to a diseased area of your body can speed the healing process. Improper breathing can be a symptom of a medical condition or disorder. For example, rapid and shallow breathing, associated with hyperventilation or overbreathing, is generally a sign of a body in stress. This type of breathing suggests the presence of a heart or lung disorder or may stem from many of the such stress-related symptoms or ailments as fatigue, headaches, asthma, angina, colitis, and panic attacks.

For all breathing, breathe rhythmically, taking as much time to inhale as you do to exhale. For example, count up to four as you breathe in, then count up to four again as you breathe out (4/4 counts).

For slow movements and exercises, use nose and mouth breathing. Breathe in through your nose for a count of four, then breathe out through your mouth for a count of four (4/4 counts). This will keep your body relaxed and ensure a regular flow of oxygen.

For exertive or rigorous activities, such as brisk walking, aerobic dancing, and swimming, practice mouth breathing using 2/2 or 3/3 counts.

With a more open and aligned posture, you can breathe more deeply and regularly. Breathing techniques are designed to bring your breathing under control, to make it more efficient, and to relax the various muscles in the body. By using better breathing techniques, you can manage or eliminate the symptoms of many health problems, such as shortness of breath, hyperventilation, or overly shallow breathing.

The breathing exercises can be used as relaxation training to cope with everyday stress, or stress caused by injury or from pain. Proper breathing techniques coupled with isometric muscle tense-and-release exercises or stretching exercises can also serve as a complete relaxation training program (see pp. 244–248). Each of the breathing techniques, from shallow breathing to belly breathing, also has its own individual purpose. Practice the following exercises during your warm-up routine as you increase your exercise intensity.

NOSE BREATHING

Breathing in and out of your nose is the most common form of relaxed breathing. While sleeping, resting, or working in the seated position or walking at a stroller's pace it is a simple yet effective relaxation technique. Nose breathing also allows nose hairs to filter, warm, and moisten the air.

MOUTH BREATHING

Mouth breathing is used for vigorous exercise when your heart rate is in the aerobic training zone. The wider opening of your mouth allows you to take in more air at a faster rate.

NOSE AND MOUTH BREATHING

Breathing in with your nose and out with your mouth is a moderately vigorous form of breathing used with such light to moderate activity as posture, range-of-motion, or isometric-strengthening exercises.

LIGHT BREATHING

Although it uses only 10% of your lung capacity, light breathing may be necessary in such special situations as when you have chest or stomach pain. If light breathing is done slowly and under the proper circumstances, it can help you more than hurt you.

PURSED-LIP BREATHING

Pursed-lip breathing is used during asthma attacks and is also recommended for heart patients who are breathing cold air. Pursed-lip breathing allows you regain your breathing function when you are breathless, and can also be used along with belly breathing (see below) to help overcome shortness of breath. You slow down your breathing to control it and to get rid of stale air trapped in your lungs.

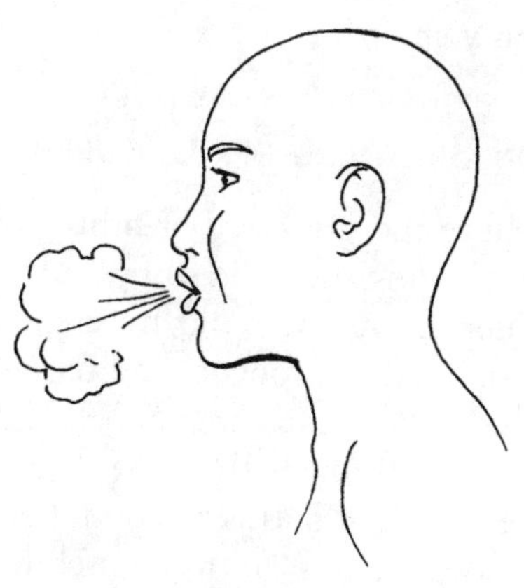

Pursed Lip Breathing

First, practice pursing your lips by puckering them until there is only a small opening through which air can pass. Breathe in slowly through your nose to avoid gulping air. Hold the air in for up to three seconds. Now, pucker your lips as if your are going to whistle. Breathe out slowly for another four to six seconds (i.e. twice as long as breathing in). (If the air is cold, you can breathe in and out of your mouth; this will help warm it. If the air is temperate, breathe in through your nose and out of your pursed lips.)

RHYTHMIC BREATHING

All proper breathing is rhythmic. You should be able to count the same number of seconds while you breathe in as when you breathe out; the brief moments or pauses between inhaling and exhaling should also have an even rhythm. It is important not to hold your breath during physical exertion, but to continue to breathe regularly.

BELLY BREATHING OR DIAPHRAGMATIC BREATHING

Belly breathing or diaphragmatic breathing is the preferred method of deep breathing that fully utilizes your lung capacity and strengthens your diaphragm and abdominal muscles.

Practice belly breathing by lying on your back. Later, you can adapt the technique to seated, standing, and moving along versions. Place one hand on your stomach and the other on your chest to feel the progress of your breathing. Inhale through your nose using your stomach muscles. The hand on your stomach should rise and the one on your chest should stay still. Purse your lips and slowly breathe out as you pull your stomach inward. Take twice as long to exhale as you take to inhale.

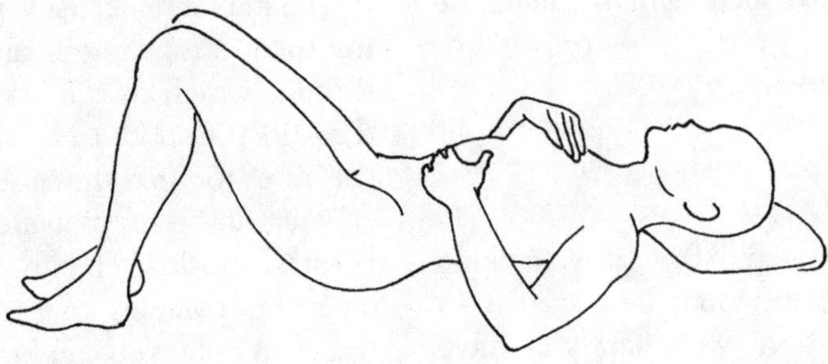

Diaphragmatic or Belly Breathing

CONTROLLED COUGHING EXERCISE

This exercise is for anyone who wants to clear mucus from airways and to save energy from excessive coughing (e.g. colds, chronic bronchitis, emphysema, asthma, and other chronic lung blockages) and it is especially useful after surgery.

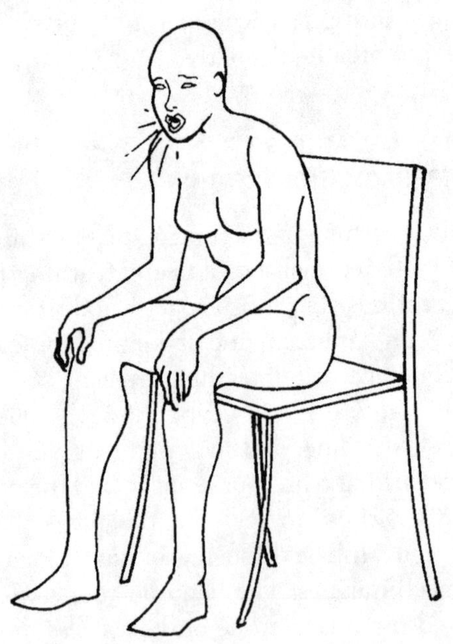

Controlled Coughing Exercise

Prepare to cough by sitting on the edge of a bed or chair, or by standing with your knees bent and hands on your thighs. If standing, be sure to lean forward and brace your abdominal muscles. If seated, place both your feet flat on the ground or one foot on the floor and the other flat on the surface of a stool.

Cough once while keeping your mouth only slightly open—this first cough will loosen any mucus. Cough again to bring up the mucus. Pause for a moment and gently sniff in air with your nose. Don't breathe deeply before you have expelled the mucus or it will slide back down again. In some cases, you will have to repeat the coughing exercise to fully clear your airway.

RELAXATION BREATHING FOR CHILDREN

You can relieve the distressed breathing of a child by first having the child sit up and lean forward. Then, have the child hyperextend the neck, stick out the tongue, and flare the nostrils as he or she tries to breathe. Have the child breathe in through the nose and out through the mouth from this position. Before any episode occurs, you can teach a child to breathe this way by having the child imitate you as in a game.

Good posture, balance, and breathing techniques keep your body aligned, reducing your chances of injury, as well as keeping your body oxygenated during slow, medium, and vigorous movement. Use the techniques to monitor and correct your body position when you catch yourself off balance. Apply the breathing techniques to keep your movements rhythmic and controlled.

Be sure to apply the basic posture, balancing, and breathing techniques you learned here as you practice the range-of-motion (ROM) exercises and warm-ups in the next chapter, as well as in all your exercise routines.

CHAPTER 8

Age Ex

Range of Motion and Warm-Ups

Range-of-Motion Exercises

Range-of-motion exercises (ROMs) are muscle-controlled moves for body parts and major muscle groups that prepare your body either for regular daily activity or for more vigorous exercise. They are designed to improve your mobility by lubricating your joints and stretching and strengthening your muscles. The slow exercise movements stimulate the secretion of synovial fluid that lubricates your joints, while the increased flow of fresh blood to local areas warms up your muscles.

If practiced as prevention, ROMs are localized warm-ups; they are stretching and strengthening exercises if practiced for rehabilitation.

Also effective as preliminary warm-up exercises, ROMs slowly raise your heartbeat. Similar to the windmill and the heel-toe roll, ROMs can also be used to improve circulation to such body areas as hands and feet that are numb, cold, or tingly. When you have been injured, ROMs function as therapeutic and rehabilitative exercises to restore body areas that have been subjected to surgery or radiation or that are still too weak from injury to begin regular stretching and strengthening exercises. When you do a number of ROMs together in a single routine, you are warming up your whole body in preparation for continuous movement exercises (see pp. 216–230).

General Range-of-Motion Principles

Do at least three to five repetitions of each exercise daily or at least every other day. Do ROMs for specific joints as needed to improve stiffness and local joint pain. Move slowly and gently. Move as many times in the clockwise direction as you do in the counter-clockwise direction. If a movement is too painful, stop and let the area rest. Also, ask your doctor for advice. Work from the neck to the toes. Take breaks between exercises if you feel especially tired, or space your exercises over the course of the day. Above all, **do not skip these exercises,** especially if you have any tendency toward arthritis or any other musculoskeletal problem.

During the course of the following two warm-up routines, you will be moving your head, shoulders, arms, legs, and feet slowly through the widest range they can safely move.

HEAD AND NECK: RANGE-OF-MOTION EXERCISES

LEVEL I

Neck ROM: Head Turns

Standing, sitting, or lying, use this exercise as a strengthening, stretching, and mobility exercise if you have aching joints (e.g. rheumatoid arthritis or osteoarthritis) or have been bedridden or immobilized for more than three days. If you are lying down, you may rest on your back with your head propped on a pillow for added comfort.

- Start with your head centered
- Turn your head slowly to the left side as far as you can with your chin parallel to your feet until you can feel the right side of your neck stretching; hold the position for a few seconds
- Return your head slowly back to center; take a brief rest
- Now, turn your head slowly to the right side until you feel the stretch in the left side of your neck
- Hold the position for a few seconds and then return to center

Repeat the movements as many times as you can up to twelve times, once or twice a day. If repeated movements are too difficult, you may space them out during the day, doing one or two repetitions at any one time. As your neck feels stronger (usually after seven days) you can proceed to the therapeutic neck ROMs (neck bends).

Neck ROM: Head Tilt

- Start with your head centered over your shoulders, eyes focused straight ahead
- Slowly tilt your head back 30 to 45 degrees, as if you are looking at the spot where the ceiling meets the wall; hold one to two seconds; return to starting position
- Now, tilt your head forward until your chin touches your chest or as far as possible; hold one to two seconds, and then return to the starting position
- Next, tilt your head to the right toward your shoulder (as if you are trying to touch your shoulder with your right ear); hold for one to two seconds, and then return to the starting position; repeat movement on left side
- Repeat the exercise

Neck ROM: Jaw Stretch

- With your mouth open, jut out your chin so your bottom teeth or jaw sticks out in front of your top teeth

- Feel the stretch in your jaw and the front of your neck
- Next, pull up your neck muscles by grimacing or further baring your teeth
- Feel the stretch in the back of your neck at the base of your skull; hold one to two seconds, and then relax

FACE

Face exercises, which can be practiced in front of a mirror, include the skin, jaw joint, face, and neck muscles.

Mouth and Jaw Joint Stretching

- Slowly open your mouth as wide as you comfortably can
- Hold one to two seconds, and then gently close your mouth
- Repeat one to five times

Smile

- Smile by baring your teeth and stretching your cheeks as wide as you can
- Pull your lips back to show your teeth and gums
- Hold one to two seconds, then gently release and close your mouth
- Repeat one to five times

BACK AND SHOULDERS

Shoulder ROM: Lying

- Start by lying on your back with your arms stretched loosely by your sides
- Slowly raise one arm over your head with your elbow slightly bent, keeping it parallel to your body; it should brush your ear as it passes overhead

Shoulder ROM: Standing

- While standing, place your hands behind your neck, move your elbows back as far as you can, and tilt your head back; hold this position for one to two seconds
- Now, bring your elbows together as you slowly tilt your head forward
- Arms lowered, raise your shoulders by shrugging them
- Move your shoulders forward, down, back, and up in a single, circular, clockwise motion

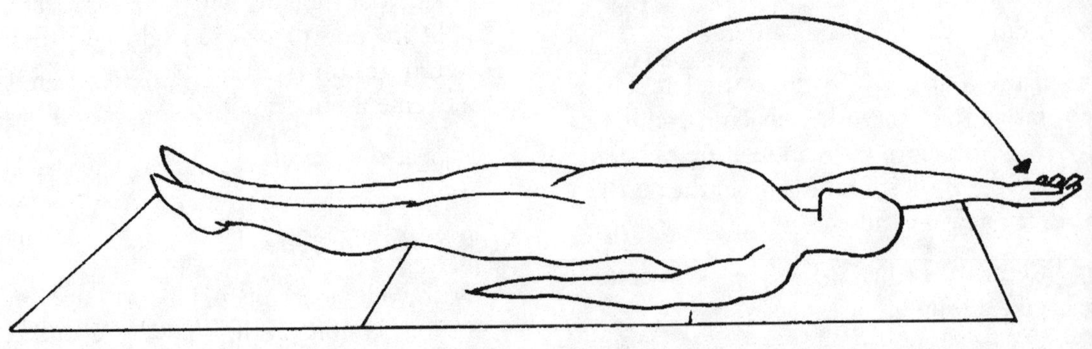

Lying Shoulder ROM

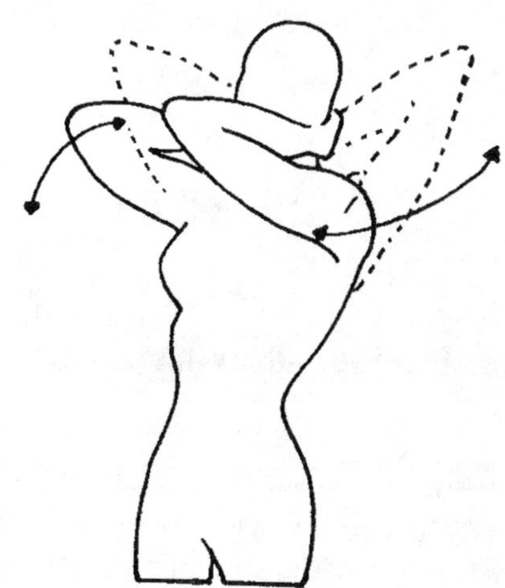

Standing Shoulder ROM

- Now change direction, moving your shoulders back, down, forward, and up in a counterclockwise motion
- Arms extended, extend your arms out from your shoulders
- Slowly rotate your arms in small, clockwise circles, moving your shoulders forward, down, back, and up
- Now change direction, making your arm circles move your shoulders back, down, forward, and up in a counterclockwise direction

Lying-Back ROM

- Lie down face-up with your arms resting by your sides
- Keep your middle and lower back flat as you raise both your arms and your right shoulder off the floor; turn your head and upper body toward your left side
- Reach out with both hands and touch the bed or the floor on the left side of your chest and shoulder; at the same time, touch your left shoulder with your chin; hold for one second, feeling the stretch in your spine and back muscles
- Rotate your head, shoulders, and arms back until you face front again; pause briefly, then continue rotating toward your right side; with both hands, touch the bed or floor on your right side while touching your chin to your right shoulder; hold for one second
- Repeat the complete left-right, right-left rotation three to eight times

Upright Back ROM

- Stand or sit with your feet firmly planted hip-width apart and parallel to one another, toes pointed forward
- Bend your elbows to 90 degrees and hold them to your sides
- Keeping your shoulders flat and chin tucked, slowly rotate your upper body and your head to the left, looking back over your left shoulder as you turn
- Pause or hold one second; feel the stretch in your upper, middle, and lower back
- Rotate your head and upper body back until you face front again; pause briefly before rotating to the right until you can look over your right shoulder; pause
- Repeat the complete left-right, right-left rotation three to five times

Windmill Exercise

The windmill is a range-of-motion exercise for the shoulder joints. It also promotes better circulation by using centrifugal force to circulate more blood to your fingers (excellent for treating Raynaud's disease).

- Extend your arms out from your shoulders and slowly rotate both or alternate arms back around your shoulder joint in eight to ten revolutions per minute (advanced exercisers may pick up the pace, but be careful not to lose muscle control of the movement); emphasize the downward swing by engaging your arm and shoulder muscles more in that phase
- Practice for one minute or until you feel warmth and sensation returning to your fingers
- When fingers are cold, stretch them wide apart while performing the windmill

Softball Pitch

This is one half of a windmill exercise.

- Pretend you are a softball pitcher; wind up, then move your arm in a circular motion down behind your body and then up and over in front of you, releasing your imaginary softball
- Practice a smooth pitch-and-release motion; avoid jerking at your shoulder, wrist, or elbow joints
- Repeat six to eight pitches per minute

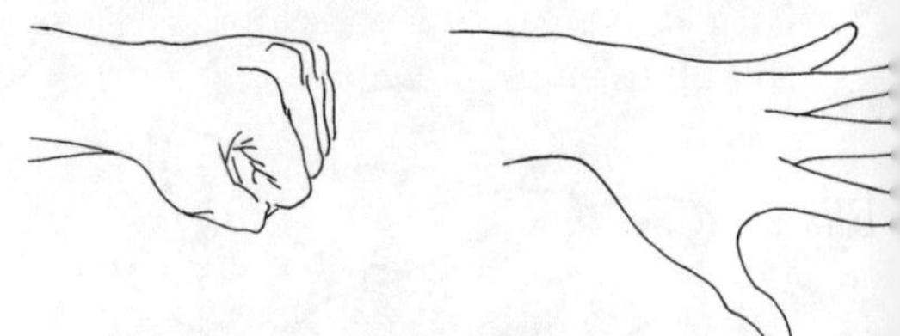

Finger Spreads

HANDS, ELBOWS, AND WRISTS

Finger Spreads

- Slowly stretch out the fingers and thumb on each hand as wide as is comfortable, then slowly bring your hand together in a loosely clenched fist; repeat one to five times

Finger Bends

- Open your hand, palms facing down (you may also rest the palm on a table or countertop)
- Bend your fingers at the hand joints (i.e. where hand joins the fingers), but keep your knuckle joints straightened
- Now, close your hand; repeat one to five times with each hand

Thumb Reaches

- Open your hand, right palm facing you (you may rest the side of your palm on a table or countertop)
- With your thumb, reach across your palm and touch the base of your little finger
- Stretch your thumb out again
- Repeat this exercise one to five times with each finger on your right hand

- Repeat one to five times touching your thumb to your left hand

Elbow ROM

- Extend one arm straight out to the side, shoulder-height
- Turn your hand palm up
- Slowly bend your elbow as you reach back to touch your shoulder with your hand

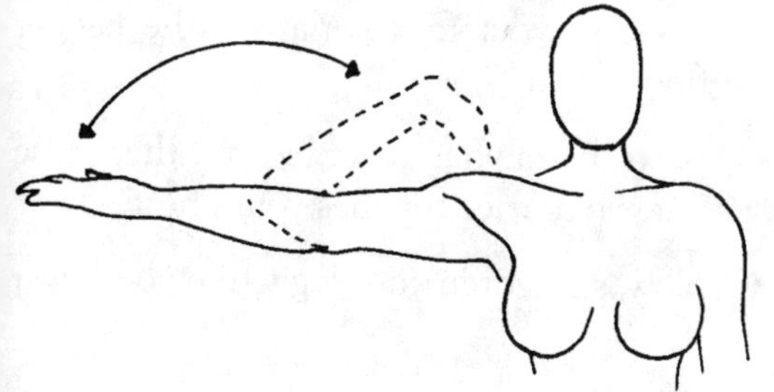

Elbow ROM

- Then, slowly return your arm back to the straightened-out position
- Now, repeat the exercise with other arm
- Alternate the arms as you continue the exercise

HIP, UPPER LEG, AND THIGH ROMS

Lying Leg-Raise Stretch

- Lie on your back with your knees bent at 90 degrees
- Raise one of your legs by pulling the knee slightly back toward your chin while straightening it out into the air above you
- Slowly bend the knee and lower the leg back to the ground
- Repeat with the other leg
- Repeat one to five times with each leg

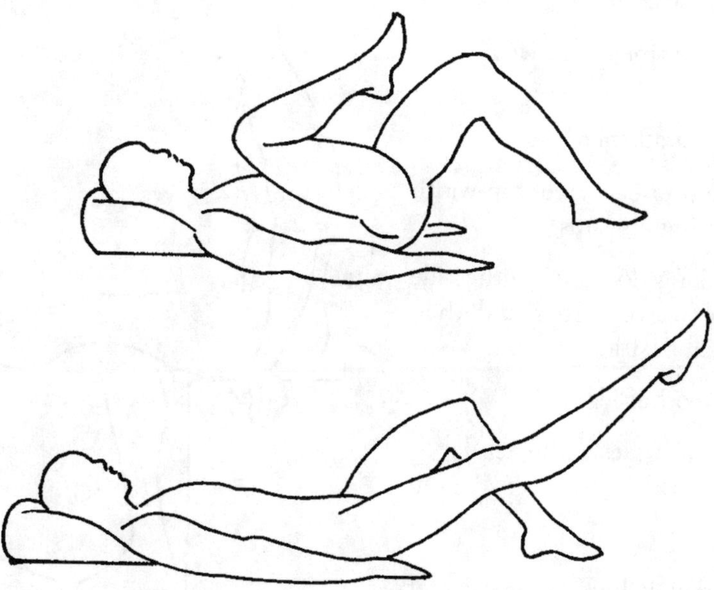

Lying Leg-Raise Stretch

Lying Hip Rotation

- Lie on your back with your feet six inches apart and legs straightened out; your knees should be slightly bent and toes pointed straight out; rest your leg on your heel
- Rotate one of your legs by rolling the foot to the outside and back to the inside
- Repeat with the other leg
- Repeat one to five times with each leg

Lying Front Thigh Strengthener

- Lie V-legged on your back, feet hip-width apart, toes pointing upwards
- Push the back of your knee against the ground as you tighten your thigh muscles; hold the contraction for two to five counts; release
- Repeat with the other leg
- Repeat one to five times with each leg

Lying Side Thigh Strengthener

- Lie V-legged on your back, feet hip-width apart, toes pointing upwards
- Slide one leg along floor out to the side another six to twelve inches and then return to original position
- Repeat with the other leg
- Repeat one to five times with each leg

Seated Leg Raise

- Sit in a chair that is high enough to let your legs swing; sit back so your knees are at the edge of the chair
- Raise one leg up, straightening your knee till it is slightly bent as you point your toes upward; do not lock your knee
- Hold the position, then lower your leg back down
- Repeat with the other leg
- Repeat one to five times

Hip and Knee ROMs

- On your back, bend one knee at a right angle so your foot is flat on the bed or floor
- Next, bend your other leg and then raise it so your knee touches your chest
- Now, straighten your leg while you lower it

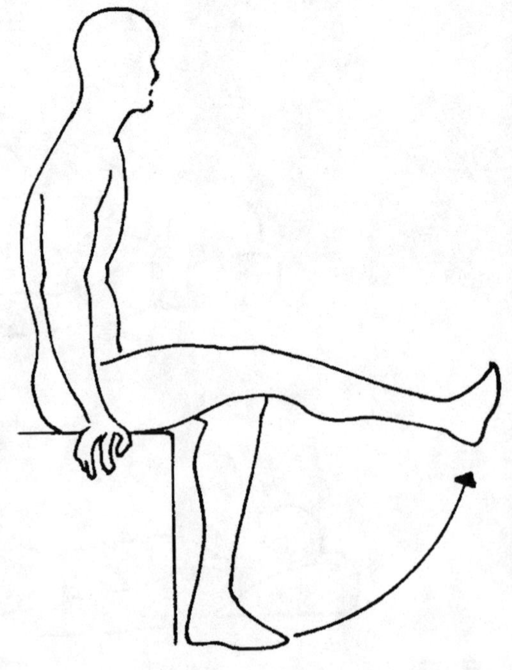

Seated Leg Raise

- Repeat the exercise one to five times, alternating legs

You can do this same exercise standing or seated, while holding on to the edge of a chair and straightening out your leg in front of you when you extend it.

FOOT AND LOWER LEG

Heel-Toe Press-Downs

- Sit in a chair or on the floor with your feet flat on the ground
- First, raise your toes and press down your heels
- Then, lower your toes and press them into the floor as you raise your heels off the ground
- Repeat one to five times

Heel-Toe Press-Outs

- Lying, seated, or standing, start by resting your feet on your heels; point and press toes away from you
- Raise your toes up and press your heels away from you
- Now, point your toes and press away from you again
- Repeat one to five times

For less emphasis on strength and more on flexibility, practice the heel-toe roll with one or both legs straightened and your feet raised up above the floor. Or, you may rest the side of your heel on the ground if you need to for this exercise.

Heel-Toe Circles

- Lying, seated, or standing, extend one leg and raise your toes off the ground
- Point your toes out and make a half-circle with your forefoot, first clockwise, then counterclockwise
- Repeat one to five times

Ankle and Foot ROMs (see illustration, p. 178)

- With knees slightly bent, raise one foot in the air
- Point your toes away from you and move your foot in a circular motion clockwise, then counterclockwise
- Now, point your toes back toward you and repeat the exercise on the other foot
- Repeat one to five times

Heel-Toe Roll

This exercise promotes better circulation in your feet and legs by pumping your calf muscles, and can be done in all positions (i.e. lying, seated, or standing). It will help with circulatory disorders, and will also lubricate the ankle and toe joints, helping to relieve arthritis.

- Whatever position you choose, keep your feet below the level of your heart to promote better lower body circulation
- Flex your forefoot up and back down toward your ankle and shin
- As you flex your forefoot up toward your shin, feel the stretch in your calf

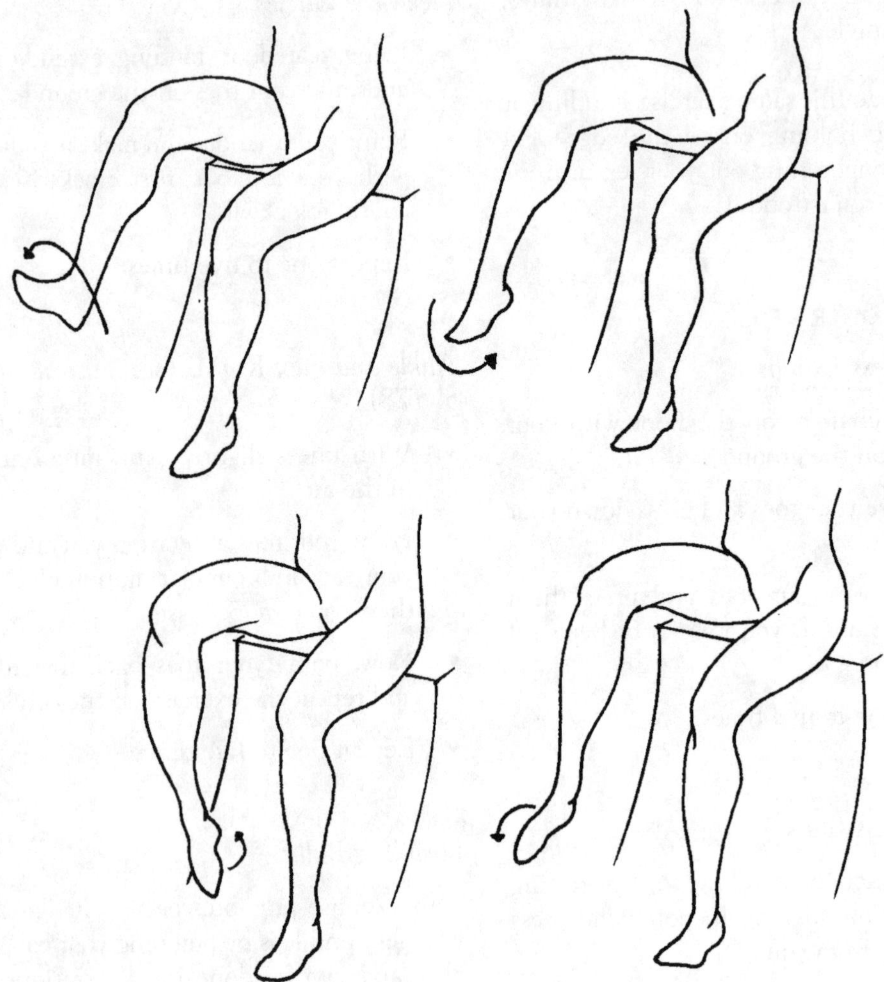

Ankle and Foot ROMs

- As you lower your forefoot, point your toes down as far as they will go and feel the stretch in your shin and the contraction in your calf
- When standing or seated, press your foot down onto the floor and raise your heels up as you roll your forefoot down
- Then, press your heels onto the ground; add your toes to the action by curling them up and down as you move your forefoot
- Repeat one to five times

Toe Bends and Spreads

- While seated or lying down, stretch out your legs and keep your toes pointing upward

- With your heels resting, slowly bend your toes up toward you, and then back down away from you
- Next, spread out your toes so they are separated, then squeeze your toes back together
- Repeat one to five times

FUTURE WARM-UPS

As you become more fit and more experienced, you will be able to vary your warm-up routine by doing slow-motion versions of the aerobic routines in Chapter Eleven.

FUTURE WHOLE-BODY WARM-UPS

- Walking (in place) warm-up (see p. 217)
- Bicycling warm-up (see p. 222)
- Swimming (in place) warm-up (see p. 220)
- Jumping jack
- Jogging (in place) warm-up (see p. 229)

Now that you have completed your warm-up, you are ready to begin the MuSkel stretching and strengthening exercises in Chapter Nine.

CHAPTER 9

MuSkel Ex

Stretching and Strengthening Exercises

Stretching and Strengthening Exercises

The MuSkel exercise prescription is made up of stretching and strengthening exercises targeted to cover all body areas surrounding your nine major joints and bones: neck, shoulders, elbows, wrists, spine, hips, knees, ankles, and toes, including related tendons, ligaments, and muscle groups. Do the exercises in the order that follows; however, if you are arthritic, injured, or disabled, follow the recommendations in Part Three for doing those exercises that apply specifically to your disorder.

The stretching and strengthening routines that follow are organized into five body areas: 1) head and neck, 2) upper trunk, 3) wrist and hands, 4) lower trunk, and 5) feet and ankles. This enables you to exercise all body areas in sequence and also find specific body weaknesses.

For each body area you can do either the lying down series or the upright series (seated or standing) depending on your condition. The standing and seated variations of an exercise are virtually the same movements, but standing usually requires more exertion. The lying down version requires the least exertion. Practice all the MuSkel stretching and strengthening routines if you have an overall weakness of the MuSkel system. If your weakness is more localized, concentrate on area-specific exercises.

Exercise Do's

The following is a list of ten basic stretching and strengthening principles designed to help you optimize your MuSkel prevention exercise routine.

1. **Stretching and Strengthening:** The first basic principle to follow is: Any muscle you strengthen must also be stretched. Stretching exercises should be done only after you have done warm-ups. Stretching a muscle also helps to strengthen it. Strengthening a muscle, on the other hand, may not always stretch it, particularly if there is little or no movement involved in the muscle contraction, such as during an isometric exercise.

   Flexible and strong muscles, tendons, and ligaments act as a cushion or shock-absorber to your joints. If muscles become fatigued, the cushioning effect is decreased and your joints and tendons begin to feel more pressure, and, consequently, are more vulnerable to injury or accidents.

2. **Balanced Use of Muscles:** Stretch and strengthen muscles equally, especially such opposing muscle groups as: biceps and triceps; front and back shoulders; chest and upper back; abdominals and lower back; front and back of thighs; inner and outer thighs; calves and shins; and the heels and forefeet.

3. **Stop When It Hurts:** Listen to your body. Catch an injury in its early stage or avoid injuries altogether by stopping when you feel any sharp pain or tenderness in your joints, tendons, and muscles. Don't resume repetitive motion until you can do it pain-free.

4. **Concentrate on Your Workout:** When exercising specific body areas, do the movements with care, concentration, and concern. Feel the sensations of your muscles stretching and contracting and make sure you can work within safe limits. Slow down the pace of your movement to focus more on your muscles.

5. **Know Your Body:** Know your inherited and developed anatomical weaknesses. Let them serve as a guide in your choices of exercise, sport, and levels of workout intensity.

6. **No Sudden Moves:** *Do not* suddenly increase the amount, speed, or work load of an exercise or move. Increase only in increments of no more than 5 to 10%.

7. **Keep Moving:** Rest when you need to but don't stop completely unless you are in pain. Hold stretches; *do not bounce*. Start by holding a stretch for three seconds, then lengthen your holding time in increments of one to five seconds up to fifteen to thirty seconds for the average stretch and up to a minute for special stretches. Work muscles slowly and continuously. Choose the number of repetitions based upon exerting yourself just beyond the point of fatigue. Start with one repetition and build up to thirty per muscle group.

8. **Don't Hold Your Breath:** Breathe slowly and deeply during all warm-up, cool-down, stretching, posture, and range-of-motion exercises. Exhale on the difficult part of a strengthening exercise, which is usually the muscle contraction; inhale on the easier part, which is usually the muscle release. Remember to breathe in through your nose, and out through your mouth when stretching. Breathe in and out through your mouth during cardiovascular or strengthening exercises.

9. **Maintain Good Posture:** Exercise with your abdominals braced (tightened) and

your back flat to avoid back strain and to strengthen your trunk.

10. **Use Resistance Devices:** Especially when exercising your arms and legs, work against resistance by pulling, pushing, or lifting with stretch cords or weights.

See Table 9.1, Schedule for Strength-Conditioning Exercises for a basic guide on where to start and how to safely build up to a higher level of exercise. Remember, when you are starting out, it is better to begin at a lower level of exertion or repetition; in this way, you can avoid overtaxing your body and causing injury.

EXERCISE DON'TS

HOLDING TIMES

Adjust the holding time for a stretch to your own body—don't slavishly follow any exercise formula. We have only suggested the ranges for the stretches and we encourage you to gradually build up the holding time for the stretches as your muscles become more flexible.

JOINTS

Avoid all sudden and extreme moves and avoid locking (hyperextending) or overbending your joints with any exaggerated movements. Locking or overbending could strain your joints and could lead to pain and injury. (Overbending movements can be found in the traditional moves of gymnastics, ballet, and yoga, so be careful when practicing these types of exercise.) Also, do not roll, swing, jerk, or rush when you are doing joint-bending moves. (Jerking and high-impact movements can be found in modern sports training and running sports.)

Arm throwing and arm and leg swinging are actions that neither strengthen nor stretch. Instead, they involve ballistic motion with little muscle action because you use your muscles only briefly and violently to initiate momentum to move your arms or legs (See Table 9.2, "Bad" vs "Good" Exercises, p. 184, for those exercises you should avoid or those that you can substitute for bad ones.)

The series of exercises that follow are organized according to such body areas as head and neck and shoulders and upper back. This lets you both exercise all body areas in sequence and find specific body areas quickly if you need to do more of an exercise on a specific weak area. They are also organized by level of difficulty with Level I being the easiest, Level II being more difficult, and Level

TABLE 9.1
SCHEDULE FOR STRENGTH-CONDITIONING EXERCISES

Level	I	II	III	IV	V
% of max rep	60–65%	65–70%	70–75%	75–80%	80–85%
Sets per session	1	2	3	4	5
Repetition (reps) per set	1–6	6–8	8–12	12–15	15+
Perceived exertion (1–5 scale)	1	2	3	4	5

Positions to Avoid

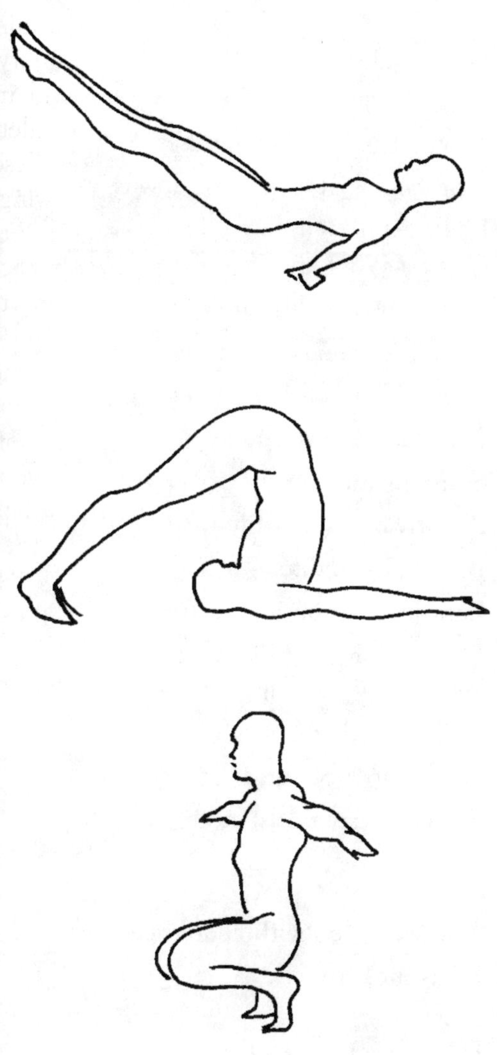

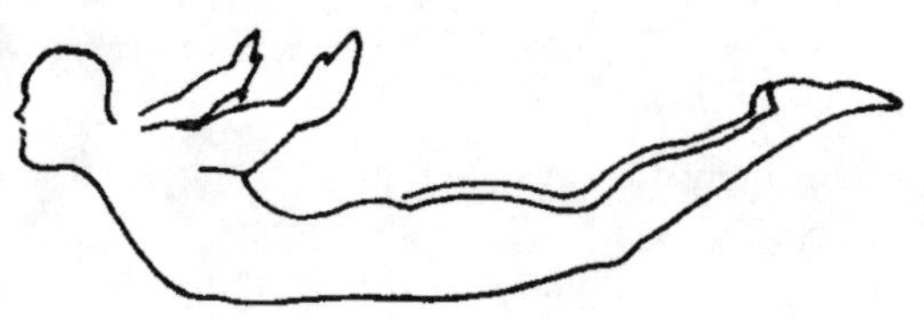

III being the hardest level. Remember, if you have weakness in a particular body part or area, start at a low level of exertion and work up to a higher level.

EXERCISE COUNTS

Practice the movement or hold the position to a level that is comfortable for you. Repeat the series of exercises one to five times. Gradually increase the number of exercise repetitions or hold counts as you move through each of the three levels.

	REPS	HOLD TIMES (in seconds)	SETS
Level I	2–7	1–2	1
Level II	8–12	3–5	2
Level III	13–20	6–12	3
Level IV	21–24	13–19	4
Level V	25–30	20–30	5

Take at least one second to execute each repetition or each hold count. Time your exercise speed by counting out a repetition or hold, adding the word "and" after each count. (1 and 2 and 3 and. . . .)

HEAD AND NECK: LYING DOWN SERIES

LEVEL I: SIDEWAYS TILT

Lying Side Head Turn

- Lie on your left side with your left leg bent for balance, and your right leg straight with the knee slightly bent; prop yourself up with your right hand on the floor, elbow bent in front of your chest

TABLE 9.2
"BAD" VS "GOOD" EXERCISES

"Bad"	"Good"
1. Standing side-bend stretches	1. Diagonal arm reach-ups
2. Back bends (arches)	2. Supine trunk and limb raises
3. Rapid arm swings	3. Arm pumps, Raises, press-downs, or rotations
4. Deep knee bends	4. Quarter (90°) knee bends
5. Trunk rotations	5. Trunk raises and bend-overs
6. Head rolls	6. Head lifts, bends, and pulls
7. Locking elbows and knees	7. Slightly bent elbows and knees
8. Shoulder stands	8. Feet and leg raises
9. Yoga "plow" (heels over shoulders)	9. Standing hang-overs
10. Locked-joint lifts	10. Slightly bent-joint lifts
11. Straight-knee/leg lifts	11. Bent-knee/leg lifts
12. Straight-knee sit-ups	12. Bent-knee sit-ups
13. Fast push-ups	13. Slowed-down bent-knee and bent-elbow push-ups
14. Straight-knee double leg lifts	14. Bent-knee double Leg Lifts
15. Toes pointed out or "pigeon-toed"	15. Parallel foot placement
16. Standing groin stretches, standing leg splits, or standing hurdler's stretches[1]	16. Seated leg split or standing lunge stretch[1]
17. Touching toes, straight-legged	17. Touching toes, with bent knees
18. Straight-legged standing hurdler's stretches and leg splits	18. Bent-knee stretches
19. Seated curl-downs	19. Leaning sideways
20. Full squats, one-legged deep squats	20. Curl-down lunge steps (quads)
21. Seated jackknifes[2]	21. Leg extensions

[1]Avoid using your full body weight to stretch the inner thigh sideways. Also avoid using over-bent knees.

[2]Also called: double leg lifts, elbows bent, hands propped jackknife; or bent-knee double leg lifts.

- Extend your left arm on the floor continuing the line of your body and rest your head on it
- Slowly raise your head, moving your ear toward your right shoulder; pause
- Slowly lower your head back down until it is about one to two inches from your resting arm; pause
- Slowly turn your head so it faces up to the ceiling; pause
- Slowly return your head to face forward; pause
- Slowly turn your head to face down; pause
- Return your head to face forward; rest
- Repeat on this side eight to twelve times according to your level
- Roll over onto your right side and repeat the sequence

LEVEL II: VERTICAL TILT

Lying Vertical Neck Stretch (Arm-Assisted)

- Lie on your back, knees bent, feet flat on the floor; interlace your fingers behind your head at ear level
- Gently pull your head forward, chin to chest
- Hold for three to five seconds, feeling the stretch in your neck and upper back; relax

Lying Vertical Neck Raise or Rotation (for Osteoporosis)

- Lie on your back with your knees bent and feet flat on the floor and resting close to your buttocks; gently flatten your neck, shoulder blades, and lower back onto the floor
- Extend your arms sideways from your shoulders, resting them palms up
- Lift your head one to three inches, chin to chest, as if you wanted to see something on the floor between your legs
- Rotate your head to the left side, chin to shoulder
- Hold for three to five seconds, feeling the contraction in the front and side neck muscles
- Lower your head back down to the starting position
- Rotate your head to the right, chin to shoulder
- Do three sets of eight to twelve repetitions
- Turn over on your stomach and prop your elbows under your shoulders with your head face down and your chin resting in your hands
- Slowly raise your head back, chin one to three inches above your hands, as you keep looking down
- Feel the muscles in the back of your neck contract
- Hold for three to five seconds; relax

Lying Rotating Neck Stretch

- Lie on your back with your arms extended straight out from your shoulders and resting on the floor palms up; keep your knees bent and your feet firmly planted near your buttocks

- Relax your neck and gently tuck in your chin, flattening your neck into the floor
- Inhale through your nose as you slowly turn your head to the left to try to look over your left shoulder
- Place your left hand on your right cheek and let the weight of your left arm gently press your head further toward the floor
- Hold for eight to twelve seconds, feeling the stretch in the right side of your neck; relax
- Repeat on the other side

Level III

Lying Diagonal Neck Stretch

- Lie on your back, knees bent, feet flat on the floor; center your head over your shoulders; extend your right arm straight down, palm down, and rest it by your side
- Place your left hand on the back part of the top of your head
- Turn your head diagonally and point your chin toward your left knee
- Rotate your head slightly toward the right so you can look forward again
- Gently pull your head forward
- Hold for twelve to twenty seconds, feeling the stretch in the back and side of your neck; relax and return your head to center
- Repeat on the right side

Lying Diagonal Head Raise

- Lie on your back, and center your head over your shoulders; extend your arms straight out from your shoulders and rest them on the floor or bed
- Turn—don't tilt—your head left, as if you were going to look over your shoulder; keep your neck straight (extended upward)
- Exhale through your nose as you slowly lift your head diagonally (in a curved path) so you can see your left armpit; your right shoulder may lift slightly off the floor; pause
- Feel the contraction in your neck muscles
- Inhale slowly through your nose as you slowly lower your head, one neck vertebrae at a time, back down to the starting position
- Repeat the exercise in the opposite direction

Head and Neck: Seated or Standing Series

Level I

Seated Side Neck Stretch (Tilt)

- Sit or stand with your arms hanging loosely by your sides or propped on elbow rests
- Tilt your head to one side, as if trying to raise your shoulder
- Hold for three to five seconds, feeling the stretch in the side of your neck; relax
- Repeat on the other side

Alternative Seated or Standing Side Neck Stretches

- Sit or stand with your arms hanging loosely by your sides
- Shrug your shoulder blades down as you push your head up and straighten out your neck
- Hold for three to five seconds, feeling the stretch in the sides of your neck; relax

Seated Chin Tuck

Please note: The seated chin tuck is a multipurpose exercise that centers your head and also stretches and strengthens your neck muscles.

- Sit or stand with your head centered, your feet hip-width apart and firmly planted on the floor, toes pointed forward; your chin should be relaxed and parallel to the ground
- Inhale through your nose as you pull your chin straight back to your neck about two to three inches; keep your chin line parallel to the ground, eyes forward, and shoulders back and down
- Pause, feeling the stretch in the front and back of your neck
- Exhale through your mouth as you slowly return your chin to the starting position
- Do one to three sets of three to eight repetitions each

Seated or Standing Side Neck Stretch (Tilt) (Arm-Assisted)

- Stand and tilt your head toward your left shoulder
- Place your left palm on the right side of your head, with your fingers touching your ear
- Gently pull your head sideways, keeping your right shoulder pressed down
- Hold for three to five seconds, feeling the stretch on the right side of your neck; relax
- Repeat on the other side

Level II

Seated or Standing Side Neck Stretch (Hand To Head)

- Sit or stand with your head centered over your shoulders; breathe gently through your nose as you do the exercises
- Tilt your head sideways to your left so that your ear is over your shoulder; continue looking straight ahead
- Place your left hand on the top left side of your head and let the weight of your left arm slowly pull your head toward your left shoulder; keep your shoulders back and down
- Extend your right arm out and reach down to the floor to feel the neck muscles stretch even more
- Hold for five to eight seconds; relax
- Repeat on the other side

Seated or Standing Vertical Neck Bend (Floor to Ceiling)

- Sit or stand with your feet parallel and shoulder-width apart, toes pointed forward; your arms should hang loosely by your sides, your head centered, chin tucked in, and jaw relaxed

- Slowly press your forehead down and forward, keeping your shoulders relaxed and chin tucked in until you are looking at the floor; pause
- Return your head to the center position; pause
- Slightly tilt your head back, then turn your head slightly to one side and then the other; pause
- Slowly bring your chin down to the starting position

Level III

Alternating Standing Back and Forth Neck Stretch

- Place your hands palms down and shoulder-width apart on a wall
- Bend your knees and bend over at the hips keeping your thighs perpendicular to the ground
- Lower your head between your arms
- Hold for five to eight seconds, feeling the stretch in your neck, upper back, and shoulders; relax

Seated and Standing Neck Bend

- Sit or stand with your feet shoulder-width apart with your head centered, arms hanging by your sides; relax your jaw (i.e. unclench your teeth)
- Slowly lower your head, right ear to right shoulder; pause
- Slowly lower your chin to your chest; pause
- Slowly bend your head, left ear to left shoulder; pause
- Slowly bring your head up to the vertical position
- Repeat eight to twelve times

Seated and Standing Rotating Neck Stretch

Please note: The seated and standing neck stretches are the same.

- Sit or stand with your feet shoulder-width apart and knees slightly bent; your arms should be hanging loosely by your sides or on top of the chair arm rests
- Turn your head to the left as if to look over your shoulder; keep your chin line parallel to the floor
- Place your left hand on your right cheek and pull it gently toward your left side; do not hunch or move your shoulders
- Hold for twelve to thirty seconds; relax
- Return your head to the starting position; repeat on the other side of your neck

Shoulders and Upper Back: Lying Down Series

Level I

Repeat each of the following Level I exercises three to eight times. Hold each stretch three to eight seconds.

Lying Shoulder and Back Stretch

- Lie on your back with your knees bent, arms extended straight out from your shoulders, elbows slightly bent
- Bring both arms across your chest, bending your elbows, and place your hands on the opposite shoulder; hug yourself
- Feel the stretch in your shoulders and upper back

Lying Shoulder Raises

- Lie on your back, arms by your sides, palms facing down, elbows slightly bent
- Slowly exhale and raise your arms to shoulder height, slowly inhale, and lower your arms back to the starting position
- Feel the contraction in the front and rear shoulders and in your upper back

Level II

Repeat each Level II strengthening exercise eight to twelve times. Hold each stretch for five to twelve seconds.

Lying Shoulder Stretch

- Lie on your back, knees bent, feet flat on the floor, arms at your sides with your palms down
- Extend your right arm above your head, palm up, keeping your left arm at your side
- Feel the stretch in your right arm and shoulder; relax
- Change sides
- Alternative: Extend both arms above shoulders

Lying Shoulder Raise

- Lie face down
- Inhale as you extend your arms forward and above your shoulders; raise them one to three inches off the floor, palms down, fingers forward as if you are starting a breast stroke
- Exhale as you slowly lower your arms down to shoulder height
- Now, turn over and lie on your back, knees bent, arms by your sides
- Inhale as you trace a large circle with your arms by slowly sliding your arms above your head and pulling them apart over your body like a double-arm back stroke
- Exhale as you slowly return to the starting position
- Feel the contraction in your back muscles; relax

Level III

Lying Shoulder Stretch

- Lie down and rest your forehead on your right arm
- Reach your left arm forward, press your palm down, and pull your hips back
- Feel the stretch in your upper back, arms, and shoulders
- Hold ten to thirty seconds
- Repeat on the other side

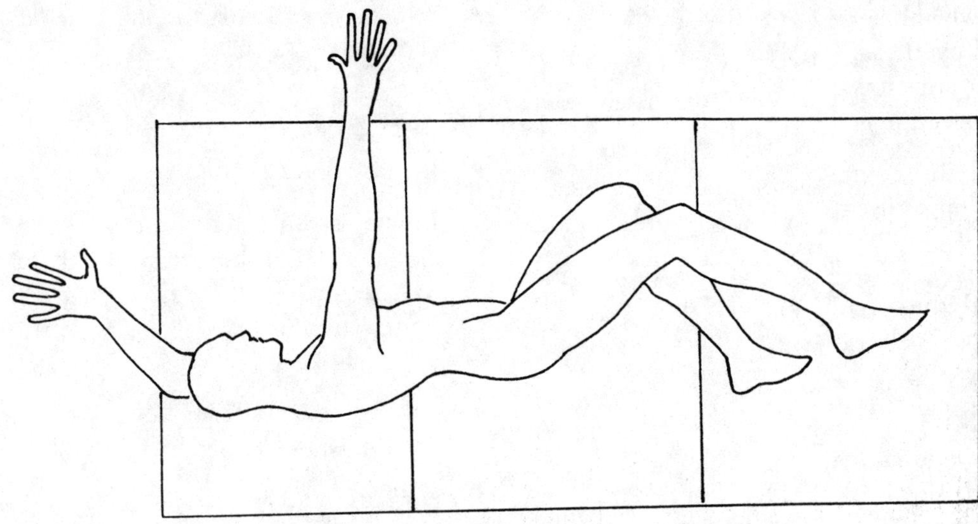

Lying Shoulder Exercise

Lying Shoulder Raise

- Lie on your back with knees bent; extend your arms straight out at shoulder level, elbows slightly bent, palms up; keep your shoulder blades back and down
- Raise your arms two to six inches off the floor
- Now, slowly circle your arms in a clockwise direction for eight to twelve counts
- Rest for five to twelve seconds
- Repeat the circles in the counterclockwise direction for eight to twelve counts
- Feel the contraction in your back and shoulder muscles

Please note: The larger your circles are, the more your back muscles will be involved.

Shoulders and Upper Back: Seated or Standing Series

Level I

Repeat each Level I and II strengthening exercise three to eight times. Hold each stretch three to eight seconds.

Seated Shoulder Stretch

- Sit or stand with your arms hanging loosely by your sides
- Shrug your shoulders up
- Feel the stretch in your shoulder and neck muscles; relax

Seated Shoulder Raise

- Sit on a chair or bench, arms by your sides, palms back, elbows slightly bent

- Slowly inhale and raise your arms up, out, and overhead, then exhale as you lower your arms forward and back to the starting position
- Feel the contraction in your shoulders and upper back

Standing Shoulder Raise

- Stand with your feet hip-width apart, knees slightly bent, arms hanging by your sides, palms facing back
- Slowly inhale as you raise your arms overhead; slowly exhale as you lower them back to the start
- Feel the contraction in your shoulders and upper back

Level II

Seated Shoulder Stretch

- Sit or stand with your fingers interlaced and your palms turned out
- Extend your arms in front of you at shoulder height
- Feel the stretch in your shoulders, back, and upper arms

Seated Shoulder Raise

- Sit at the edge of a chair or bench or stand with your arms hanging straight down at your sides. (Optional: hold weights, palms in.)
- Inhale as you raise your arms or weights to shoulder height (not greater than a 90-degree angle from your body); keep your arms straight
- Pause, then exhale as you lower your arms back down the same way to the starting position
- Feel the contraction in your front and side shoulder muscles; relax

Standing Shoulder Stretch

- Sit or stand and put your left hand on your right shoulder
- Pull your left elbow with your right hand across your chest toward your right shoulder
- Feel the stretch in your left shoulder and the back of your upper arm; relax, then repeat on the other side

Standing Shoulder Raise

- Stand or sit with your elbows raised to shoulder height and pointed away from your body, forearms dangling
- Extend your forearms out; relax

Level III

Repeat each Level III strengthening exercise eight to twelve times. Hold each stretch twelve to thirty seconds.

Seated Shoulder Stretch

- Sit or stand with your fingers interlaced above your head and your palms turned upward
- Push your arms up and behind your head
- Feel the stretch in your shoulders, back, and arms; relax

Seated Shoulder Raise

- Sit on a chair and place your hands on the side of the chair or the arms (you can also sit back on the floor in a recumbent position)
- Keep your knees bent and shoulders down as you start and continue the exercise
- Inhale as you slowly lift yourself straight up from your seat by pushing down on the chair and straightening out your arms; keep your feet flat on the ground and lean forward slightly as you go up; pause
- Now, exhale as you slowly lower yourself down onto the chair again
- Feel the contraction in your shoulder blades; relax

Standing Shoulder Stretch

- Stand and bend your head sideways toward your left shoulder
- Gently pull your right arm down, behind, and across your back with your left hand (as shown)
- Feel the stretch in your shoulders and neck; relax

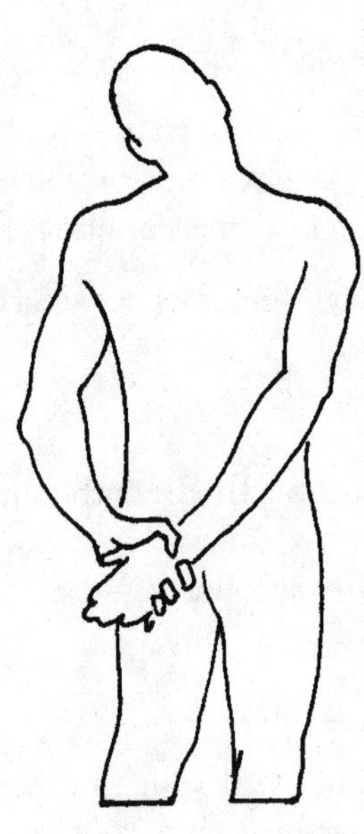

Standing Shoulder Stretch

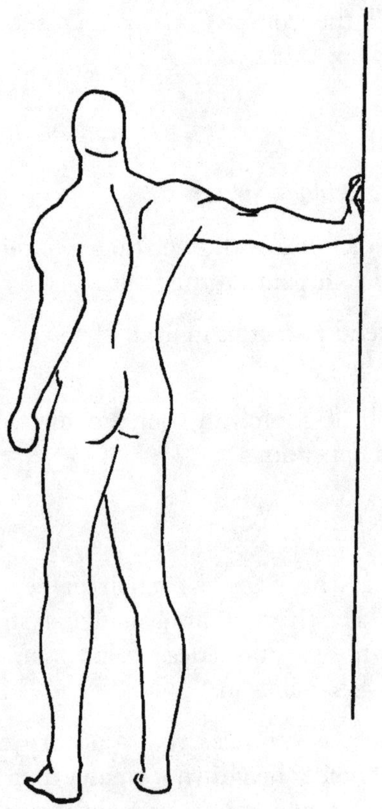

Alternative Position

Alternative Standing Shoulder Stretch

- Stand with your right side at an arm's length from a wall
- Extend your right arm out, fingers back, palm out, against the wall
- Turn your whole body to the left, moving your feet from the wall; keep your head centered and chin parallel to the floor
- Feel the stretch in your right shoulder and upper back
- Repeat this stretch with your left arm

Standing Shoulder Raise

- Stand or sit; raise your arms to shoulder level and inhale as you reach forward, bending your elbows, and turning your palms toward you as you would to hug somebody; pause
- Exhale as you extend your forearms to the side and pull your elbows back as you try to touch your forearms behind you
- Feel the contraction in your shoulders and upper and middle back muscles

Alternative: Shoulder Raise

- Stand, or sit at the edge of your chair, knees bent at 90 degrees, upper body bent forward and parallel to the floor
- Let your arms hang over the outside of your knees and your head hang down; your back should look as if it is shaped like a turtle shell
- Inhale and reach forward as you slowly raise your arms and head until they are parallel to the ground
- Exhale as you slowly bring your arms back to your sides and return to the starting position
- Feel the contraction in your shoulder and back muscles

Chest and Triceps: Lying Down Series

Level I

Lying Chest Stretch

- Lie on your back, legs straight, knees slightly bent; extend your arms overhead,

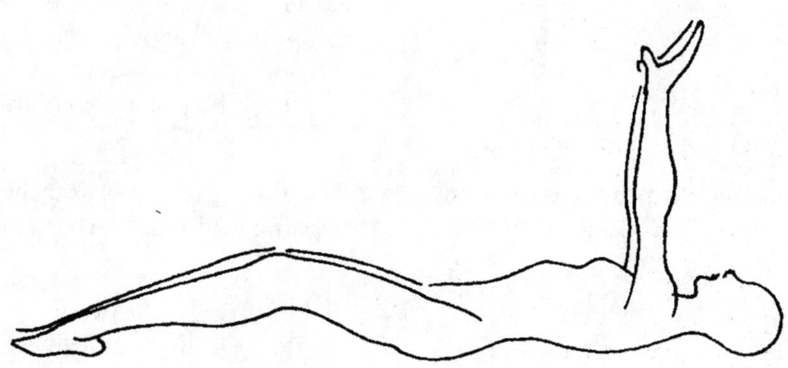

Lying Chest Stretch

palms up, fingers extended, toes pointed down

- Push your hands up and heels down
- Hold for three to eight seconds, feeling the stretch in your arms, chest, and legs

Lying Chest Press

- Get down on all fours: kneel on the floor and put your hands palms down; your hands should be chest- to shoulder-width apart, on the floor in front of you
- Keeping your knees bent and upper body rigid, slowly lower yourself until your chest is above the floor in line with your elbow joints; keep your elbows in and head up so it is in line with your back
- Pause, then push back up to the starting position
- Inhale as you go down, exhale as you push up
- Feel the contraction in your chest, arm, and shoulder muscles
- Repeat eight to twelve times

Level II

Lying Chest and Arm Stretch

- Lie on your back, knees bent, feet flat
- Interlace your fingers behind your head and press your elbows and shoulders down
- Hold for three to eight seconds, feeling the stretch in your chest and arms; rest

Lying Chest Press

- Lie face down with palms down on either side of your chest, elbows up and in
- Your legs are straight out, propped on the balls of your feet, knees slightly bent
- Keep your body rigid and head up as you push up with your hands until your arms are extended, elbows slightly bent; pause
- Lower your body slowly back down until your chest just touches the floor but does not rest there
- Inhale as you go down, exhale as you go up
- Feel the contraction in your chest, triceps, shoulders, and upper back; rest
- Repeat eight to twelve times

Level III

Lying Chest Stretch

Please note: This exercise is particularly useful for correcting rounded shoulders and relieving menstrual cramps. As a specific prescription for cramps, you can hold this position for as many as five to fifteen minutes.

- Kneel on all fours, thighs perpendicular to the floor, hands placed directly under shoulders, elbows bent; avoid arching your back by placing your arms well forward
- Rest the right side of your head on your forearms and pull in your stomach muscles
- Hold for twelve to twenty seconds, feeling the stretch in your rib cage; relax

- Repeat by resting your head on your left side

Lying Chest Press

- Lie on your back, arms straightened and extended out to the sides at shoulder height, palms up
- Exhale as you raise your arms up above your chest bringing your palms together
- Inhale as you lower your arms back to the starting position
- Feel the contraction in your chest muscles
- Repeat three to twelve times
- Alternative: Holding a barbell or weight in each hand, press them straight up from your chest and straighten out your arms

CHEST AND TRICEPS: SEATED OR STANDING SERIES

LEVEL I

For all levels, repeat each strengthening exercises three to six times. Hold each stretch twelve to thirty seconds.

Seated Chest and Arm Stretch

- Sit on a sturdy chair, buttocks planted firmly, or on the floor, tailor-fashion
- Extend your left hand to the floor; raise your right hand and lift up your rib cage to the left without bending your waist while bracing your weight with your left hand
- Feel the stretch on your right side and arm
- Repeat on your left side

Seated Chest Press

- With your feet flat on the floor, sit on the edge of a chair or bench and hold firmly on to the arm rests, palms down, fingers forward
- By straightening your arms, raise your body off the bench or chair; pause
- Lower your body down again; feel the contraction of your chest and triceps muscles; relax

Standing Chest and Arm Stretch

- Stand or sit with your feet planted hip-width apart, knees bent, stomach muscles braced
- Extend both your arms above your head and align them with your ears, palms facing in, shoulders back and down; reach up high without shrugging
- Feel the stretch in your rib cage and arms; relax
- Reach diagonally right without bending your waist; feel the stretch; relax
- Reach diagonally left without bending your waist; feel the stretch; relax

Standing Chest Press

- Stand facing a wall, an arm's length away
- Place your palms at chest level and shoulder-width apart on the wall, fingers up
- Slowly bend your elbows and lean into the wall as far as you can control the weight; pause

- Slowly push away from the wall, straightening out your arms
- Feel the contraction in your chest, triceps, and shoulders; relax

LEVEL II

Seated Chest Stretch

- Sit or stand with your arms hanging down by your sides, elbows bent and pointed behind you
- Gently push your elbows together behind your back and squeeze your shoulder blades together; keep your head and chest up
- Hold for eight to twelve seconds
- Feel the stretch in your chest

Seated Chest Press

- Sit on a floor, knees bent, in the recumbent position
- Lower your upper body back a few inches, bending your elbows
- Straighten out your arms to raise yourself back to the starting position
- Feel the contraction of your chest and triceps muscles
- Repeat three to eight times

Standing Chest Stretch

- Stand with your hands resting above the back of your hips, elbows bent, and pointing back
- Slowly press your hands into your hips as you push your elbows back and together
- Hold for eight to twelve seconds, feeling the stretch in your chest; relax

Standing Chest Press

- Stand with your feet shoulder-width apart; extend your arms and place your hands on either side of a door frame
- Lean forward bending your arms; keeping your body rigid, lower your body through the door frame; keep your head aligned with your upper body; pause
- Return to the starting position while maintaining proper alignment
- Feel the contraction in your chest, triceps, and lower back
- Repeat three to eight times

LEVEL III

Seated Chest Stretch

- Sit on a chair, reach behind you, and clasp your hands together
- Bend your elbows and gently push them toward each other as you lean your head back slightly
- Hold for twelve to twenty seconds, feeling the stretch in your chest, arms, and front shoulders

Seated Chest Press

- Sit on a chair or bench and hold on to the edge, palms facing down, feet flat on the ground
- Bend your arms and rest your body weight on your palms

- Straighten out your arms to raise your body; pause
- Bend your arms to lower your body back down
- Feel the contraction in your chest and triceps
- Repeat twelve to twenty times
- Inhale as you lower your body; exhale as you raise it up

Standing Chest Stretch

- Stand with your knees slightly bent, and either hold the ends of a towel or place your hands at shoulder level on both sides of a door frame
- With the towel, first straighten out your arms in front of you, and then lift them up and behind your head slightly
- With the door frame, push your upper body forward
- Keep your chest and head up
- Hold twelve to twenty seconds, feeling the stretch in your chest and arms; rest

Standing Chest Press

- Stand with feet hip-width apart, hands resting at an arm's length on a sturdy desk or table top
- Keeping your body fully straightened, slowly lower it forward until your chest just touches the desk or table
- Pause, then raise your body until your arms are straightened out
- Feel the contraction of the chest, arm, and shoulder muscles; repeat twelve to twenty times; rest

ARMS: LYING DOWN SERIES

A general note about arm exercises: Choose one of the three positions below (i.e. lying, seated, or standing) for your arm exercise series. Before doing the biceps curl (p. 198), repeat the stretching exercises for the chest and triceps, pp. 195–196. Beginners should exercise one arm at a time. Advanced exercisers can exercise both arms. By squeezing your elbows into your sides, you can also work your chest muscles.

By turning your wrist from palms out to palms up, you can have a combination of exercises using biceps, triceps, and chest with hand, wrist, and forearm exercises. For example, when you grasp the bar and turn your wrist during the biceps curl you work hand, wrist, and forearm. You also stretch the triceps muscles. When you do a triceps extension you stretch the biceps muscle. For these reasons, when we refer to arms in this exercise section, we mean biceps, triceps, forearms, elbows, and wrists, unless specified otherwise.

LEVEL I

Lying Arm Curls and Extensions

- Lie on your back, knees bent, with your arms by your sides, palms down
- Keep your elbows flat on the floor and bring them into your sides as you bend your right elbow and slowly raise your right arm up toward your shoulder; at the

same time, turn your wrist palms up and out; feel the contraction in your biceps and forearms; pause

- Lower it back down; slowly turn your wrist clockwise palms in, then down, and finally outward
- Feel the contraction in your triceps; relax
- Repeat the exercise with your left arm (you can also do biceps curls with both arms simultaneously)
- Do one to three sets of five to eight repetitions for each arm

Level II

Lying Biceps Curl

- Lie back on a bench with your arms hanging to the floor, wrists turned palms in; you may also hold three- to ten-pound weights in each hand
- Inhale as you slowly curl up your arm, turning your palms toward your head as they pass your thighs and reach your shoulder level
- Feel the contraction in your biceps muscles; pause
- Exhale as you slowly lower your arm to the starting position turning your wrist from palm up to palm in as you pass by your thighs
- Keep your elbows tucked in throughout this exercise
- Do one to three sets of eight to twelve repetitions

Arms: Seated or Standing Series

Level I

For all levels, do one to three sets of five to eight repetitions for each exercise.

Seated Arm Curl and Wrist Turn

- Stand or sit on the edge of your chair or bench with your feet firmly planted on the floor, arms hanging by your sides, palms outward; you may also hold a one- to three-pound weight in each hand
- Keep your elbows slightly bent and bring them into your sides, turning your forearms away from your body
- Inhale as you curl your arms up, turning your palms up as they pass your thighs
- Just as your palms reach shoulder level (and not before), turn your wrist, palms out; pause
- Feel the contraction of your biceps
- Exhale as you lower your arms back down to the starting position turning your wrist from palm out, to up, to in; relax

Standing Biceps Curl

- Stand with your feet hip- to shoulder-width apart, feet parallel, and toes pointed forward; hold your arms by your sides, elbows slightly bent, palms in; you may also hold a one- to three-pound weight in each hand
- Keep your upper arms close to your sides as you inhale and slowly curl your arm up to your shoulder, turning your wrist palm up as it passes your thigh and palm out as it reaches your shoulder; pause

- Exhale as you slowly lower your arm, wrist turning from palm out, to up, to in, and finally out
- Feel the contraction in your triceps as you turn your palm out away from your body
- Feel the contraction in your biceps muscles

Please note: If you do not wish to use weights, you can use one-arm wall push-ups. See Level III below.

Level II

Seated Biceps Curl

- Sit sideways to your left side on the edge of a chair, legs apart, your right knee pointing forward and bent out at 45 degrees, feet flat on the floor
- Point your left knee down to the left side, bent at 45 degrees with your foot firmly planted on its ball
- Brace your left hand by your left side on the chair seat; you can hold a three- to five-pound weight in your right hand, palm up, and hanging between your legs, elbows slightly bent
- Inhale as you curl your arm up toward your shoulder turning the wrist out at the top; pause
- Feel the contraction of your biceps muscles
- Exhale as you slowly lower your arm through the same path back to the starting position

Standing Biceps Curl

- Stand with your feet shoulder-width apart, arms at your sides, palms facing front; you may also hold a stick or barbell with your hands shoulder-width apart and resting on your upper thighs
- Keep your lower back flat, head up, elbows in, and shoulders back and down as you do the exercise
- Curl your arms or the bar upwards in a semicircular motion, bringing your hands toward your shoulders; if you are not using weights, turn your wrists out
- Feel the contraction in your biceps; relax

Level III

Standing One-Arm Wall Push-Ups

- Stand facing a wall, keep your head up, back straight, shoulders down, and knees slightly bent
- With your palms and fingers up against the wall, slowly bend your elbows and lean toward the wall as far as your arms can control the weight
- Slowly push yourself back up to the starting position; relax

Please note: You can also practice this exercise at different angles to the wall: facing front, sideways, and at a diagonal.

CHAPTER 10

Meta Ex

Duration and Lower Trunk Exercises

BALANCE IS KEY TO YOUR META SYSTEM

Just as balance is the ongoing theme for the metabolic system, it is also the standard for its most beneficial exercise. Moderate-paced, weight-loaded, lower trunk stretching and strengthening exercises are the best to help your metabolic system. Vigorous exercise is not recommended because it can cause dramatic swings in your blood sugar level and can substantially increase your appetite. Low-intensity exercise, on the other hand, does not burn off enough fat to make a difference. The Meta exercises in this book, however, use routines that help regulate your body's energy expenditure and nutrient balance by stimulating the middle area of your body (i.e. the lower trunk), the body's center of gravity where most of the metabolic organs are located and function. Adding weight or resistance to any exercise is the fastest way to change your body composition and shift the imbalance of too much fat to a little more muscle.

HOW TO DETERMINE YOUR MINIMUM ACTIVITY LEVEL

Unless you are severely obese (seventy-five pounds or more over your "ideal" weight), you will most likely start to exercise before committing to a diet. You should condition your body before beginning the process of weight reduction, and then build up to the activity level that will help you maintain your ideal weight.

The key to maintaining the healthiest body composition for your age is to live an active life. Use Table 4.2, p. 67, Ideal Body Weight, to determine your daily activity level target and meet it by following these six steps:

1. Determine what your healthiest "ideal" weight should be from the age and body build column: _____ pounds.
2. Next, choose one of these multipliers, based on your level of physical activity: 14—Not very active; 15—Somewhat active; 16—Active; 17—Very active. Multiply your normal weight by the correct multiplier to determine the amount of calories you need to maintain that weight: _____ calories.
3. Now, weigh yourself and place your current weight here: _____ pounds.
4. If you weigh more than the ideal weight for your age, subtract the ideal weight from your actual weight: _____ pounds. This is the number of pounds you are overweight. If you weigh less than the ideal weight, you are underweight and should consider trying to gain weight by adding extra calories to your daily intake.
5. Convert the difference in pounds to activity calories by multiplying each extra pound by 3,500 calories: _____. This is the total calories you will need to burn during the period you have designated to lose the excess weight.
6. Divide the total number of calories you need to burn by the number of weeks you plan to use increased levels of activity to burn off the extra weight: _____. For example, let's say that you want to lose ten pounds in twelve weeks. The first calculation is to find the total number of calories that you will need to burn. For this number you will multiply the number of extra pounds (10) by 3,500 calories. This equals 35,000 calories. You then divide 35,000 by the number of weeks that you are going to try to lose the weight (12). 35,000 divided by 12 equals 2,917 calories per week. Because it is easier to deal in round numbers, you round this number up to 3,000. This is amount of calories that you should burn up each week for twelve weeks in order to lose the ten pounds. The example that follows is a typical scenario:

Joan is a medium-framed, 5'6" tall woman who is thirty-five-years old.

- Her normal weight should be 136 pounds
- She is not very active, so she will need 136 × 14 or 1,904 calories of fuel to maintain this weight
- Her current weight is 146 pounds
- 146 – 136 = 10 pounds overweight
- She needs 10 × 3,500 calories = 35,000 extra calories to burn off those extra 10 pounds
- She has set a five-week goal; 35,000 ÷ 5 = 7,000 extra calories worth of exercise each week to attain this goal

How Many Calories Must You Burn to Lose or Maintain Your Weight?

To maintain your weight, you must burn about 1,200 to 2,000 activity/exercise calories per week. This translates to twelve to twenty miles of walking (about three to four hours), fifteen to thirty-five miles (two to three hours) of cycling, twenty-seven to thirty-six laps (one and a half to two and a half hours) of swimming, or various combinations. To lose weight, you will need to build your maintenance exercise routine one-half to four times above this level to achieve your weekly weight-loss goal of one-half to two pounds per week. One-half pound of body fat loss takes an additional 1,200 calories of exercise or double the time spent per week; two pounds of body fat loss takes 7,000 calories of exercise a week or about three times the maintenance level. Of course, after you have begun to exercise regularly, your resting metabolism rate will go up, too, adding between eighty and 200 calories burned per day while resting. You will feel more energetic and be more enthusiastic about doing such physical chores as home repair, gardening, climbing stairs, and running errands on foot—activities that can burn another 100 to 500 calories per day.

The type of exercise you do is also significant. For example, if you are only doing leg exercises, stepping, or cycling, you can almost double the rate of calorie burn by simultaneously moving your arms and increasing your step length as you walk.

EXERCISE COUNTS

Practice the movement or hold the position to a level that is comfortable for you. Repeat the series of exercises one to five times. Gradually increase the number of exercise repetitions or hold counts as you move through each of the three levels.

	REPS	HOLD TIMES (in seconds)	SETS
Level I	2–7	1–2	1
Level II	8–12	3–5	2
Level III	13–20	6–12	3
Level IV	21–24	13–19	4
Level V	25–30	20–30	5

Take at least one second to execute each repetition or each hold count. Time your exercise speed by counting out a repetition or hold, adding the word "and" after each count. (1 and 2 and 3 and. . . .)

HIP, PELVIS, AND GROIN: LYING DOWN SERIES

LEVEL I

Lying V-Legged Stretch

- Lie V-legged on a bed, floor, or mat, with your knees bent and out to the sides so the soles of your feet are together
- Relax your legs and hips, and let gravity do the stretching
- Hold for three to ten seconds, feeling the stretch in your groin and hips

Lying Wall Leg Split Stretch

- Lie on a floor mat beside a wall; bend your knees and turn your body around so it is at a right angle to the wall
- Raise both your legs and slide your buttocks against the wall; back away from the wall one to two feet if your buttocks are too close; slowly spread your heels apart
- Hold for three to ten seconds, feeling the stretch in your groin, hips, and inner thigh

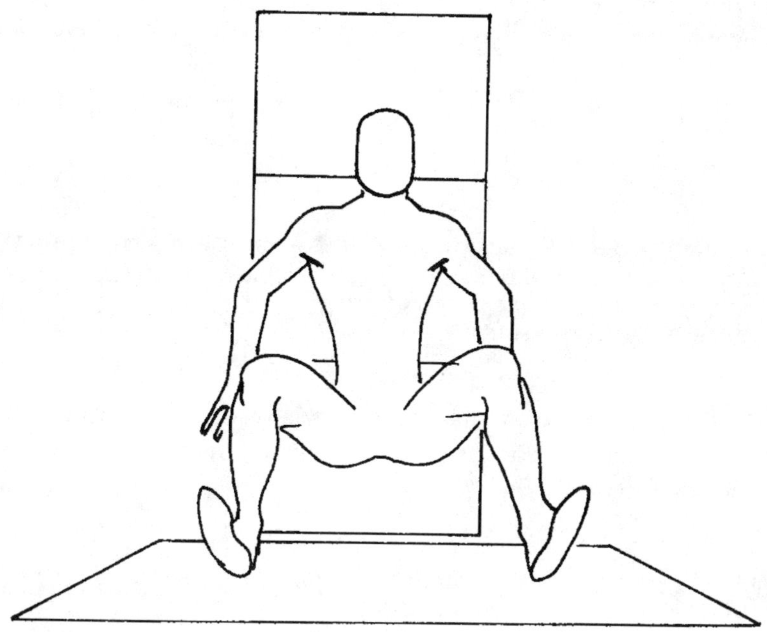

Lying Wall Leg Split Stretch
(view from above)

Lying Pelvic Tilt (Hip Curl)

- Lie on a firm bed or a floor mat
- Bend your knees and slide your feet back so your heels are near your buttocks; press your toes down
- Rest your arms out to your sides at shoulder height
- Tighten (brace) your abdominal muscles; pull your abdomen up and in at the same time as you flatten your pelvis and lower back to the ground; continue to press your toes down
- Slowly tighten your buttocks and curl your hip up off the floor one to four inches
- Hold for one to two seconds
- Slowly uncurl until your buttocks are flat to the ground again
- Repeat two to three times

Please note: You can combine this exercise with the Lying Kegel exercise, p. 204.

Lower Abdominal Exercise

Do this series of exercises to strengthen the muscles of the lower abdomen and to help you do the pelvic tilt.

- Lie with your back flat and feet flat against the bed or floor
- Pull your abdomen up and in as if to tuck it under your rib cage

- Now, lift your right foot off the floor and bring your right knee toward your chest pointing it at your chest
- Keep your back flat and lift the left foot and left knee to the same position; stop if your back arches
- Lower your right leg to the starting position
- Lower your left leg to the starting position
- Repeat the exercise five to ten times with each leg, starting the sequence with the alternate leg each time

Lying Abdominal Exercise

Repeat the prior exercise lifting each foot until the thigh is vertical or is at a 90-degree angle with the ground

Lying Kegel Exercise

Please note: Do this isometric exercise to strengthen pelvic floor muscles and help with bladder and bowel leaking, constipation, and pelvic and rectal pain. Pelvic floor muscles stretch from your pubic bone underneath and around your groin up to your coccyx or tailbone. They include the sphincter muscles that surround your anus and the perineal muscles underneath your bladder, which help control bowel movement and your urine flow. When doing this exercise, pretend you are trying to stop and start the flow of urine and the flow of gas.

- Lie down face up
- Do not tighten your abdominals or buttocks
- As you tilt your pelvis slightly, tighten your sphincter muscles, and then tighten your perineal muscles; for women, the perineals are also called the vaginal muscles
- Hold for one to ten seconds
- As you begin to lower your pelvis back down, slowly relax these tightened muscles
- Relax for ten to twenty seconds
- Repeat the contract/relax phases five to ten times

LEVEL II

Lying Cross-Legged Hip Pull Stretch

- Lie on your bed or a floor mat; bend your knees and cross your right leg over your left knee
- Stretch your arms to shoulder height or interlace your fingers behind your head
- Keep your shoulders, upper back, and elbows flat on the bed or floor
- Use your right leg to gently pull your left one toward the floor; feel a mild stretch in your hips and lower back

Lying Bent-Knee Across Chest Raise

- Lie face up with your knees bent at 90-degree angles and your arms extended to shoulder level
- Raise one leg and, with knee still bent, pull it across your chest to the opposite shoulder, then return it to the starting position
- Raise your other leg, knee bent toward

your chest, then return it to the starting position

- Alternate raising and lowering each leg twelve to twenty times

LEVEL III

LYING CROSS-LEGGED HIP PULL

- Lie on a bed or floor mat with your legs straight out, knees slightly bent
- Bend your right knee, extend your right arm straight out to shoulder height
- Use your left hand to pull your right knee to the left, across your body, while you turn your head toward your right arm
- Keep your upper back and shoulders flat on the floor
- Hold for ten to thirty seconds, feeling the stretch in the side of your hip and lower back
- Repeat on your other side

Lying Side-Leg Raise

- Lie on your right side with your right arm extended above your shoulder and under your head
- Extend your left leg and bend your right knee bringing it slightly forward of your body
- Place your left hand on the floor next to your chest
- Raise your left leg one to three feet toward the ceiling while keeping your leg straightened, foot flattened, toes pointing forward
- Feel the contraction in your outer hip
- Repeat the leg raise eight to twelve times on each side

HIP, PELVIS, AND GROIN: SEATED OR STANDING SERIES

LEVEL I

Seated V-Legged Stretch

- Sit on a floor mat with the soles of your feet pressed together
- Grab your feet and gently pull forward while keeping your back straight
- Hold for fifteen to thirty seconds, feeling the stretch in your groin, inner thigh muscles, and lower back

Seated Pelvic Tilt (Buttocks Bounce)

- Sit on a chair or floor mat
- Slowly squeeze your buttocks muscles and tuck them under your pelvis

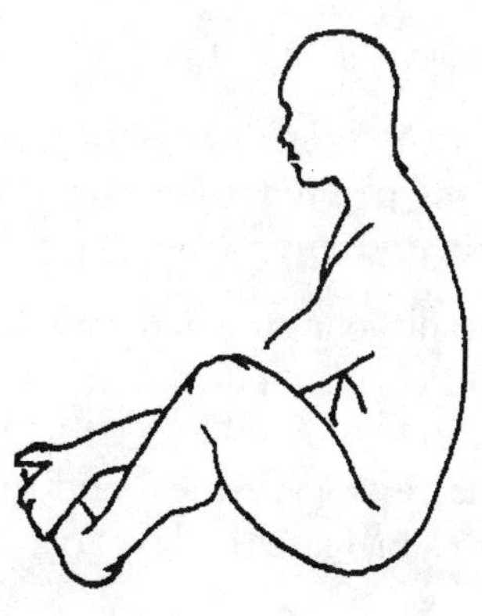

Seated V-Legged Stretch

- At the same time, tighten your abdominal muscles; let your thighs turn outward as you do this
- Hold a moment, then relax
- Now, repeat the exercise in one-second intervals as you try to bounce your body up and down in your chair
- Feel your buttocks and abdominal muscles as you contract and release them
- Repeat two to three times

Standing Bent-Knee Across Chest Pull

- Stand sideways to a wall or chair and hold on to it with your inside hand; your feet should be shoulder-width apart, toes pointed straight ahead; keep your heels flat and your knees one-quarter bent
- Grasp your inside knee with the outside hand and pull it across your chest
- Hold position for three to ten seconds, feeling the stretch in your hips, hamstrings, calves, and ankles
- Repeat with other leg

Standing Pelvic Tilt (Hip Curl)

- Stand with your feet shoulder-width apart, toes pointed straight ahead, and knees slightly bent
- Slowly pull your stomach muscles in as your tighten your buttocks muscles and tilt your pelvis under your body; you can also squeeze your perineal and sphincter muscles to increase the level of difficulty
- Hold for one to ten seconds, feeling the full contraction of the abdominal, buttocks, and pelvic floor muscles
- Repeat two to three times

LEVEL II

Seated Cross-Legged Stretch

- Sit on the floor with your legs straight out in front of you, knees slightly bent
- Bend your left leg and cross it over your right leg, placing your left foot on the outside of your right knee
- Grab your left knee with your right hand and pull it across your body toward the right shoulder
- Hold five to twenty seconds, feeling the stretch on the side of your hip and hamstrings
- Repeat with the other leg

Seated Bent-Knee Across Chest Raise

- Sit up on a bed or chair with your hands braced on either side of your body
- Alternately raise each leg, bringing your knee across your chest; lift the right knee up and over to the left side of the chest and then lift the left knee up and over to the right side; try not to assist the movement with your hands
- Feel the contraction of your groin and outer hip flexor muscles
- Repeat ten to twenty times with each leg

Standing Groin Stretch

- Stand with your feet shoulder-width apart, feet pointed straight ahead

- Bend your left knee slightly and turn your right hip downward and toward the left knee
- Hold on to the back of a chair for extra balance
- Hold the stretch for five to fifteen seconds, feeling the stretch in your groin

Standing Front and Back Straight-Leg Raises (Swings)

- Stand sideways to a wall or chair back with your feet hip-width apart, knees slightly bent; place your hand against the wall or chair back
- Raise and lower your outer leg forward, backward, sideways, and across your body
- For forward leg raises, lift and lower your straightened leg from knee to hip height; keep the knees slightly bent
- As you raise up, sink down slightly on your standing leg
- Extend your leg behind your body, lean forward with your upper body, and sink down by bending your standing leg as your leg swings back
- Feel the contractions in your front hips and groin; your abdominals and lower back muscles should act as stabilizers
- Repeat each leg raise five to fifteen times

LEVEL III

Seated Cross-Legged Twist

- Sit on the floor with both legs out in front of you, knees slightly bent
- Bend your left leg and cross it over your right leg; place your left foot on the outside of your right knee
- Place your left hand behind your left hip on the floor
- Bend your right elbow and rest it on the outside of your left knee
- Turn your head over your left shoulder and rotate your upper body to the left
- Hold for five to thirty seconds, feeling the stretch in the side of your hip, lower back, and neck
- Repeat the stretch on your other side

Seated Straight-Legged Heel-To-Chest Pull

- Sit on the floor with your back against a wall; your right leg should be straight out in front of you; support your back by placing a pillow between it and the wall
- Your left knee should be bent and your left forearm is cradling the back of your knee; grab your left ankle with both hands
- Slowly pull your whole leg toward your chest until you feel a light stretch in the back of your upper leg; slightly rotate your upper leg to stretch both hamstring muscles; be sure not to overstress your knee
- Hold for ten to twenty seconds

Seated Half V-Legged Stretch

- Sit on the floor with your legs straight, or on a chair with legs bent and feet flat and shoulder-width apart
- Bend your right leg at the knee and place the foot and heel against the opposite

thigh; (on top of the opposite thigh if you are seated in a chair)

- In either the chair or on the floor, extend your arms forward as you slowly bend forward toward the straightened leg
- Keep your back straight and avoid dipping your head forward as you stretch
- If you are in a chair, grab your top knee and ankle and pull yourself forward; if you are on the floor, wrap a towel around the foot of your straightened leg to help pull yourself forward
- Hold for five to fifteen seconds, feeling the stretch in your hamstrings and hips

Standing Raised-Leg Stretch

- Stand with your feet shoulder-width apart, toes pointed toward a sturdy chair or table that should not be higher than your hips
- Place the heel of your left foot on the raised surface
- Straighten out your raised leg as you slightly bend your standing knee
- Grasp your raised knee with both hands
- Lean forward slightly
- Hold for twenty to thirty seconds, feeling the stretch in your the back of your hip and hamstrings; advanced exercisers can add a slight rotation or oscillation
- Change legs

Standing Leaning Forward Leg Lift

- Stand with your left side to a wall or the back of a chair; balance yourself with your left hand
- Extend your right arm out to the side for balance
- Lean forward as you bend your left knee and raise your leg up to your chest
- Hold a moment and extend your leg down and back as you straighten it out behind you
- Bend your knee again as you bring your leg back under your body and your knee to your chest
- Feel the contraction in your front hip and abdominals in the forward lift, and feel it in your back hip and hamstrings on the backward extension
- Change legs and repeat the stretch
- Repeat eight to twelve times on each leg

Side Leg Raise Variation

- Return to the same starting position as in the standing leaning forward leg lift (above) with knees slightly bent
- Raise your left leg straight out to the side
- Lower it down again
- Feel the contraction in your hip and outer thigh
- Exhale as you raise your leg, inhale as you lower it
- Repeat twelve to twenty times on each leg

Standing Quarter Bent-Knee Squat

- Stand with your feet hip-width apart; turn feet and legs outward at a 45-degree angle (V-footed), knees slightly bent, feet flat on the ground
- Place your hands on your hips or hold onto the back of a chair to balance yourself
- Slowly sink down until your knees are quarter-bent, tucking your buttocks under and keeping your lower back flattened
- Slowly raise your body up and return to the starting position by straightening out your legs
- Feel the contraction in your thighs as you sink down, and feel it in your inner thighs, hamstrings, and buttocks as your raise your body up

Abdominals, Lower Back, and Hamstrings: Lying Down Series

Level I

Lying Bent-Knee to Chest Pull

- Lie on a floor or bed, face up, with your right leg straight and left leg bent
- Grasp your left thigh with both hands and gently pull it toward your chest
- Hold for five to thirty seconds, feeling the stretch in your hips, lower back, and hamstrings
- Change legs

Lying Hip Roll

- Lie down, face up, knees bent, feet flat and firmly planted, hip-width apart
- Place your arms out to your sides at shoulder height
- Keep your shoulders and hips flat and in contact with the floor
- Lower both your legs to the left side of your body until your left outer thigh touches the bed or floor
- Inhale as your raise your leg, exhale as you lower it
- Return to the start and repeat on the right side
- Use your abdominals to help control movements

Lying Stomach Curl

- Lie face up on the floor with knees bent and feet flattened and anchored, placed on a chair, or against a wall
- Slide your buttocks close to the wall or chair so your knees are at a 90-degree angle with the floor
- Cross your arms over your chest, or place your hands, with fingers interlaced, behind your head
- Curl your upper body up toward your knees; raise your body only as high until your shoulder blades clear the floor; concentrate the work on your abdominal muscles; don't swing your body or pull yourself up from behind your neck
- Return your body slowly to the starting position

- Feel the contraction in your abdominal muscles, exhaling on the way up, inhaling on the way down
- Repeat three to twenty-five times

Lying Pelvic Raise

- Lie on a floor mat or a firm bed, knees bent, feet flat
- Keep your arms by your sides and flat on the floor as you lift up your hips
- Hold for a moment, then lower your hips back down to the starting position
- Exhale as you lift up, inhale as you go down
- Repeat three to eight times

Lying Back Stretch

- Lie on your back and rest your feet on top of a chair, bed, foot stool, or sofa that is as high as your thighs are long
- Slide your buttocks toward your resting feet so your hips are forward of your knees
- Relax your arms by your sides
- Hold for five to ten minutes, feeling the stretch in your hamstrings and lower back

LEVEL II

Lying Bent-Knee to Chest Stretch Out

- Lie face up on a floor mat with your knees bent at 90-degree angles and your arms by your sides
- Stretch your arms out over your head and extend your legs out on the mat, knees slightly bent, turning your feet so the toes are pointing away from your body
- Hold the stretch for three to ten seconds
- Feel the stretch throughout the muscles of the front of your body, but especially in your abdominals, chest, legs, and shoulders

Lying Bent-Knee to Chest Raise

- Lie face up on a floor mat or firm bed with your knees bent at 90 degrees, feet planted flat, and close to your buttocks
- Keep your back flat as you pull your left knee toward your chest

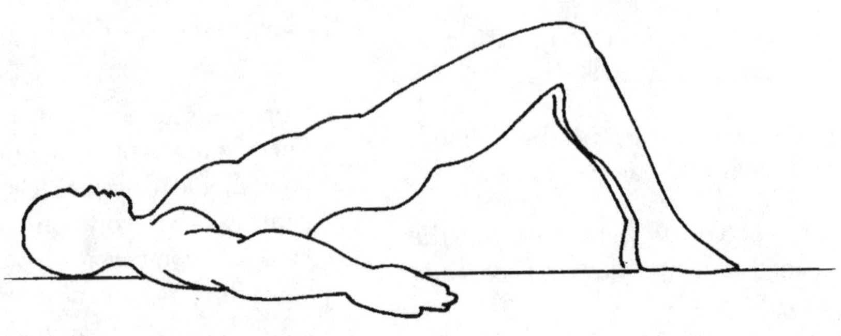

Lying Pelvic Raise

- Keeping both your knees bent, lower your left leg to the starting position
- Repeat the exercise with your right knee
- Inhale as you raise your legs up, exhale as you lower your legs down
- Keep your back flat on the ground as you feel the contraction in your lower abdominals
- Repeat the exercise eight to twelve times

Please note: Never lift both legs at the same time. Use your hands and lift only one at a time. Raise and lower one leg at a time.

LEVEL III

All Fours Arm and Leg Raise

- Kneel on the floor, legs hip-width apart, with your hands propped in front of you; your thighs and arms should be parallel to each other and perpendicular to the floor
- Simultaneously, lift your right arm and left leg to form a straight line with your body
- Hold for two to three seconds and return to all fours
- Inhale as you raise your arms and legs, exhale as you lower them
- Feel the contraction in your lower back
- Repeat with your left arm and right leg

All Fours Back Arch

- Kneel on the floor, legs hip-width apart
- Bend down and rest your body on your forearms on the floor in front of your head with palms down
- Keep your thighs upright at a right angle to the floor
- Press your chest down as close to the floor as possible
- Hold for three to eight seconds, feeling the stretch in your lower back, upper back, and shoulders

Lying Double Knee to Chest Pull

- Lie with your back flat on the floor, legs straight, knees slightly bent
- Bend your legs, grab behind your knees and gently pull your knees up to your chest, one at a time
- Hold for fifteen to sixty seconds, feeling the stretch in your lower back, hips, and hamstrings
- Return to the starting position

Lying Back Leg Raise

- Lie face down on your bed or floor with your arms folded and your head resting on your arms
- Raise your left leg from the hip, two to three inches
- Lower your leg back to the starting position
- Feel the contractions in your buttocks and lower back
- Inhale as you raise up, exhale as you go down

Abdominals, Lower Back, and Hamstrings: Seated and Standing Series

Level I

Seated Bent-Knee to Chest Pull

- Sit on a chair with your shoulder blades touching the chair back, or on a floor mat in the recumbent position with your elbows at your sides to prop you up
- Slide your pelvis forward on the chair, or if on the floor, lean back, and clasp your right knee with both hands
- Gently pull your knee as close to your chest as possible
- Hold for three to eight seconds, feeling the stretch in your lower back and hamstrings
- Repeat on your left leg

Seated Pelvic Raise

- Sit on the edge of a chair with your legs extended, feet flat on the floor
- Grasp the side of the seat or the chair arms
- With elbows bent, raise yourself off the chair one to three inches
- Slide your pelvis forward so your upper body is leaning back at a 45-degree angle
- Lift your hips up, hold briefly, and lower them back to the starting position
- Feel the contraction of your abdominal muscles
- Repeat three to eight times

Standing Bent-Knee to Chest Pull

- Stand with your feet shoulder-width apart, toes pointed straight ahead; keep your heels flat and your knees bent
- Bend forward and grasp your knees
- Hold position for five to ten seconds, feeling the stretch in your hamstrings, calves, and Achilles tendons

Standing Bent-Knee to Chest Raise

- Stand sideways to a chair back or wall, holding on for support
- Place your feet parallel and shoulder-width apart, bend your knees slightly
- Lift your outside leg and raise the knee toward your chest without any assistance from your arms
- Hold a moment, feeling the contraction in your hip flexor muscles as you raise your leg and in your lower back muscles as you slowly lower your leg
- Exhale as you raise your leg, inhale as you lower it
- Change legs
- Repeat three to eight times

Supported Pelvic Tilt or Standing Back-Pain Rest

Please note: All pelvic tilts are effective for scoliosis sufferers.

- Stand with your back to a low wall,

bureau, kitchen sink, or sofa and rest your forearms on it

- Tilt your pelvis under your body and pull in your stomach
- Hold five seconds to one minute, feeling the stretch in the lower back

LEVEL II

Seated Torso Bend Over Stretch

- Sit upright on a chair or floor mat, feet flat, legs extended, knees bent at a 120-degree angle
- Slowly bend over from the hips as you run your hands down the outer side of your legs
- Grasp your ankles and pull until your chest touches your thighs
- Hold for five to thirty seconds, feeling the stretch in your lower back muscles

Seated Torso Raise

- Sit back on a chair with your thighs supported and your torso upright; if you choose to sit on a floor mat, make sure to keep your back against a wall, knees bent at a 90-degree angle, with your feet flat
- Grasp the arm rest or sides of the chair or place your hands on the floor mat on either side of your hips
- From the upright position, slowly bend over from your hips until your chest touches your thighs
- Hold a moment, feeling the contractions in the abdominals as you go down and in the lower back muscles as you go up; slowly raise your torso back to the upright position
- Exhale as you raise up, inhale as you go down
- Repeat eight to twelve times

Standing Bend Over Stretch (Back)

- Stand with your feet shoulder-width apart, toes pointed straight ahead, heels flat, and knees slightly bent
- Slowly bend forward at the hips reaching as far as you comfortably can to the floor below you
- Hold for five to thirty seconds, feeling the stretch in your hamstrings and lower back
- Roll up the spine to resume the starting position

Standing Torso Bend Over

Please note: Do the seated version if you have back discomfort, back injury, or if you are unfit.

- Stand with your feet shoulder-width apart and toes pointed forward
- Beginners: stand facing the back of a sturdy chair
- Keep your back straight by turning your pelvis under; pull your stomach in and relax your shoulders back and down
- Slowly bend forward until your upper body is bent between a 45- and 90-degree angle (i.e. a 90-degree angle is parallel to the floor)

- Slowly raise your upper body to the starting position
- Exhale as you bend over, inhale as you straighten up
- Beginners: keep your knees slightly bent; advanced: keep knees straightened

LEVEL III

Standing Curl and Unfurl

- Stand with your feet shoulder-width apart, toes pointed straight ahead, arms hanging down loosely by your sides, elbows and knees slightly bent
- As you curl down your spine, one vertebrae at a time, slowly sink down until your knees are bent halfway; at the same time, extend your arms in front of your body for better balance
- Hold for five to fifteen seconds, feeling the stretch in your lower back, calves, and front thighs
- Return to the starting position, rolling your lower back up one vertebrae at a time while slowly straightening your arms and legs, feeling the contraction of the calves, hamstrings, and lower back
- Repeat three to eight times

Seated Combined Torso Cross Turn and Stretch

- Sit on a chair or floor mat with your feet hip-width apart, knees bent at a 90-degree angle with your feet flat; let your arms hang by your sides with elbows bent at 90 degrees
- Keep your torso upright and shoulders square as you turn your upper body to the right side, tuck your arms and elbows in to your sides while you rotate your arms and torso as a unit
- Repeat the turn on each side twelve to twenty-five times or alternate left and right turns
- Feel the stretch in your lower back as you turn
- Exhale as you turn out, inhale as you turn back in

Standing Cross-Legged Stretch

- Stand with your feet shoulder-width apart, knees bent and feet parallel, arms hanging loosely by your sides
- Place your hands on your hips (you can also hold on to a wall or chair back if you are standing sideways to it)
- Cross your right leg over your left leg and firmly flatten it down distributing the weight equally on both feet
- Bend over from the hips keeping your knees locked
- Let your upper body and arms hang down toward your feet; for a greater stretch, slide your hands down the outside of your leg, grasp the back leg and pull
- Hold the stretch for five to thirty seconds, feeling the stretch in your lower back, hips, and hamstrings
- Change legs and repeat

Standing Torso Reach Down

- Stand with your feet parallel and shoulder-width apart
- Keep your back straight, head up, and knees slightly bent
- Extend your arms by your sides, elbows slightly bent; you may also grasp a broomstick or barbell in front of your thighs with your hands chest-width apart
- Bend over at the hips and slowly lower your hands, stick, or bar to the floor
- Hold a moment, feeling the stretch in your lower back muscles
- Slowly return to upright position, feeling the contraction in lower back muscles
- Repeat eight to twelve times

CHAPTER 11

Cardio Ex

Aerobics and Continuous Movements

The Most Effective Exercises for Your Heart

The five major muscle groups that generate the greatest amount of blood flow from the heart and air flow from the lungs, are (1) the calf muscles; (2) the thighs and buttocks muscles, (3) the upper arms, (4) the shoulders, and (5) the upper back muscles. Although they are also important for circulatory and respiratory health, your abdominals and lower back cannot generate as much continuous blood flow as these five major muscle groups. The arms, shoulders, upper back, legs, buttocks, thighs, and calves work all the other major muscle groups.

The five major muscle group movements that contribute the most benefit to circulatory stimulation are (1) stepping for calves and shins, (2) kicking for thighs and buttocks, (3) rotating the torso for abdominals and lower back, (4) stroking (swimming or rowing movement) for arms, chest, and upper back, and (5) arm raising for arms and shoulders. These movements when done in a continuous fashion, work your largest muscle groups to produce a steady flow of blood to and from almost all of your working muscles and vital organs.

To improve air flow and develop and maintain the breathing capacity of your lungs is to breathe in and out of your mouth while vigorously exercising at a rate of approximately twenty to thirty deep breaths per minute. This is the best breathing technique for Cardio exercise. Forty breaths or more per minute is too fast and will lead to hyperventilation. Twenty to thirty breaths allow the maximum amount of air to flow into your body.

;ARDIO PREVENTIVE EXERCISE

:he basic Cardio preventive health prescrip- ion is circulatory exercise, continuing major nuscle movements for thirty to sixty minutes er day, five to seven days a week. For the najority of people, this translates into 1,200 ɔ 2,000 calories of exercise per week. The urpose is to increase your blood flow and air ow. The best respiratory health prescription aerobic exercise, which strengthens your eart and lung volume and improves your reathing function.

IONITORING YOUR HEART RATE

/hether you have heart disease or not, you ill need to know the right level at which to art exercising your Cardio system. You will ɔ this by measuring how your heart rate and eathing rate responds during continuous ıysical activity using your major muscle oups. The safest way is for your doctor or ealth club to administer a fitness test. If you ıve been diagnosed as healthy, you can give urself a simple walking, stationary cycling, water-movement test.

Before treating yourself, you should learn w to monitor your heart rate. As a healthy ult you should be able to raise your heart te from seventy to eighty beats per minute rest to 130 to 160 beats per minute during ercise. Maintaining your heart rate contin- usly in that range is the ultimate test of ıether any exercise, sport, or continuous ɔvements qualify as Cardio exercise. While ıny do qualify, as you will see in Part Three, ey may also have unwanted side effects.

Heart monitoring can both establish your rting level of exercise and help you mea- e the results. If your heartbeat is irregular if you have been inactive for more than twelve months you should seek medical evaluation.

CARDIO EX

Cardio exercise is a "continuous, rhythmic, and coordinated" motion of the arms, legs, and trunk muscles. These exercises raise your heart and breathing rates substantially above your resting rates and also increase the flow of oxygenated blood to most of your major muscles groups and to your extremities (i.e. hands, feet, and head). These exercises, when practiced at a heart-training rate that is higher than resting heart rate—up to 60% of the maximum heart-training rate (also called VO_2 max)—are called "circulatory" exercises. When practiced at 60 to 85% of the heart-training rate, they are called aerobic exercises. Above 85%, they are called anaerobic exercise.

WALK, BIKE, SWIM

Of the more than seventy-five sports that are practiced as exercises, the three best Cardio exercises for low-injury risk and ease of practice are walking, stationary cycling, and water exercise. These three can be combined or also practiced separately as standing, seated, and prone exercises. (Also see Sports and Exercise Injuries List, pp. 152–154).

BETTER WALKING TECHNIQUES

Walking is not only the most popular exercise, it is also the easiest and most accessible. Combined with arm swinging or arm pumping, walking offers total body coverage—arms, trunk, and legs—simultaneously together in a smooth, rhythmic motion. It can be done at a variety of slow to moderate to fast paces. When you take a walking step, the impact is measured at one to one and a half times your body weight; when you take a running, jogging, or jumping step, the impact is four to five times greater than that of a walking step. The difference in higher levels of impact forces is especially important when the movement is repeated continuously.

The essentials of proper walking technique are:

- Walk with proper posture
- Your head and back should be erect
- Your shoulders should be pulled back (not slumped) and relaxed
- Your upper and lower body joints should be properly aligned
- Viewed sideways, your ear should be aligned with your shoulder, hip, and ankle joints, connecting an imaginary straight line that is perpendicular to the ground
- Viewed from the front or back, your shoulders should be pulled back slightly
- Your stomach and buttocks muscles should be tightened and pressed in support your lower back
- Avoid tilting your head forward
- Your chin should be parallel with the ground and tucked in
- Your eyes should be focused at least fifteen feet ahead of you on the ground
- Your feet should be hip-width apart and parallel with toes pointing forward
- Step forward by landing on your heel firs and rolling your foot forward and to th outer edge
- Swing your arms in a natural arc as yo walk
- Each arm should swing forward with th opposite leg to counterbalance your for ward motion
- To walk vigorously, bend your arms to 90-degree angle and pump them instea of just swinging them

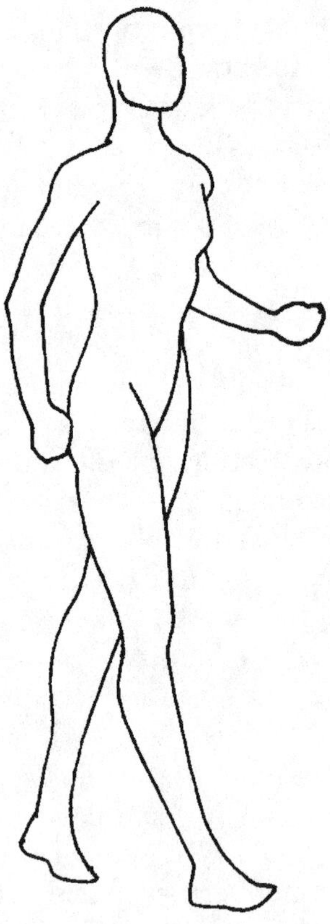

Basic Walking Technique

TABLE 11.1
CARDIO EX WALKING/CYCLING SCHEDULE

Levels	*Beginner*	*Advanced Beginner*	*Low Intermediate*	*High Intermediate*	*Advanced*
Intensity					
heart-training rate	50–60%	60–70%	70–80%	80–90%	90+%
METS	3–5	5–8	8–12	12–15	17–22
Speed					
(steps/leg rotations/arm swings/rotation of arms per mile)	30–45	45–60	60–90	90–100	100–120
Minute miles	60–30	30–20	20–17	17–15	15–10
Miles per hour	1	2–3	3–3.5	3.5–4	4.5–6
Duration (minutes per session)	1–5	5–15	15–30	30–45	45–60
Distance (miles per week)	2–4	4–8	8–12	12–18	18–20
Calories burned (per week)	200–400	400–800	800–1200	1200–1800	1800–2000
Frequency (times per week)	1–2	2–3	3–4	5	6–7

Table 11.1 provides a schedule of arm and leg repetitions that you should use to monitor and increase the speed and intensity of a cardio walking and cycling program. Note that the repetitions for walking and cycling are the same.

Start at the level of exercise that corresponds to your current physical condition and increase your workout level of intensity every six to twelve weeks. If you are not sure about your starting level, start at the "beginner" level, using it to measure your exercise response. If it feels challenging, stay at that level. If it feels easy, progress to the "advanced beginner" level and test out your response to that level before moving on until you reach a level that feels challenging.

WATER-SUPPORTED EXERCISES

Water's buoyancy provides a safer exercise environment that is free from falls and is less apt to allow jerking and jolting movements that might crack or break bones, pull muscles, or stress joints. Water also provides a naturally even and easy source of resistance in all the directions you can move your arms, legs, and trunk. Warm water helps to relax the tension in your muscles.

Swimming has long been regarded as one of the safest and most beneficial exercises because it works many muscle groups in a balanced and low-impact way. Swimming strokes are rhythmic and can be practiced continuously. Surprisingly, however, swimming has produced a higher than acceptable number of shoulder, knee, and lower back injuries when practiced regularly. Over a given year, at least 25% of all swimmers experience shoulder, knee, or lower back injuries. To reduce shoulder injuries, you can shift up to 50% of the shoulder work load to your legs by wearing fins. (Kicking without fins only accounts for 10% of the work load).

To avoid knee pain caused by whip-kicking during the breast stroke, vary the kicks and strokes—wearing fins also helps by smoothing out each kick and reducing the ballistic or "snapping" action of the kicks. To avoid lower back pain from overarching your back during the breast stroke or crawl, switch to a back and side stroke. Yet another alternative is upright water exercise.

Water exercise is an upright version of swimming that takes the pressure off your back and shoulders and incorporates walking, jogging, dancing, and calisthenic movements adapted to water. You take advantage of the water's natural buoyancy. Water also provides a cushion for painful, injured, or overloaded joints.

The upright position in water is also safer for doing swimming strokes and for converting shorter kicks into smoother stepping movements. The upright position allows you to keep your back flat while doing the breast stroke or crawl or you can alternately raise and lower your legs in a kicking action that resembles a march step.

You can soften the impact of most high-risk sports movements by doing them in knee- to shoulder-high water. Depending on the speed of the move, water will cut the impact force from 20 up to 90%. Both the ground impact and the ballistic forces are significantly diminished. The impact caused by such high-risk leg moves as jogging and jumping steps can be reduced by 75 to 90%. Such high-risk arm moves as raises, strokes, and pushes are slowed down and smoothed out thereby diminishing the chance for injury. Such risky postures and positions as high knee raises are also made safer in water by improving your balance and reducing your

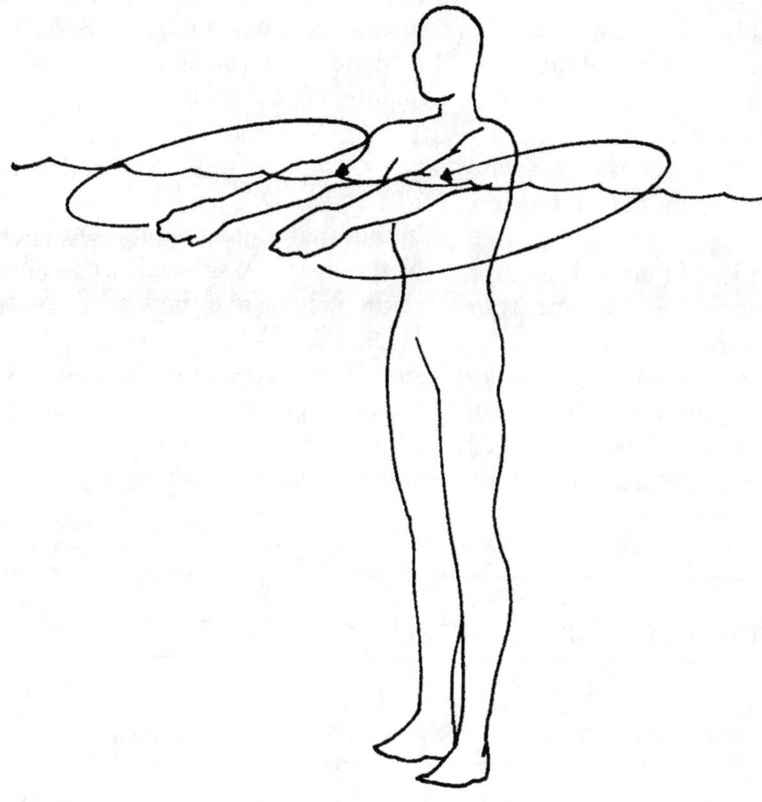

Standing

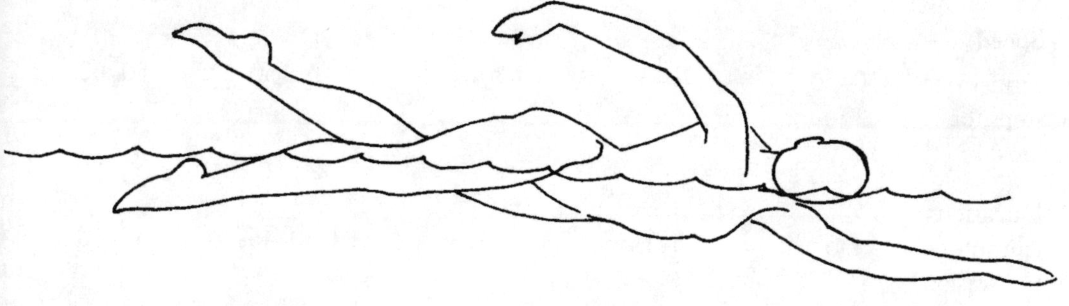

Swimming

Water-Supported Exercise

risk of falling. Even when you tip over, the water prevents or slows down the fall and cushions the impact. For extra stability, you can also hold onto the edge of the pool.

Our basic recommendation: Practice by repeating your favorite exercise or sports moves under water as a personal water exercise routine.

Use Table 11.2 to build up and monitor your Cardio water exercises. Measure your speed and progress by the number of simultaneous arm and leg repetitions you can do. Adjust and monitor the intensity, speed, duration, or frequency of your program based on your level of fitness. When an exercise level feels like it is too easy, move up to the next level. After you have reached the intermediate level, you can stay at that level as a maintenance program.

Better Cycling Techniques

Traditional outdoor bicycling poses some health risks. As a result of the heightened traffic volume and the lack of special bicycle lanes, the risk of injuries from falls or collisions has been greatly increased. We recommend using a trike (a three-wheeled bicycle) to reduce the possibility of falling as one injury-avoidance technique.

TABLE 11.2
WATER-SUPPORTED CARDIO EXERCISE SCHEDULE

Levels	*Beginner*	*Advanced Beginner*	*Low Intermediate*	*High Intermediate*	*Advanced*
Intensity (heart-training rate)	50–60%	60–70%	70–80%	80–90%	90+%
METS	3–5	5–8	8–12	12–15	17–22
Speed (armstrokes, steps, or kicks)	10–20	20–30	30–45	45–50	50–60
Duration (minutes per session)	1–5	5–15	15–30	30–45	45–60
Frequency (per week)	1–2	2–3	3–4	5	6–7

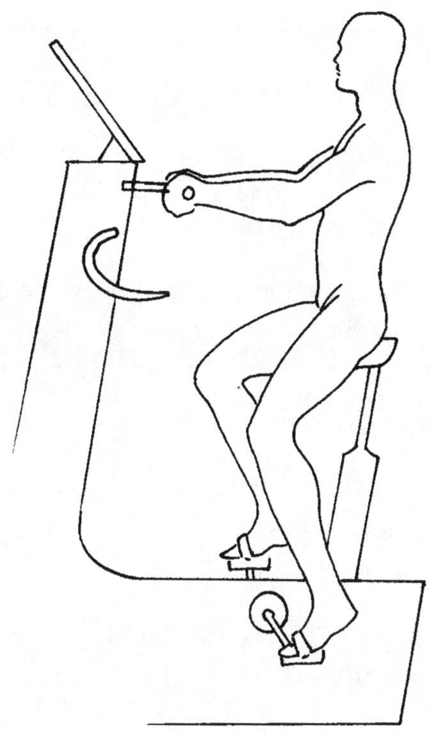

Upright-Stationary Bike

Collisions and falling from bicycling outdoors notwithstanding, stationary cycling and arm rowing are far better than traditional bicycling because they support your body and therefore reduce the number of injuries while also improving the body coverage of the exercise. Stationary cycling offers the best seated aerobic and circulatory exercise.

To cycle means to move in circular motion around a central point. Arm cycling—also called arm ergometry or arm rowing—involves rotating your arms around your shoulder joints as you bend and extend them. Leg cycling or bicycling involves rotating your legs around your hip joint as you bend and extend your knee joint.

Practice good cycling techniques by maintaining a proper seated posture. Maintain an upright seated position or a recumbent (i.e.

Forward Leaning-Racing Bike

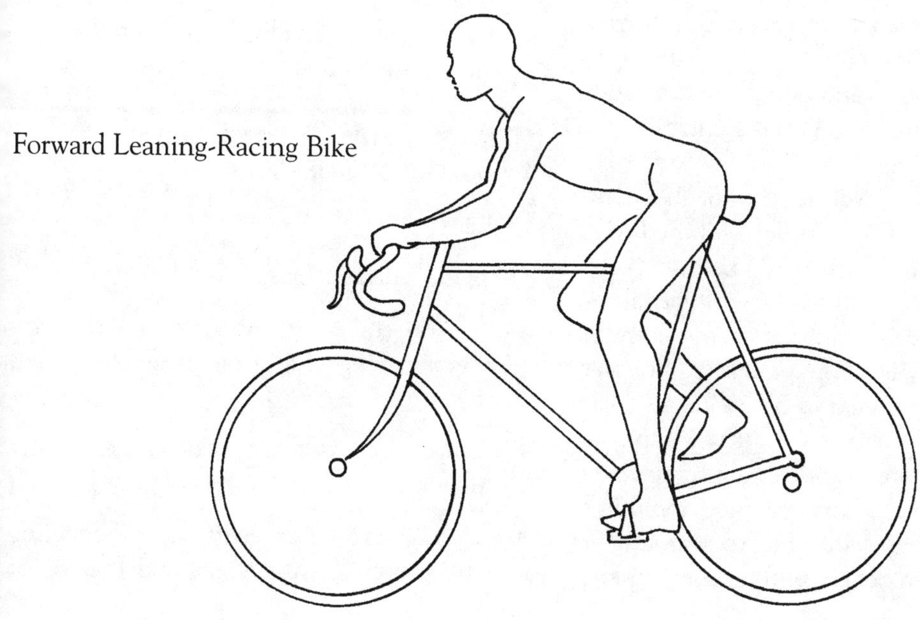

Cycling Technique

seated leaning back position). Avoid the forward leaning position because it can place too much pressure on your hands and wrists, which can cause nerve damage, carpal tunnel syndrome, and can also strain your lower back.

For arm cycling, your arms should be shoulder-width apart, palms and fingers forward and thumbs parallel. For leg cycling, your feet should be parallel, toes forward. To avoid knee and hip joint strain, set your bicycle seat high enough (109% of your inseam length or 100% of the distance between your hip bone and the floor). You should be able to pedal without rocking your hips or fully straightening out your leg. Maintain the leg rotation by pressing your heel and forefoot down. Roll your foot forward and back in a smooth circular motion, called ankling.

Keep your feet planted on the pedals and push down forward or backward in a circular motion. Use foot straps to anchor your feet so you can push and pull using all your leg muscles as well as your abdominal and lower back muscles. You can also use hand straps to engage all your arms and upper trunk muscles in a similar rotary motion on the ergometer or arm cycle machine.

Arm and leg cycling cannot be combined, but leg cycling can be combined with arm rowing. Some brands of exercise cycles allow you to pump arm sticks while pedaling. You can also simulate this action free-handed or combine it with arm pumping. Practice arm ergometry separately while sitting upright at a stationary cycle, or you can supplement arm ergometry with walking or water exercise section. Many people, including paraplegic patients, are able to an achieve anaerobic training effect with arm ergometry alone.

EXERCISE COUNTS

Practice the movement or hold the position to a level that is comfortable for you. Repeat the series of exercises one to five times. Gradually increase the number of exercise repetitions or hold counts as you move through each of the three levels.

	REPS	HOLD TIMES (in seconds)	SETS
Level I	2–7	1–2	1
Level II	8–12	3–5	2
Level III	13–20	6–12	3
Level IV	21–24	13–19	4
Level V	25–30	20–30	5

Take at least one second to execute each repetition or each hold count. Time your exercise speed by counting out a repetition or hold, adding the word "and" after each count. (1 and 2 and 3 and. . . .)

CALVES, SHINS, ANKLES, AND FEET: LYING DOWN SERIES

LEVEL I

Lying Calf and Achilles Stretch

- Lie on the floor and extend your arms overhead with legs straight, feet together, resting on heels
- Point your toes and bend your forefeet down
- Hold for three to eight seconds, feeling the stretch in your shins and the top of your foot; relax

- Bend your toes and forefeet back, pressing your heels forward
- Hold for three to eight seconds, feeling the stretch in the calves and the arch and ball of foot; relax

LYING FOOT CIRCLE STRETCH (OR SQUARE TRACING)

Please note: "Circle" is a misnomer. You are actually tracing a square with the lying, seated, and standing foot circle exercises.

- Lie on your back with your knees slightly bent, legs extended downward propped on your heels, your feet should be shoulder-width apart, with your arms extended sideways, palms up
- You may do this exercise one foot at a time or together—move your right foot clockwise and your left foot counterclockwise; keep the heel of your moving foot anchored on the floor or bed throughout the exercise
- Bend your toes down; pause
- Turn your toes outward (i.e. turn your right foot out to the right, your left foot out to the left); pause
- Bring your feet back to the starting position; pause
- Turn your toes inward; pause
- Feel the stretch in the tops of your feet and in your ankles
- Repeat this sequence three to eight times clockwise and three to eight times counterclockwise

LEVEL II

Lying Lower Leg Stretch

- Lie on your back and bend your left knee; keep your feet and lower back flat
- Lift your right leg straight up from the hip
- Pull back the toes of your right foot
- Hold five to twelve seconds, feeling the stretch in your calf and hamstrings; relax
- Repeat with the other leg

Lying Heel-Toe Roll

- Lie on your back, knees bent, and heels placed close to buttocks, arms resting at sides
- Raise your heels and roll both feet forward
- Press down with forefeet and toes; pause
- Roll both of your feet back to the heels, pulling up your toes; pause
- Feel the contraction in your calves and shins
- Repeat three to eight times

LEVEL III

Lying Calf Stretch

- Lie on your back, bend your legs, and place your feet flat against a wall or chair edge
- Press down with your heels
- Hold for eight to twelve seconds, feeling the stretch in your calves

Calves, Shins, Ankles, and Feet: Seated or Standing Series

Level I

Seated Calf and Ankle Stretch

- Sit on the floor with your legs straight out in front, both knees bent, or sit on a chair with knees bent and feet flat; if seated on a chair, raise right leg up in front
- Bend your body forward, pulling in your abdominal muscles; rest your left forearm on your left knee
- Lean forward and grasp the ball (not the toes) of your right foot with your right hand
- Gently pull your forefoot back and try to straighten your leg
- Hold for three to five seconds, feeling the stretch in your calf and forefoot muscles; relax
- Repeat on the left leg

Seated Calf and Achilles Stretch

- Sit on a chair (or kneel on the floor) and place your right foot forward and left foot back, balancing on the ball of your left foot
- Lean to the left and rest both arms crossed on your left thigh; gently press down on your thigh and lean forward keeping your left heel raised
- Hold for three to eight seconds, feeling the stretch in your left calf and Achilles tendon; relax
- Switch legs

Seated Foot Circle (Square Traces)

- Sit on a chair or on the floor in the recumbent position, propped up on your arms
- For one leg circle, cross your right leg over your left knee so that the right lower leg is dangling; for both legs, simultaneously bend your knees and prop your heels on the floor
- Circle your right foot counterclockwise by raising your toes back; pause
- Turn to the left side; pause
- Flex your toes downward; pause
- Turn to the center; pause
- Circle your left foot; pause
- Turn your forefoot to the left side; pause
- Push your toes down; pause
- Turn your foot inward to the starting position
- Feel the contractions in your calves, shins, and the sides of your lower legs
- Repeat the sequence three to eight times clockwise and three to eight times counterclockwise on each foot separately or together in opposite directions

Standing Calf Stretch

- Stand with your feet hip-width apart
- Step straight back with your left leg, planting your left foot flat, toes pointed forward
- Bend your right knee and lean forward; in your mind's eye, a long diagonal line forms from the back of your head to the back of your left heel and then to the floor

- Brace both your hands, arms at shoulder height, on your front thigh or on a wall or counter for more leverage; press your heel back down onto the ground
- Hold for three to eight seconds, feeling the stretch in your calf and Achilles tendon as your weight is shifted forward; turn in your left foot to increase the stretch
- Repeat on the other leg

Standing Foot Circle

Please note: Do this exercise one leg at a time.

- Sit or stand with your feet hip-width apart, knees slightly bent
- Move your left leg out to the side and prop it on its forefoot
- Keeping your left foot propped on the ball, trace a square with your heel
- On your right, raise your heel straight up; pause
- Turn your right heel out to the right; pause
- Lower your heel back to the floor; pause
- Slide your heel back to the center position; pause, feeling the contraction in the back of your calves and the sides of your legs
- Repeat the tracing motion three to eight times clockwise and three to eight times counterclockwise for each foot

LEVEL II

Seated Heel-Toe Roll

- Sit on the edge of a chair, feet hip-width apart and slightly forward of your knees; prop your hands on your thighs
- Roll forward on your forefeet and toes as your heels are raised up
- Lean over your knees and rock your upper body to shift your weight forward; pause
- Roll back onto your heels and backward to shift your weight there; raise your toes and forefeet off the floor, pressing down with your heels
- Feel the contraction in your shins and calves
- Repeat the sequence eight to twelve times
- Press your hands down on your thighs on the forward and backward shifts to gain additional leverage

Seated Lower Leg Strengthener

- Sit on a chair or floor and bend your left knee; grab your ankle with your right hand, your forefoot with your left hand, and turn your forefoot sideways, sole out, toes up
- Gently rotate the foot around the ankle clockwise and then counterclockwise eight to twelve times
- Repeat on the other foot
- At the end of each exercise, you can also stretch your toes by gently pulling each one toward you, holding the stretch for three to eight seconds; you can also massage the sole of your foot by pressing with your thumb and massaging up and down the arch and side of your foot

Standing Calf and Achilles Stretch

Please note: This transfers more weight to the lower leg muscles you are stretching.

- Stand facing a wall; lean your upper body forward and rest palms on the wall, arms slightly bent
- Step back with your right foot and place it firmly flat on the floor, toes pointing forward
- Bend your left knee and bring that leg behind you, hooking the forefoot behind your right ankle
- Keep your right heel pressed to the floor
- Hold for eight to twelve seconds, feeling the stretch in lower right leg
- Repeat on left foot

Standing Heel-Toe Roll

- Stand sideways to a wall, a chair back, or a counter, feet hip- to shoulder-width apart, arms extended or in front of you, and brace yourself with one hand
- Rock back and forth on the outer edge of the soles of your feet
- Bend your knees and roll up onto the balls of your feet bringing both arms behind for counterbalance; pause
- Roll back onto your heels and raise your toes up as your arms are brought forward in front of your body
- Feel your calves and shins contract
- Inhale as you roll forward, exhale as you roll back
- Repeat the sequence eight to twelve times

LEVEL III

Seated Foot Stretch

- Sit on a chair and stretch your legs in front of you; cross your left leg over your right and prop your left heel on top of your right forefoot
- Bend forward and reach with both hands to grasp your left forefoot; gently pull your forefoot toward you as you straighten both legs
- Feel the stretch in your calves and bottom of the foot; relax
- Repeat on the right leg

Standing One-Footed Heel-Toe Rolls

- Stand next to a wall or chair back so you can hold on to it for balance
- Bend your left knee at a 90-degree angle and raise your lower leg up; keep your right knee bent at a one-quarter angle
- Slowly raise your right heel off the floor and roll up onto the ball of your foot, straightening (but not locking) the knee as you go up; pause
- Lower your heel back to the floor, feeling the contraction in your calf and shin
- Repeat twelve to thirty times
- Change legs and repeat sequence

Please note: For increased ROM and added difficulty, stand on the edge of a stair, toes pointing toward the next stair up, arches and heels hanging over the edge of the step. Slowly and carefully, press your heels down for a really good stretch. Be sure to hold on to stair rail for stability.

Standing Slow-Motion Jumping

- Stand sideways to a chair back with your feet hip-width apart, toes pointed forward; keep your upper and lower body aligned throughout the moves (if needed, hold on to the chair for extra balance while doing the jumps)

- Let your arms hang loosely by your sides raising them up and forward slightly as you lift off and back down as you land (see Posture Position Guide, p. 157)

- Bend your knees, sink down to a quarter knee bend, and lean slightly forward

- Push up evenly on both legs as you begin to straighten your legs and raise your heels, first rolling all the way up to your toes before letting your feet leave the ground; as you push off, your legs should be straightened with your knees slightly bent

- Land on your forefeet first, making sure to let your feet roll down to heels before rolling up to forefeet again to initiate next jump

- Feel the contraction in your calves and quadriceps

- Repeat twelve to twenty jumps

A Safer Running Technique

While you may not win a marathon practicing this technique, you will reduce the average impact by 33 to 66% on your ankles, knees, and hip joints. Normal joggers have a ground impact of within three to five times their body weight. By using this technique, you will reduce this to **one and a half** to **two and a half** times your weight. By reducing the impact, you minimize the risk of injury.

Here's how to practice safer running:

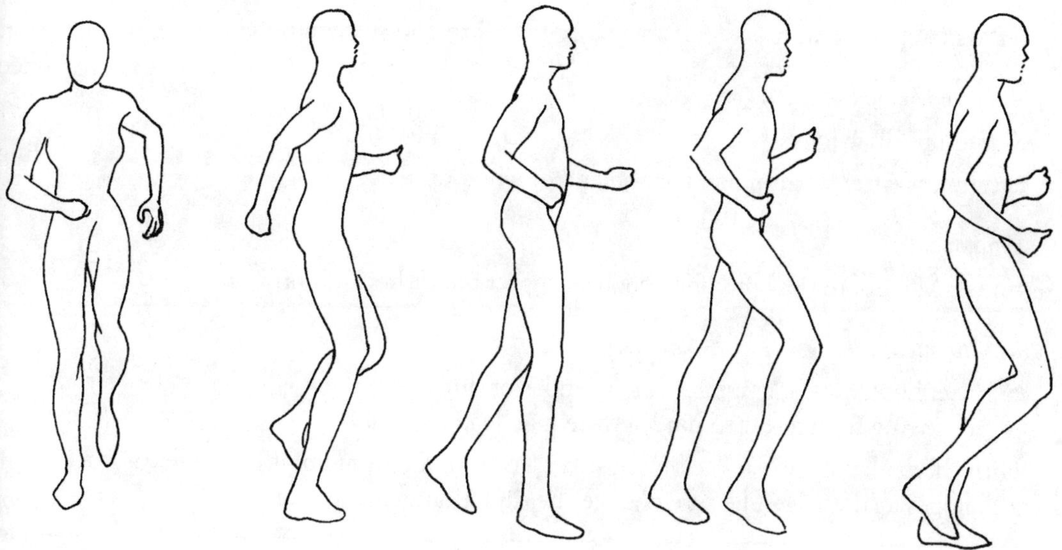

Safer Running Technique

Start out by jogging slowly. Practice keeping your hip and leg joints aligned by running with your feet parallel and three to five inches apart. After reaching a comfortable pace, pull your foot up so you are landing on your heel, and your toes are at a 45-degree angle to the ground as you land. This angle produces a smoother landing than regular jogging; it is similar to the way an airplane touches down, first landing on the rear wheels, then touching the front wheels to the runway. Once you've landed on your heel, roll all the way to your toes on the outer edge of your foot before pushing off for the next step. This method will ensure that you spend a reduced amount of time airborne, and thus you will hit the ground with less force than you would in a conventional running style. Finally, pump your arms back and forth, keeping them close to your body. This will give you an upper body workout, increase your heart rate and exercise intensity, and help to propel you forward.

TABLE 11.3
RUNNING PRESCRIPTIONS

Safety Range	
Daily miles	1 to 3 miles/day
Weekly miles	7 to 15 miles/week
Exercise Speed/Repetitions	
Top speed	4 to 6 miles/hour
Top pace	9 to 12 minute miles
RPMs (steps)	120 to 150 steps/minute

Practice Method

Warm-up: Slow jog

Stretches: After warm-up and at the end of workout

Equipment

Shoes: Make sure they provide adequate support and shock absorption

Environment

Surface: Look for a soft surface like a cinder or dirt track; there is some evidence that changing from a soft to hard surface may lead to injury

Hills: If you have a weak back or legs, keep hills to a minimum; if the street or track slopes at the edges, be sure change the direction every few days

CHAPTER 12

Psyche Ex

Cool Down and Muscle Relaxation

Relaxation Techniques

The best relief for chronic muscular tension is relaxation techniques. By fully contracting a muscle, it can be more easily relaxed. This is the basic principle of isometric exercise. Stretching and massage can also be used to release partially contracted muscles. Cardio exercise can also relieve muscle tension by bringing a fresh flow of blood and nutrients to tense body areas. Finally, rest can also relieve muscle tension by relieving postural muscles of their work in holding you upright or in one position.

The Role of Exercise in the Psyche-Immune System

In a similar way that warning signals alert you to the needs of your car (e.g. out of gas, low oil, engine temperature), your Psyche-Immune system also warns you of impending dangers and unhealthy situations.

Just as your blood pressure controls your Cardio health, stressful reactions control your Psyche-Immune health. The role of exercise in the Psyche-Immune system is to gain physical control of your stressful reactions. Being in a constant state of fatigue or muscular tension can produce headaches and cause muscle spasms. When muscles go into spasm, they pinch nerves and pull at joints and tendons, causing joint and back pain. Such organs as your colon and bowel can also be affected by muscular tension. Your body can be permanently damaged if you allow your stressful reactions to persist.

Exercise improves your mental and emotional health and strengthens your immune system, increasing your ability not only to fight off infectious diseases, but also to cope with the trauma of hearing a diagnosis of a life-threatening disease.

Psyche-Immune Preventive Exercises

Psyche-Immune exercises are designed to squeeze residual tension out of your muscles by stretching, fully contracting, and circulating fresh blood to them. You can do these exercises during the cool-down portion of your preventive exercise routine, and then practice them as intervention therapy during periods of peak stress.

EXERCISE COUNTS

Practice the movement or hold the position to a level that is comfortable for you. Repeat the series of exercises one to five times. Gradually increase the number of exercise repetitions or hold counts as you move through each of the three levels.

	REPS	HOLD TIMES (in seconds)	SETS
Level I	2–7	1–2	1
Level II	8–12	3–5	2
Level III	13-20	6-12	3
Level IV	21-24	13-19	4
Level V	25-30	20-30	5

Take at least one second to execute each repetition or each hold count. Time your exercise speed by counting out a repetition or hold, adding the word "and" after each count. (1 and 2 and 3 and . . .)

Fingers, Forearms, Hands, and Wrists: Lying Down Series

Level I

Lying Finger Lift

- Lie down on your back; hold your hands in front of you with each finger touching slightly
- Round your knuckles, keeping your fingers relaxed, slowly press the tips of your fingers together, thumb to thumb, index finger to index finger
- Feel the contraction in your finger muscles
- Repeat the sequence three to eight times.

Please note: You may do this exercise in a standing or seated position also. When sitting, pull your elbows in to your sides.

Lying Hand Stretch

- Lying on your back, extend your arms in front of you, palms down
- Gently separate and straighten your fingers while bending your hands up
- Hold three to eight seconds, feeling the stretch in your fingers and wrist; relax
- Repeat one to three times on each hand

Please note: You may do this exercise in a standing or seated position also.

Level II

Lying Finger Circles

- Lie down and hold your arm in front of you, elbows bent, palms down

- Circle each outstretched finger three to ten times clockwise, and then three to ten times counterclockwise; repeat entire exercise one to three times

Please note: You may do this exercise in a standing or seated position also.

Kneeling Forearm Stretch

- Kneel on all fours with your thumb out and fingers pointed back toward your knees
- Gently flatten your palms and lean back
- Hold for eight to twelve seconds, feeling the stretch in your wrists, forearms, and biceps; relax

LEVEL III

Lying Forearm Lift

- Lie on your left side with your right forearm palm facing down
- Slowly raise your forearm off the floor turning your palm out
- Hold and lower it, elbow anchored; repeat eight to twelve times
- Repeat on the other side with left forearm

FINGERS, FOREARMS, HANDS, AND WRISTS: SEATED OR STANDING SERIES

LEVEL I

Seated Hand Lift

- Sit or stand; extend your arms out in front of you, palms up; bend your arm at the elbow and place it on a table or on your thigh
- You will move your hand through four positions: 1) up, center; 2) down, center; 3) right, center; 4) left, center
- Hold your hand straight out without bending your wrist
- Slowly lift your fingers, keeping them extended and together, toward the top of your forearm; pause; return to the starting position
- Slowly bend your hand down until it forms a right angle with your forearm; pause; slowly lift your hand up and return it to the starting position
- Turn your hand to the right side; pause; return to the starting position
- Slowly turn your hand to the left side, feeling the contraction of your wrist and forearm muscle; pause, then return to the starting position
- Repeat the sequence three to eight times with each hand (you can also exercise them simultaneously)

Please note: This exercise can also be done in a lying down position.

Seated Forearm Stretch

- Sit or stand and rest your elbow on a table
- Hold your forearm off the table, palm down, fingers together and extended or curled
- Slowly turn your palm upward as far as it can go
- Hold for three to eight seconds

- Slowly turn your palm down and outward as far as it can go
- Hold for three to eight seconds, feeling the stretch in your forearm, wrist, and fingers; relax
- Change hands
- Repeat three to eight times with each arm

Standing Hand Press

- Stand over a table with your arms hanging loosely by your sides; bend your arms and hold your hands forward, palms on a table top
- Extend and close your fingers
- Slowly open your fingers wide apart; pause
- Slowly close them together into a fist; pause
- Slowly open your fingers and curve your palms and fingers as if you were holding a baseball; pause
- Slowly flatten your palms down on the table

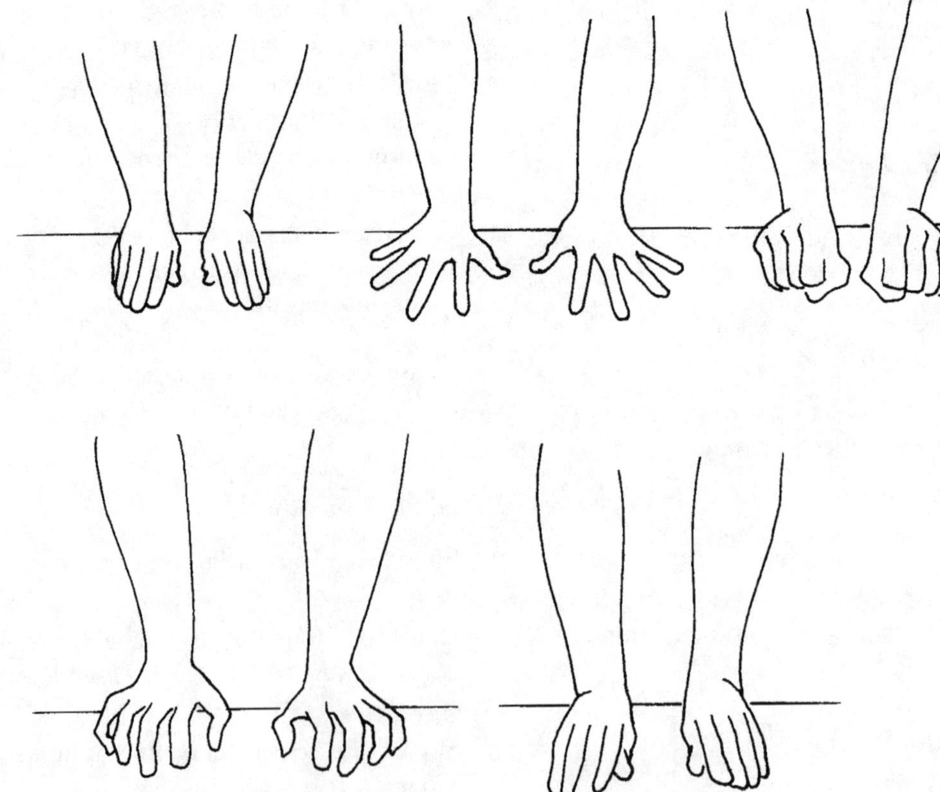

Standing Hand Press

- Feel the contraction in your wrist and forearms
- Repeat the sequence three to eight times with both hands (you can also do them simultaneously)

Standing Forearm Stretch

Please note: This exercise is particular effective in treating the overuse of the wrist by holding or gripping something too long and hard (e.g. tennis racquet, bike handlebars, typing).

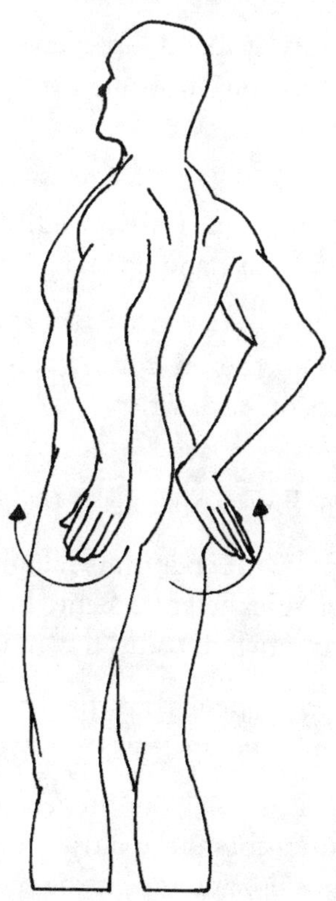

Standing Forearm Stretch

- Stand with your shoulders back and down; place your hands on the back of your hips below your waist, fingers pointing down; avoid arching your back
- Push your palms against your hips, put your fingers together and extend them upward
- Press in with your thumb and rotate your arms down and back
- Hold for three to eight seconds
- Feel the stretch in your forearms, wrist, and fingers; relax

LEVEL II

Seated Hand Circles

- Sit with your elbows on a table; bend your right arm in front of you, hand extended, palm down (if you are standing

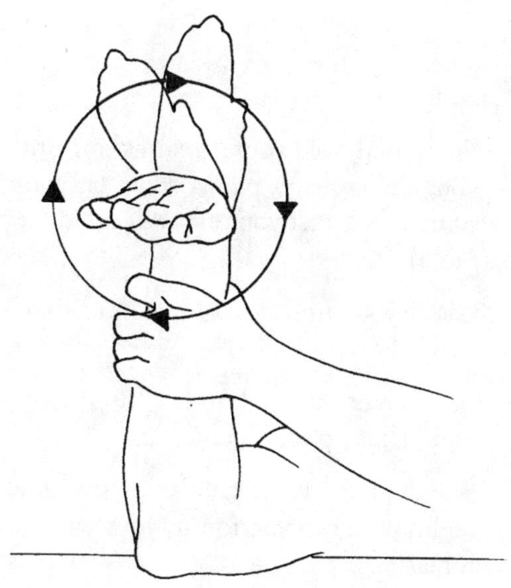

Seated Hand Circles

or lying down, rest it at the side of your chest)

- Close your fingers
- Hold your right forearm with your left hand
- Make clockwise circles with your hand, feeling the contraction of your wrist and forearm muscles
- Repeat the hand circles three to eight times clockwise, then counterclockwise three to eight times
- Switch hands and repeat the sequence

Seated Forearm Stretch

- Sit or stand, interlace your fingers in front of you, and turn your palms out
- Slowly extend your arms out at the wrists to chest level, feeling the stretch in your fingers, wrists, and arms

Standing Hand Twists

- Stand and hold your forearms in front of you, elbows bent, palms down (if you sit or lie down, rest your elbows on a desk or table)
- Close your fingers together and extend them
- Slowly turn your hands, thumbs apart and palms upward; pause
- Slowly turn your hands, palms down, feeling the contraction in your wrist and forearms
- Repeat the sequence eight to twelve times

Standing Arm Stretch

- Stand or sit; interlace your fingers above your head, palms up
- Straighten your arms up above your head, feeling the stretch in your fingers, wrists, and arms
- Hold for eight to twelve seconds

LEVEL III

Seated Wrist Curls

- Sit bent over with your right elbow propped on your thigh, arms bent, palms up; extend your fingers or hold a weight in each hand
- Curl your hand up; pause, feeling the contraction in your wrist and forearm muscles
- Lower your hand back down to the starting position (Advanced: Continue to move your hand down so fingers point to the floor)
- Repeat the exercise twelve to twenty times on each wrist

Standing Finger Spreads

- Stand with your arms hanging loosely by your sides, elbows bent; hold your forearms forward, palms down, fingers curled
- Slowly open your fingers and extend them as far apart as they will go; pause
- Slowly close your fingers together and tighten them into a fist; turn your hands, palms up, and repeat the sequence
- Practice each sequence eight to twelve times

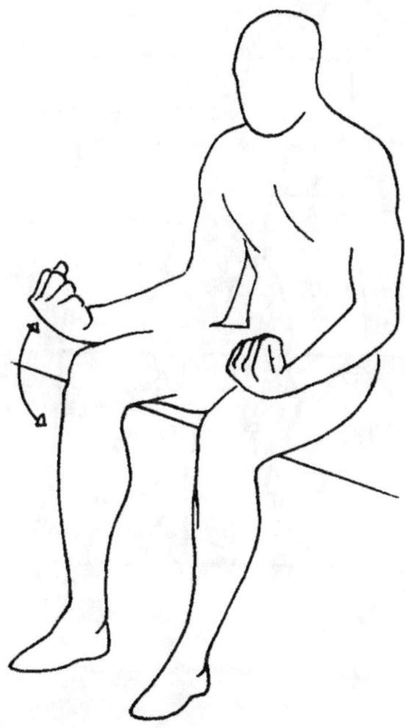

Seated Wrist Curl

LEGS AND THIGHS: LYING DOWN SERIES

LEVEL I

Lying Thigh and Ankle Stretch

- Lie on your right side and rest your head in the palm of your right hand; pull your left knee toward your chest and hold the top of your left foot with your left hand
- Gently pull your left heel toward the left buttock; hold your stomach in
- Hold for three to five seconds, feeling the stretch in your front thigh, shin, and ankle; relax
- Change sides and repeat

Alternate Lying Face Down Thigh and Ankle Stretch

- Lie face down on your stomach
- Reach behind you with your left hand and grab the front of the ankle of your right foot
- Gently pull your right heel toward the middle of your buttocks, keeping your thighs flat on the floor
- Hold three to five seconds; relax
- Change legs

Lying Leg, Knee, and Thigh Extension

- Lie on your back with your knees bent at a 90-degree angle and extend your arms out from your shoulders on the floor, palms down
- Slowly raise your right foot three to six inches off the floor, and extend it to the straightened position with your knee slightly bent; hold, feeling the contraction in your right thigh
- Slowly bend your lower leg back down and lower your thigh three inches, but don't let it rest on the floor
- Repeat the sequence three to five times on the right leg and again on the left leg

LEVEL II

Lying Hamstring Stretch

- Lie down on your back, legs extended, knees slightly bent
- Raise your right leg
- Raise your body up and lean forward to grab hold of your right knee with your right hand and your right ankle with your left hand
- Gently pull your leg as a single unit toward your chest

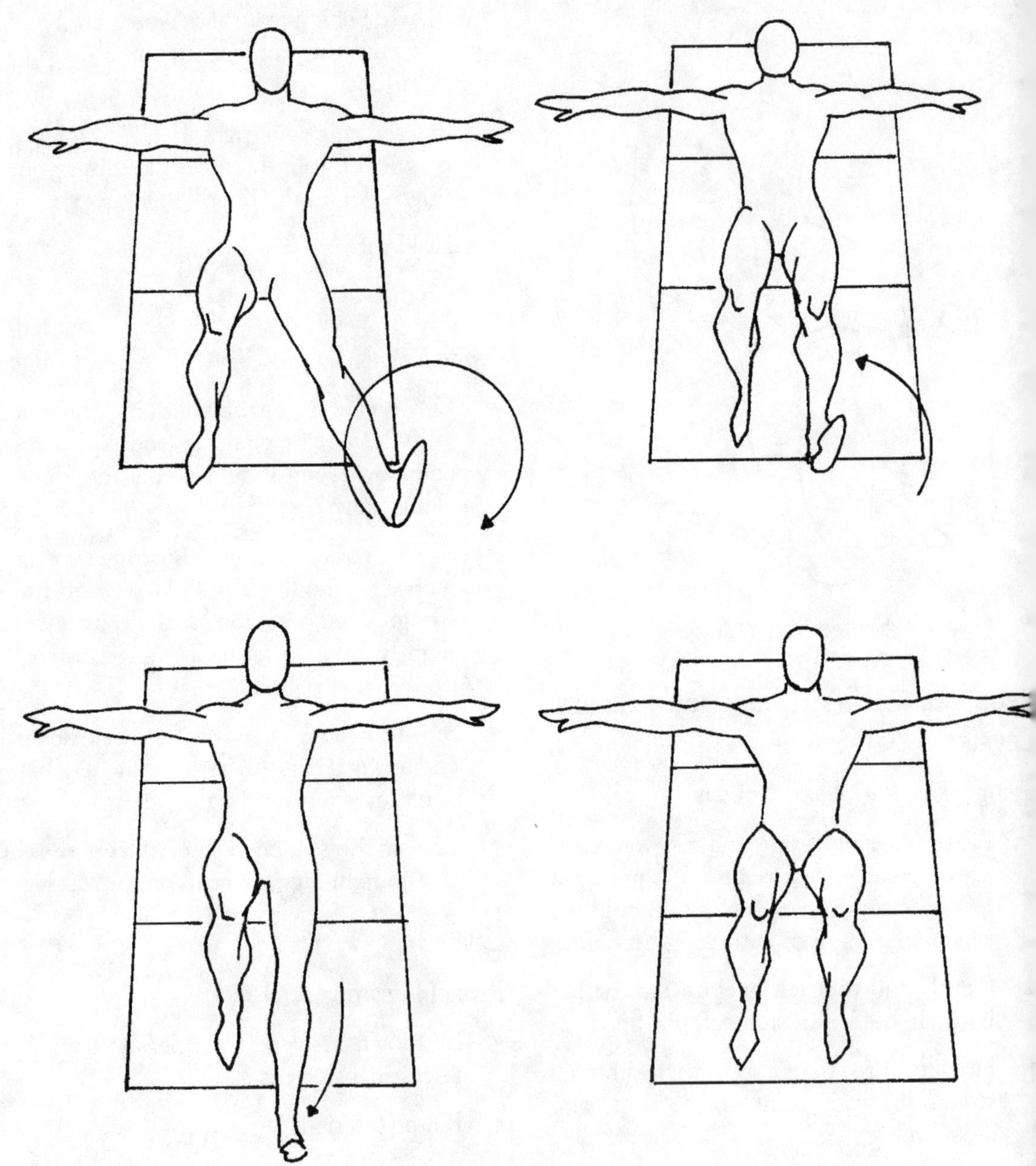

Lying Leg Circle

- Hold five to twelve seconds, feeling the stretch in your hamstring and buttocks
- Repeat with the other leg

Lying Leg Circle

- Lie on your back with arms resting at your side, shoulder level, knees bent, feet flat near your buttocks
- Tighten your buttocks and lift your pelvis
- Lift up your left leg and extend it vertically from your hips
- Feel the contraction in your front thigh; pause
- Open it out to the left in a downward circle; pause
- Cross it back to the right while simultaneously bending your knee; pause
- Return it to the vertical position and straighten your knee; lower it back down so it is parallel to your right thigh
- Repeat this sequence twelve to twenty times
- Bend your left leg
- Put your left foot down next to your right
- Repeat the sequence with your right leg

LEVEL III

Lying (All Fours) Quadriceps and Hamstring Stretch

Please note: If your knees hurt, do the Alternate Lying Stretch or the Seated Stretch (both in Level III) instead.

Hamstring and Quadriceps Stretch

- Kneel down and place your hands on the floor in front of you
- Move your left leg forward so your left knee is between your arms and under your chest; straighten your right leg back out; keep your left knee directly above your ankle joint
- Shift your weight onto the toes and ball of your right foot; keep your left foot flat
- Hold for eight to fifteen seconds
- Feel the stretch in your hamstring, groin, and hip; relax
- Shift your weight to your right knee
- Reach back and grab the top of your right foot with your left hand; bend your right leg and gently pull your right heel toward the middle of your buttocks
- Hold for eight to fifteen seconds, feeling the stretch in your right quadriceps muscles; relax
- Change sides and repeat the same hamstrings and quadriceps stretch sequence with your right leg forward

Alternate Lying Straight-Legged Stretch

- Lie on your back, legs straightened, knees slightly bent
- Bend your left leg and bring your thigh to your chest; your right leg should remain straight down, heel touching the floor
- Hug your left leg with both hands wrapped around the knee

- Slowly straighten out your left leg—don't lock your knee—and hold your thigh as close to your body as you can
- Move your hands along your leg to your calf muscle, pulling your leg from there toward your head
- Hold for eight to twelve seconds, feeling the stretch in your hamstrings

Legs and Thighs: Seated or Standing Series

Level I

Seated Thigh Stretch

- Sit bent forward on the floor with both legs bent at a 90-degree angle
- Wrap both arms around your left leg under the knee (as shown) and bring it forward
- Try to straighten out your leg
- Hold three to five seconds, feeling the stretch in your hamstrings; relax
- Repeat on the right leg

Seated Leg Extension

- Sit back in a chair and hold on to the sides or arm rests; your knees should be bent and feet planted on the floor
- Raise your left leg three inches, and straighten it out to the slightly bent position; hold, feeling the contraction in your front thigh muscles
- Lower your thigh three inches as you bend your knee back down
- Slowly repeat the sequence three to eight times before resting
- Change legs

Standing Thigh Stretch

- Stand with your left side to a wall so you can lean your hand against it for balance
- Shift your weight to your left leg and bend your left knee slightly
- Bend your right leg and raise your right knee in front of you, then grab your foot around the top part with your right hand

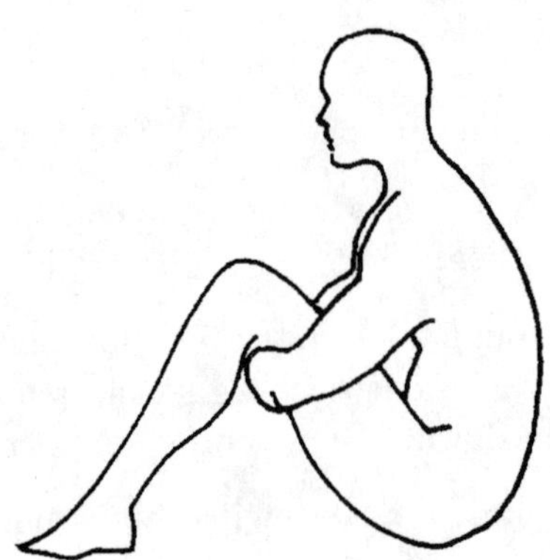

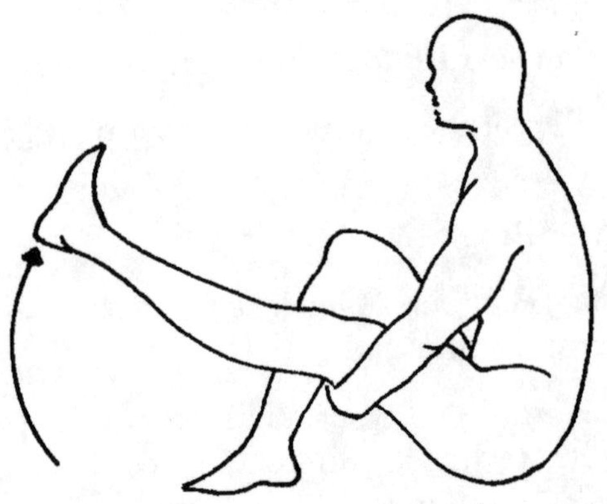

Seated Thigh Stretch

- Slowly pull your right leg behind you with knee pointing down
- Hold for three to five seconds, feeling the stretch in your right thigh
- Change sides and repeat

Standing Leg Extension

- Stand sideways with your left side facing a wall; to maintain your balance, hold on to a chairback with your left hand, arm extended
- To reach the starting position, bend your left leg and lift your knee about three to six inches in front of you
- Extend your left lower leg forward to a straightened position with your knee slightly bent
- Feel the contraction in your front thigh muscles; pause
- Bend your lower leg back down, but do not lower your thigh
- Raise your thigh three inches and repeat the motion; pause
- Bend your lower leg back and lower your knee only three inches; rest
- Repeat the exercise three to eight times
- Change legs

LEVEL II

Seated Hamstring Stretch

- Sit on a chair or floor with both feet planted on the floor
- Grab the front of your left knee with both hands
- Gently pull it toward your chest to the left shoulder
- Hold for five to eight seconds
- Feel the stretch in your hamstrings
- Repeat with your right leg

Seated Leg Circle

- Sit back in a chair or on the floor in the recumbent position with your knees shoulder-width apart
- Lift your left leg, knee bent, and open it toward the left; pause
- Straighten your left leg out horizontally; pause
- Cross it toward the right until it is parallel with your right leg; pause
- Repeat the sequence eight to twelve times before resting your left leg, then repeat the sequence with your right leg

Standing Hamstring Stretch

- Stand in the proper posture position, feet straight forward and hip-width apart
- Hold your stomach in, sink down in your knees, and bend over at the hips with your arms hanging down
- Place your palms on the floor in front of your feet and let your head hang down; if your hamstrings are too tight, put your hands on a telephone book
- Slowly straighten your legs, one at a time or simultaneously
- Hold eight to twelve seconds, feeling the stretch in your hamstrings

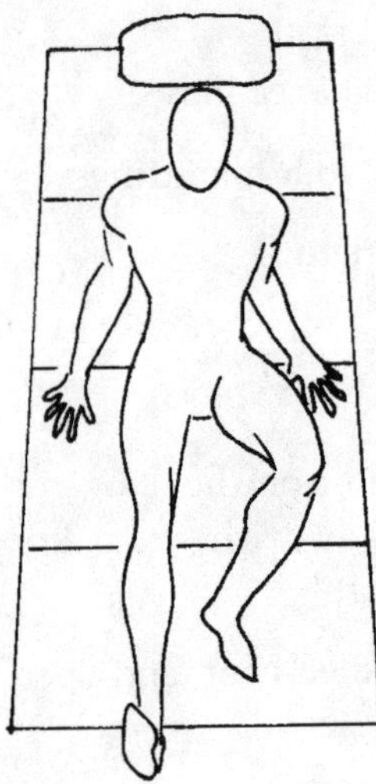
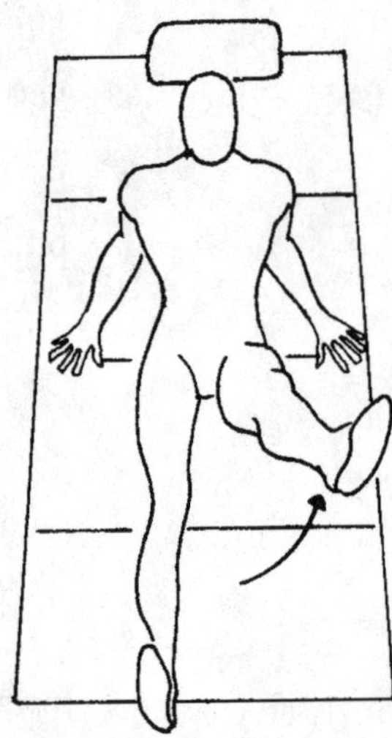
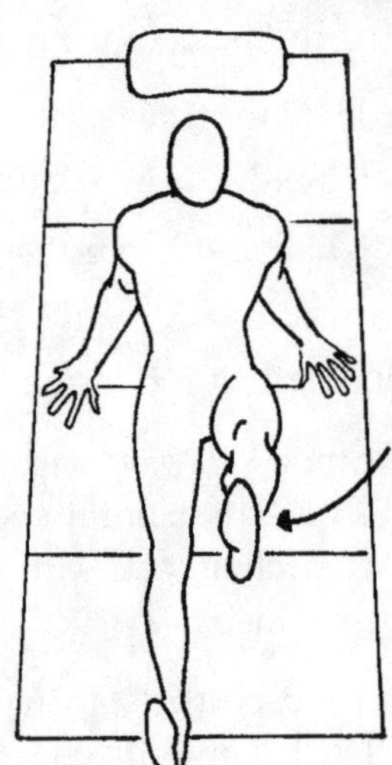

Seated Leg Circle

Standing Raised Leg Thigh Stretch

- Extend your foot in back of you, resting the top of it on a sturdy surface; keep your standing leg toes forward and knee slightly bent
- Pull your resting leg forward against the surface resistance
- Hold for eight to twelve seconds, feeling the stretch in your front hip and thigh
- Change legs

Standing Back Leg Circle

- Stand facing a wall or chair back so you can brace yourself for better balance
- Hold on with your right hand and bend your left leg to lift your foot up six to twelve inches behind you
- Draw a circle with your left foot about six inches in diameter
- Do three to six clockwise repetitions and three to six counterclockwise
- Lower and rest your leg
- Change sides and repeat sequence

LEVEL III

Standing Raised Leg Hamstring Stretch

- Place your left foot on a sturdy raised surface (e.g. a chair, a wall); keep your right (supporting) leg straight, knees slightly bent, toes pointed straight ahead
- Place your hand(s) on a wall or on your hips for balance and support
- Bend your left knee and move your hips forward

- Hold for five to twelve seconds, feeling the stretch in your hamstrings and front hips; relax
- Change legs.

Seated Thigh Stretch (Modified Hurdler's Stretch)

- Sit on the floor with your left leg bent and lying on its left side, knee pointed out
- Extend your right leg, knee slightly bent
- Lean forward at your waist and reach for your right ankle with your left hand; you may place your right palm on the ground for support
- Hold for eight to fifteen seconds, feeling the stretch in your right hamstring muscle and the left side of your back
- Switch legs and repeat

Seated Wall Seat Squats

- Stand with your back and feet about sixteen to twenty inches away from a wall

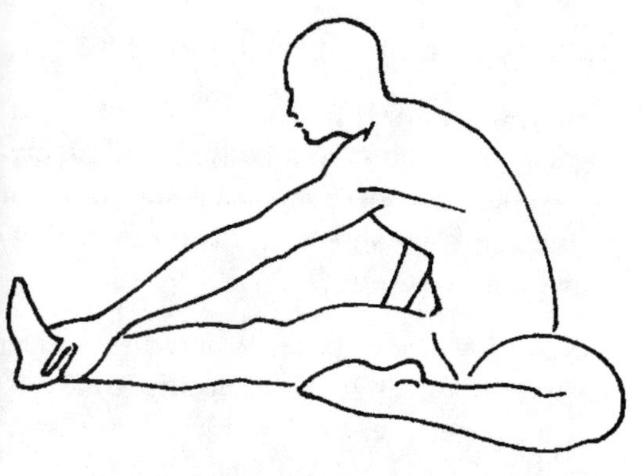

Seated Thigh Stretch

- Place your feet shoulder-width apart, hands on your hips or crossed over your chest
- Lean back against the wall and slowly sink down into the one-quarter to one-half squat position; knees remain over the ankles, not moving forward over the toes; pause
- Return back up to the starting position; use the wall to guide your descent and ascent, but avoid leaning
- Keep your head up, eyes forward, chin tucked in, and stomach held in throughout the exercise; if done properly, you should not feel any tension in your back (Hint: Place a ball in the small of your back to reduce the sliding friction and stress on your knee joints)

Standing Groin Stretch

- Standing with your left foot on a chair or bench, place your hands on your hips; keep your right leg straight, knee slightly bent, toes pointing sideways
- Bend your left leg (knee) and move your hips forward
- Hold for eight to twelve seconds, feeling the stretch in your groin and upper leg; relax
- Change legs

Standing Back Lunge Steps

- Stand with your feet shoulder-width apart, toes pointed forward, feet parallel; your arms should be extended out from your shoulders, palms down for balance;

(hold on to a sturdy chair back, counter or wall with your left hand for better balance)

- Step straight back with your right foot about two to three feet and land on the ball of your foot
- Bend your back knee while keeping your front leg aligned with your knee directly over or behind your ankle, your back straight, and your shoulders aligned over your hip joint
- At the same time, bend your knee and slowly sink down, keeping your forward foot flat to the floor; you can kneel down with your back leg, but don't touch the floor with your knee; pause
- Feel the contraction of your front quadriceps and rear calf
- Push off with your rear foot to return to the starting position; pause
- Lunge-step back with your left foot; repeat the sequence
- Alternate right and left lunge steps twelve to twenty-four times

Alternate Standing Quarter Squat and Side Leg Lift

- Stand in front of a sturdy chair with your feet shoulder-width apart, hands on your hips, by your sides, or extended out sideways at shoulder level
- Lean forward and slowly sink down in your knees until they are one-quarter to one-half bent; if half-bent, your buttocks should slightly touch the chair; pause
- Raise your arms out sideways and slightly forward to shoulder height for better balance
- Straighten your legs, raising your right leg out to the side, lifting it six to twelve inches above the ground
- Both legs should be fully straightened at this time
- When your right leg is fully straightened, lower it back down to shoulder-width; pause
- Sink down into the quarter-bent knees squat; pause
- Your raised leg should be lowered back to the floor when your knee is one-quarter bent
- Straighten your legs again, and this time, extend your left leg out to the side
- Repeat three times building up to twelve

Relaxation Training Exercises

You can learn to relax your body with the following long-term and short-term exercise techniques.

Program 1: Long-Term Techniques

1. Adopt a relaxed posture. Whenever you get a chance, rest your body. Avoid sitting on the edge of your seat, standing in lines, or lying with your head propped in awkward positions.
2. Slow down your pace. When you notice you are rushing about, losing track of things, getting tired easily, slow down your pace and use deliberate, continuous, and controlled movements.

3. Seek out and do exercises and activities that bring you joy and make you feel less competitive. The choice is an individual one. One person's chore is another's treat.

4. Pace your daily activities and take short exercise breaks. The more stressed-out you feel, the more frequent your breaks should be—normally ten minutes every hour, but sometimes fifteen minutes or even a half hour may be necessary to restore your equilibrium.

5. Relax when you feel pain or pressure. Don't let pain mount up. It can, if it's not attended to. You can avoid longer bouts of pain by relaxing in the wake of smaller episodes. Practice the appropriate relaxation exercise for overall or body area-specific symptoms.

PROGRAM 2: DEEP BREATHING EXERCISES

For stress such as anxiety and panic attacks, do deep breathing to counteract the rapid shallow breathing and rapid heart rate which result from these episodes. They are the Psyche-Immune equivalent of a muscle spasm.

Ex 1: Breath Control

Purpose: Take control of your exaggerated, out-of-control (hyperventilation) breathing and heartbeat by breathing deeply and rhythmically, slowing down the pace of your breathing and relaxing your whole body in the process.

Symptoms and conditions: Apprehension, confusion, dizziness, palpitations, breathlessness, chest tightness, choking, faintness, fatigue, hot flashes and sweating, muscular tension, nausea, numbness and tingling, panic. Psyche conditions: anxiety, fear, phobia, worry and fear, pain and suffering from acute traumatic and chronic diseases. Uncontrolled symptoms often contribute to the severity and duration of the symptoms.

Breathing control exercise: Very slowly, breathe in through your nose counting 1 and 2 and 3 and as long as you can. Mentally note how many counts you achieve. Hold for a brief second. Breathe out through your mouth taking as many counts as you did to breathe in. Repeat this breath control exercise one to six times. If your symptoms persist, practice a second set of breath control exercises until you have normalized your breathing rate to two-second breathing (Each second is 1 and 2 count breath.

Ex 2: Diaphragmatic or Stomach Breathing

Expand your capacity for staying relaxed by developing an expanded breathing capacity. As you continue to practice breath control, expand your stomach by pushing it out as you breathe in. This allows your lungs to fill with more air and slow down your rate of breath even further. (Up to five seconds per breath). A slower breathing rate also slows down your heartbeat.

Ex 3: Paper Bag Breathing

If your panic attack or hyperventilation is severe, practice breathing into a paper bag or cupped hands. Do not use a plastic bag! You are using a paper bag to increase the level of carbon dioxide that has been reduced because of your overbreathing. The bag lets you rebreathe the carbon dioxide-laden air you just breathed out.

Practice this exercise by holding the empty paper bag tightly over your nose and mouth with both hands, leaving no holes for leakage. Breathe in and out for a maximum of ten breaths until the unpleasant sensation of overbreathing ceases.

Program 3: Deep Muscular Relaxation

As with deep breathing exercises, these tension-release exercises can help you bring exaggerated muscle tension under control by tensing your muscles even further through isometric contraction in order to allow for a full release.

Moderately tense muscles can be relaxed by doing regular stretching and strengthening exercises but severely tense muscles will not fully relax even from regular exercise. Practice the following set of tension-releasing exercises for one to five seconds of tension and as many seconds of muscle relaxation. For example, if you tense a muscle group for three seconds, relax for another three seconds before moving on to the next muscle group.

In this series, you will be tensing and relaxing the muscle groups of your body starting with your hands and arms, and continuing through your shoulders, feet, legs, thighs, buttocks, lower and upper trunk, and head. Continue breathing through each contraction.

Practice these relaxation exercises in a prone or seated position. You can also practice these exercises in a series or selectively in one body area whenever you feel particular muscles getting tense.

Body Area Muscular Tension Exercise

Ex 1: Hands

Clench both your fists with your knuckles facing out. Hold for a count of one to six seconds. Breathe in and out slowly. As you breathe out, slowly release the grip of your fingers and let the blood circulate to your fingertips as you feel your hands grow heavier for another set of three to six seconds.

Apply the tightening and releasing procedure you used on your hands to your remaining body areas. Breathe rhythmically.

Ex 2: Arms and Biceps

Bend your arms at the elbow. Keep your hands loose, tighten your biceps, hold for one to six seconds. Relax your biceps as you lower your arm to the straightened out position.

Ex 3: Arms and Triceps

Straighten your arm fully, tightening your triceps, release.

Ex 4: Shoulders

Shrug your shoulders, raising them as if to touch your ears.

Ex 5: Feet

Scrunch your toes together, then release.

Ex 6: Front leg

Flex your feet downward by pointing your feet away from your body. Try to make them parallel to your legs, hold, then release.

Ex 7: Back of legs

Flex your feet upward, pressing your heels down. Hold, then release.

Ex 8: Thighs

Tighten the front of your thighs by pressing your knees down, then release.

Ex 9: Buttocks

Squeeze your buttocks together. Hold, then release.

Ex 10: Abdominals

Tighten or brace your stomach. Hold, then release.

Ex 11: Lower back

Flatten and press the small of your back against the ground. Hold, then release.

Ex 12: Chest

Breathe in as you tighten your chest muscles. Hold, then release.

Ex 13: Neck

Tilt your head back pointing your chin up. Hold, then release. Tilt your head forward. Try to touch your chin to your chest. Hold, then release. Continue breathing. Release your mouth and jaw. Pucker your lips and clench your teeth. Hold, then release.

Ex 14: Eyes

Squeeze your eyelids together. Hold. Continue breathing as you release.

Ex 15: Forehead

Raise your eyelids and wrinkle your forehead. Hold. Continue breathing. Release.

Ex 16: Scalp

Push your ears back, smoothing out the lines in your forehead. Hold, then release.

Ex 17: Face

Scrunch all your facial muscles together—eyes tight, lips to nose. Hold, then release.

ROMs and Stretching Exercises

The head, neck, and back are the areas where muscular tension starts. Selectively practice range-of-motion and stretching exercises to relieve the tension soon after it occurs. (For head tilts and neck stretches, see pp. 171, 184–188, for back stretches, see pp. 209–210, and for torso bends, see pp. 213–214.)

Yoga Alternative

Yoga is a 5,000-year-old system of exercise that is the mother of many of our exercise techniques and forms including postural training, breathing exercise, progressive muscle relaxation, range-of-motion exercise, stretching, Kegel, and back exercises. Yoga offers over 200 different exercises in beginner, intermediate, and advanced forms. However, some of these exercise positions can put too much stress on your neck and lower back. It is difficult to learn yoga without the assistance of an instructor. It is also risky to selectively practice individual yoga exercises apart from a balanced and complete regimen.

Yoga has a good reputation for providing many health and medical benefits. However, many health claims still need to be substantiated. For example, it is believed yoga postures and exercises may help redirect the flow of blood to such organs as the heart, brain, and colon as well as to joints. Breathing routines may increase or relieve pressure on the colon and thyroid glands. Yoga stretching exercises may help increase the blood flow to disks and joints. Some studies show that yoga practice has at least a temporary effect on body functions including blood pressure, perhaps by relaxing the muscles that control the diameter of blood vessels.

PART THREE

REHABILITATION RX

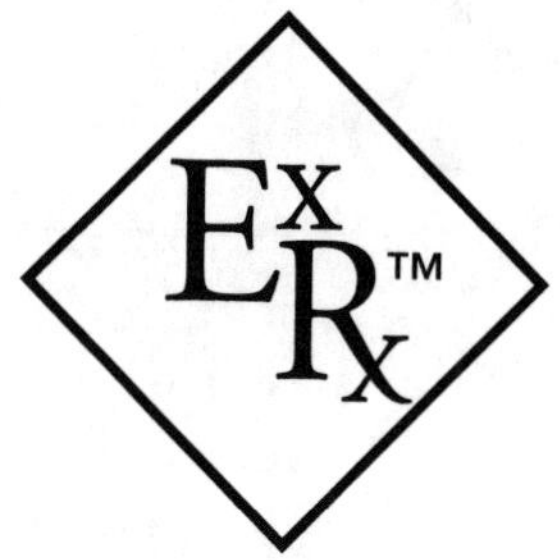

Introduction to Rehabilitation Rx

How to Use Rehabilitation Rx

Use the Rehabilitation Rx section of the book to find the specific exercise prescriptions in Part Three for more than 500 major diseases and disorders. There are two ways to locate the correct exercise prescription for you: (1) you can locate and find the disease or symptom by using the index (p. 473) or (2) you can use your medical profiles for the five body systems, which were completed in Part One. When health problems involve two or more systems, practice the exercise prescription in Part Three for each system.

Each chapter in Part Three contains alphabetical lists of disease descriptions including symptoms and exercise prescriptions for the five different systems. There are also a series of comeback stories that will inspire you to use exercise to manage your health or the health of the person in your care.

Similar to surgery, many injuries involve rehabilitative exercise of a local or general nature. If the injury is localized, as with a broken arm, you must try to exercise the rest of your body while the arm heals. Then, after the cast comes off, the muscles in your broken arm can be retrained with range-of-motion, stretching, and strengthening exercises.

Each of the five chapters in Part Three contains an Exercise Rx section. This section is divided into three phases; each phase includes exercise for both your whole body system and specific weakened body areas (e.g. knee, neck, back, and so on). Depending on the severity of the injury or disease, you will start at one of the three phases: Most Severe (Phase I), Moderately Severe (Phase II), Mildly Severe (Phase III). Each phase is designed to restore basic body functions and to get you, your child, or your patient up and moving. The exercises are often done seated or lying down, but always should include some effort to stand up, and regain balance and equilibrium.

PHASE I

Most Severe covers the initial period after surgery or treatment for the most severe level of a disease (e.g. bone fracture, cancer surgery, heart attack, stroke). Phase I is usually done with the assistance of a doctor or physical therapist and can run from a few days to a few weeks, depending on the severity of the disability or injury. Some of the Phase I exercises are depicted or described here, but the major portion are Phase II and III exercises because these can be done at home.

PHASES II AND III

Moderate and Mild are exercise treatments designed to rehabilitate or restore basic body systems, functions, and body areas that have been damaged or immobilized. You will follow Phase II or III exercises from two to twelve weeks, depending on the body system or area you need to rehabilitate. If you have to start at a lower-level phase, finish that phase and then go on to the next phase.

All exercises designed to restore body function from a disease or disability are called rehabilitative. Some diseases and disorders, however, cannot be completely rehabilitated (e.g. Parkinson's disease, multiple sclerosis). In these cases, you use the same rehabilitative exercises (usually Phase II or III) to slow down the progress of the physical disability and provide relief from various symptoms.

Even chronically ill and disabled patients should exercise as much as they can to reduce the risk of stroke and cardiovascular disease, which is greater in the sedentary, physically disabled person than in an able-bodied person. Disabled athletes have led the way and now many physical improvements are possible with exercise training.

If you are in the rehabilitative mode, you will not be able to practice any of the Preventive exercises in Part Two until you have completed the exercise regimen in Phase III, (Mild) in Part Three, or unless you are specifically referred to those exercises as part of your program.

CHAPTER 13

Age Rx

Exercise Solutions for Nervous and Sensory Systems

NERVOUS AND SENSORY SYSTEMS

This section of Exercise Rx covers your nervous system and sensory system. The body areas covered are: head, neck, spine and lower back, ears, and eyes. The primary symptoms and physical conditions for which Age Rx offers help are those that involve the loss of movement and muscular control, the loss of such sensory functions as seeing and hearing, and the loss of such mental functions as the ability to concentrate and remember.

Nervous neuromuscular and sensory system disorders are included in Age Rx because they share many of the same physical characteristics and conditions that characterize aging—namely the decline of balance, coordination, agility, mobility, hearing, and visual acuity. Although the aging process also includes loss of muscular strength and cardiorespiratory capacity, these are conditions that are experienced across all age groups.

Nervous system and sensory loss are dominant in older-age groups and are also the first priority in age rehabilitation. For example, without minimum balance and coordination it is not easy to engage in strength and aerobic conditioning. Of course, if you suffer from other such symptoms of aging as incontinence or arthritis you will find the exercise solutions in other chapters in Part Three, such as Chapter 15, Meta Rx for incontinence or Chapter 14, MuSkel Rx for arthritis. If you are unsure where to find a specific injury or disorder, consult the index, p. 473.

The exercises included here are warm-ups, range-of-motion (ROM), posture, and balancing exercises. The head and neck area contribute most to the rehabilitation of the nervous and sensory systems. They are the body areas most associated with balance, coordination, and muscular control. Exercise at the level appropriate to the severity of your symptoms and physical disabilities as evaluated by your doctor and physical therapist.

When you have settled on the correct level you need, look up your specific disease, disorder, or injury in the descriptions that follow and then practice the specifically recommended exercise routines. Be sure to always practice any exercise in a supported position, especially if balance and sensory loss are a problem.

The major portion of this chapter is broken down into five distinct areas, which are: (1) nervous system diseases, disorders, and injuries, (2) head and neck diseases, disorders, and injuries, (3) ear diseases, disorders, and injuries, (4) eye diseases, disorders, and injuries, and (5) lower back injuries. Each of these five areas is followed by an alphabetic listing of the diseases, disorders, or injuries found under that category. Symptoms are then described for each disease, disorder, or injury, which is followed by an ExRx for that specific ailment. You will note that some of the more common, more rehabilitative diseases and injuries have many exercises associated with them, while other diseases (e.g. Alzheimer's disease, multiple sclerosis, muscular dystrophy) will have only a few exercises associated with them. If you feel you want more exercise than what is given with any ExRx, consult Parts I and II of this book and practice those preventive exercises that are associated with the body system or area that you are rehabilitating. Remember: Always start at a lower level and work your way up to your own personal optimum level. Do not turn your rehabilitative exercise therapy into a competition with anyone—including yourself. That is the surest, fastest way to injury, pain, and setbacks on the road to recovery.

Some of the injuries covered in the five areas are caused by overuse. Overuse injuries are more easily prevented by safer exercise techniques and also more directly affected by therapeutic and rehabilitative exercise. Rehab usually begins directly after the injury. There are various levels of injury, ranging from moderate to severe, the most common being bruises, sprains, and strains. A bruise is an injury that usually causes a rupture of small blood vessels, which in turn causes discoloration without a break in the surrounding or overlying skin; a sprain is a partial or complete tear of the ligaments surrounding a joint; a strain is an injury to the muscle or tendon. Sprains and strains may heal without surgery; most bruises require a minimum amount of therapy. For most of these types of injuries, doctors and physical therapists will use the following protocol: Rest, ice, compression, and elevation (RICE), and medical attention for more severe injuries; medications will include acetaminophen, ibuprofen, or aspirin for mild to moderate injuries; for severe injuries, doctors will prescribe bed rest with analgesics and anti-inflammatory drugs.

WARNING: Although many over-the-counter and prescription pain relievers are prescribed for reduction of pain in sore muscles, bones, joints, and skin, do not take any pain relievers before exercising as they tend to mask pain, which can cause further injury resulting from overexercising or overusing an injured body area or part. Take the medication as directed, after exercise and when you are more stationary. Awareness of an injury is key to healing it!

AGE RX SYMPTOMS AND CONDITIONS LIST

- headache
- sensory loss
- eye pain
- ear ache
- throat soreness
- neck pain and stiffness
- back pain
- loss of musculoskeletal control
- muscle weakness

EXTREME SYMPTOMS AND CONDITIONS LIST

- seizures
- faintness and fainting
- facial paralysis
- tremor
- numbness and tingling
- loss of sense of smell or taste
- vision loss, spots, blurring
- eye drooping
- deafness, buzzing

THERAPEUTIC EXERCISE PRESCRIPTIONS

- Warm-up ExRx—For painful, numb, tingling, and fatigued body areas by increasing blood and oxygen flow
- Range-of-motion ExRx—To improve coordination, muscle control, and strength; therapy for tenderness and painful areas
- Balancing ExRx—To reestablish muscle control and reduce trembling
- Head–Eye ExRx—To strengthen eye and neck muscles along with eye-head coordination
- Posture ExRx—To take excessive pressure off nerves and muscles by aligning nearby body areas

REHABILITATIVE EXERCISE PRESCRIPTIONS

- Stretch and strengthen damaged or weakened eyes, jaws, neck, and spine muscles

Nervous System Diseases, Disorders, and Injuries Rx

The nervous system is the body's information gathering, storage, and control system. It is divided into two parts. The first is the central nervous system, which is the brain and spinal cord. The second is the sensory nervous system, including such sense organs as the eyes and skin, which, through the nerves, inputs information to the brain and spinal cord and then returns processed output information to the skeletal muscles, organs, glands, and skin.

Disorders of the nervous system result from damage or dysfunction of either or both of these two component parts. If you are suffering from fatigue, disorientation, forgetfulness, inability to concentrate, declining muscle control, insomnia, lack of coordination, memory loss, language ability loss, or higher susceptibility to infection, Age Rx can help you regain control of your muscles and motor sensory functions through ROM, stretching, and strengthening exercises. Many nervous system diseases are induced by stress, fatigue, and overstimulation and thus respond to relaxation and deep breathing exercise as well.

AGING

The natural deterioration of body tissues, and therefore functions, as the result of the passage of time.

Symptoms:
Increased susceptibility to infection, muscle wasting and weakness (especially after age fifty), also more prone to accidents.

ExRx:
At least one study shows that exercise reduces the age-related decline in both T-cell function (T cells defend against infection and cancer cells) and production of cytosine (a component of DNA), while also reducing muscle deterioration and weakness (especially after age fifty), increasing neural coordination, and improving the quality of life for the aged by increasing flexibility, strength, and mobility.

ALZHEIMER'S DISEASE

Deterioration of mental function. There is no cure for Alzheimer's—exercise or otherwise. Exercise can help manage symptoms, however. Patients may be taking antidepressants, hypnotics, and neuroleptics. The prevalence of Alzheimer's increases with age: 0.5% in those under sixty-five, 3% in those that are sixty-five to seventy-four years of age, and 10% in people aged eighty-five years or older.

Symptoms:
Fatigue, confusion, disorientation, lack of coordination, incontinence, sometimes a high level of agitation, as well as limited mobility.

ExRx:
Exercise should be carefully planned, closely supervised, and executed with consistency and patience. Choose exercises and activities that are familiar to the patient. Walking, rocking in a chair, sanding wood, folding laundry, or gardening are good examples. Range-of-motion and strengthening exercises should also be emphasized along with various forms of recreational and occupational therapy. Exercise at the beginning of the day when the patient's energy level is highest, and avoid exercise at day's end when agitation (known as "sundowning") is highest.

These exercise prescriptions that are given for Alzheimer's disease are for the patient's care giver. The care giver should reduce the sources of stress that come from:

1. A change of routine or a change of environment
2. Fatigue
3. Excessive demands
4. Illness and pain
5. Overwhelming stimuli
6. Too much medication

An easy, but structured and repetitive, exercise program of a therapeutic nature (less difficult as the disease progresses) will help the patient relax and become more reality-centered. A daily exercise schedule should be written down with specific day-by-day instructions. Exercise devices or equipment should be labeled and put in the same position to provide as little opportunity for confusion as possible.

The overall exercise goals of an Alzheimer's patient are to maintain basic fitness and reduce the anxiety associated with the disease with relaxation techniques.

ELROY BERKOWITZ

DIAGNOSIS: DEGENERATIVE SPINAL DISEASE

Aging is often attended by a host of degenerative diseases. Elroy Berkowitz, seventy-one, has undergone a variety of surgeries, all of which stemmed from calcifications and degeneration in his spine, heart, hip, and shoulder.

Elroy went into these operations healthy. "I'm a runner. I have been my whole life. I'm basically a healthy person."

Elroy's first operation, a lumbar lamenectomy to repair his lower spine, took place in 1987. He was up and walking the day after the surgery. Elroy "walked his way up," beginning with short walks on flat ground and then worked his way up to hills. In rehab, which he attended twice a week, the therapist prescribed flexibility and strengthening exercises. Together, they worked on stretching exercises, electricity therapy, and finally weight lifting. Elroy calls that part of his therapy a "get started" activity.

On his own, Elroy continued to practice other activities he'd been doing his entire life, such as playing racquetball, rowing, swimming, and especially deep-water running. He has regularly done this sort of cardio training four to five times a week. Elroy says it took him six months to fully recover from the lumbar lamenectomy.

His therapy was virtually the same for his other three surgeries. In 1989, Elroy underwent open heart surgery involving an aortic valve replacement. The next surgery, in 1994, was a total left hip replacement. The last, completed in November of 1995, was a repair of his left rotator cuff. Elroy had a four- to six-month recovery period after each of these three operations. "Most people are impressed with my recovery," he says.

His plan for each recovery began with walking and then, after he was somewhat healed, he would get in the pool. Elroy says, "Deep-water running is the single-best exercise. . . . Water is a gravity-free environment. It has no concussion. Water is twelve times denser than air." This makes deep-water running not only a great cardio workout, but also effective resistance training. Deep-water running was not introduced to Elroy in rehab. He has been doing it for "years and years." It was his participation in competitive running that introduced him to the exercise.

"Major runners spend as much time in the water as they do on the road," he has said.

Elroy advises those taking up deep-water running to use some sort of support, such as "a flotation device."

As to his current health, Elroy says, "Nothing impedes my activities." He still works out four to five times per week.

Amyotrophic Lateral Sclerosis (ALS; Lou Gehrig's Disease)

This is the most common form of progressive neuromuscular disease. Weakness and atrophy can occur in any of the skeletal muscles but usually starts with your hands and feet. Onset begins between ages forty and seventy, and is rapidly fatal.

Symptoms:
The disease proceeds at a steady rate without remission and is accompanied by spasticity leading to disability, diminished breathing ability, and speech loss. Poor balance, lack of motivation, and occasional urinary urgency are also associated with ALS.

ExRx:
Patients are encouraged to keep active but also to rest frequently and avoid excessive overexertion. The goal should be to maintain a higher level of functioning ability for as long as possible. Exercise can help the portion of muscle weakness that comes from the disease or inactivity but will not slow down or reverse the disease progression. Exercise helps maintain the patient's functioning ability including improved muscle strength and endurance. Range-of-motion and stretching exercises also help minimize the pain from joint stiffness. The patient should be supported during exercise when necessary. Eventually all exercise levels will decrease as a result of the loss of functional capacity.

Brain Aneurysm

Dilation of arteries in the brain.

Symptoms:
Headache, stiffness (neck, back, legs), and nausea.

AGE RX: LIST OF ADDITIONAL NERVOUS SYSTEMS DISEASES, DISORDERS, AND INJURIES BENEFITED BY HEAD AND NECK REHABILITATIVE EXERCISE

- Bell's palsy
- brain tumor
- bruise (or contusion)
- encephalitis
- hydrocephalus
- Huntington's disease
- meningitis
- osteosclerosis
- radiculitis (pinched nerve in neck)
- Reye's syndrome
- skull fracture
- speech disorders
- spina bifida
- spinal impact injuries
- spondylosis (spur formation)
- thyroid cancer
- torticollis (wryneck)
- trigeminal neuralgia

ExRx:
Bed rest and head and neck stretching exercises. (See neck and facial exercises, pp. 171–172.)

Cerebral Palsy (CP)

The most common cause of crippling and underdevelopment of affected limbs in children. A neuromuscular disorder whose causes include prenatal complications, birth trauma, forceps delivery, and brain infection.

Symptoms:
Range from mild motor impairment (exhibited only during such strenuous physical activ-

ties as running) to seizures, speech disorders, and mental retardation. Also, sharp, jerky movement, lack of coordination, spasticity (increased muscle rigidity), alternating muscle contraction and relaxation. Children with spasticity walk on their toes with a scissors gait and have uncoordinated muscle movements.

ExRx:
Exercise can help reduce the risk of stroke and cardiovascular disease. Range-of-motion exercises to minimize muscle contraction and maximize muscle relaxation can help with spasticity along with graded stretching and strengthening exercises for balanced muscle development. It is extremely important to receive physical therapy to prevent rapid and uncontrollable muscle contractions or joint contractures and joint destruction. Aerobic capacity and endurance can be increased with lower and/or upper limb ergometers (in a wheelchair). Walking with crutches and/or a wheelchair pusher six to fifteen minutes once or twice a day, three to five days per week at 40 to 85% of the maximum heart-training rate is an excellent aerobic and strengthing exercise. Practice strengthening exercises with free weights or weight-lifting machines two sessions per week. Practice stretching all joints (whether diseased or not) after ROM warm-up at beginning and end of exercise session.

EPILEPSY

Abnormal electrical discharges in the brain resulting in seizures, body tingling, twitching, and loss of consciousness.

Symptoms:
Recurrent seizures, low blood sugar, and excessive fatigue. It is triggered by flashing lights, breathing too quickly, loud noise, odors, among others. A partial seizure is when one limb stiffens or jerks and has tingling sensations. A general seizure is when the person's body falls to ground, stiffens, then alternates between muscle spasms and relaxation.

ExRx:
Rest and relaxation, reduction of stimuli, deep-breathing exercise, and relaxation techniques all can help. Avoid such dangerous activities as swimming alone or climbing ladders. Aerobic, stretching, and strengthening exercises can reduce the frequency of seizures. In a recent medical study, fifteen women with pharmacologically intractable epilepsy did aerobic dancing with strength training and stretching for sixty minutes, twice weekly, for forty-five weeks, which led to a reduction of seizures and complaints about muscle pains, sleep problems, and fatigue. **BUT CARE MUST BE TAKEN,** because 5% of epileptics run the risk of exercise-induced seizures.

FRAILTY

Frailty is the physical decline associated with advanced aging that can be found across the entire age spectrum. The fastest growing population segment is over age eighty-five. Frail persons have a variety of medical problems—especially metabolic.

Symptoms:
Confluence of slightness, weakness, and vulnerability and the lack of ability to perform daily activities required for independent living.

ExRx:
Maintaining physical activity is critically important for delaying metabolic disorders.

Past exercise history and preferences are important in determining a starting point. These can best be achieved by increasing muscular strength and endurance as well as aerobic capacity. To avoid fatiguing too quickly, take more time to build up to a steady rate of exercise. This means very gradual increases in speed and duration. Bicycling and water exercise is preferred over walking for those people with degenerative joint disease and joint replacements. Strength training should include ankle, hand, and wrist strengthening. Warm-ups should concentrate on balancing exercises, hand to eye coordination, and prevention of falls. Practice seated and supported exercises when there is a danger of a fall or fracture from osteoporosis, perceptual deficits, or balancing difficulties. Finally, monitor the frail patient for symptoms of dehydration (i.e. thirst, pallor, faintness) and insulin insensitivity. Emergency procedures should be planned and set up in advance. Walking may be the best exercise. But water exercise and such seated exercises as bicycling and chair calisthenics are better for those with degenerative joint diseases and knee and hip replacements. Participation is more important than regulating exercise coverage or intensity and ROM strengthening exercises are more important than aerobic exercises.

Guillain-Barré Syndrome

Immunological attack on nerve cells—stripping off their sheaths and causing muscle weakness and sensory loss, along with mild motor and reflex loss. Peripheral nerve degeneration (nerves outside the brain and spine) prevents them from sending messages back to the brain. Recovery is spontaneous and complete in 95% of people.

Symptoms:
Numbness, muscle weakness, and sensory loss starts in arms and legs and prevents movement; later extends to face.

ExRx:
Learn to walk short distances with a cane or walker, or to lift your body from your wheelchair by using your arms. Muscle massage and ROMs will not slow down muscle weakening but will delay atrophy.

Headaches

Usually a symptom of another underlying disorder. Although 90% of headaches come in two forms, the mild tension headache and the migraine, 10% come from disorders in the skull (e.g. eyes, teeth, ears, tumors). Cluster or tension headaches come from muscular contractions; migraines are linked to arterial contractions in the head. Other factors include fatigue, emotional stress, diet, alcoholic hangover, menstruation, environmental stress (e.g. loud noises, bright lights, cramped living spaces).

Symptoms:
Severe or persistent head pain, head tightness, tender spots on neck, and vision impairment.

ExRx:
Practice relaxation exercises, facial and neck stretching and massage. Tension headaches can be prevented or relieved by stretching the muscles of the face, forehead, scalp, neck, and shoulders. Range-of-motion exercises for these areas also increase blood flow and relief. Also, muscle relaxants and psychotherapy for emotional distress can help. Vascular headaches (including migraines) require greater care

including avoiding certain "trigger" foods and abstaining from aerobic exercise during migraines. Medical studies show, however, that aerobic exercise provides long-term benefits in the management of classic migraine symptoms. Cluster headaches (90% occurrence in men) can often be exercised away with vigorous exercise. (Also see Psyche-Immune Rx, p. 427.)

HEAD INJURY

Traumatic head injuries, mostly from auto accidents and gunshot wounds, occur approximately 500,000 times per year, and are as prevalent as heart attacks. These injuries are classified as mild, moderate, and severe. Head injuries can be similar to stroke in the extent of brain damage. They can also cause secondary injuries including edema, ischemia, and metabolic disorders.

Symptoms:
Physical disabilities such as locomotion problems including paralysis can occur. Mental and emotional problems such as agitation, confusion, compulsiveness, inattention, learning deficits, and memory disturbances are also fairly common symptoms.

ExRx:
Exercise, supervised by a care giver, can help patients become more independent and improve their mobility. Watch out for seizures and hyperventilation induced by exercise. Slower walking and cycling (thirty to sixty spm/rpm) speeds with gradual progression to faster speeds (sixty to ninety spm/rpm) are preferred. For those in wheelchairs, use arm ergometers or special cranks that are attached to wheels. Practice coordination and balance exercises to improve neuromuscular function as well as extra stretching and strengthening of the injured side of the body. (Also see Stroke, p. 269.)

JET LAG

A disturbance of the normal rhythm of the nervous system.

Symptoms:
Fatigue, sleeplessness, muscle tension, dizziness, loss of balance, stiffness, dehydration, and sensitivity to light are all symptoms.

ExRx:
Various exercise approaches including walking, stretching, balancing exercises, ROMs, and napping. Exposure to sunlight is also believed to help. Sometimes, twirling your body clockwise, then counterclockwise three to eight times, will also help adjust your body clock.

LOU GEHRIG'S DISEASE: SEE AMYOTROPHIC LATERAL SCLEROSIS, P. 258

MIGRAINE: SEE HEADACHES, P. 260

MULTIPLE SCLEROSIS (MS)

Disease of the brain and spinal cord that impairs nerve-impulse transmission. Onset usually begins between ages twenty and forty, with 70% leading active lives with prolonged remission. Flare-ups of muscle weariness and lack of motor coordination may be triggered by overwork, fatigue, pregnancy, or respiratory infection.

Symptoms:
Emotional stress, fatigue, acute respiratory infections, eye disturbance, muscle weakness,

ZOE KOPLOWITZ

DIAGNOSIS: MULTIPLE SCLEROSIS

Zoe Koplowitz has multiple sclerosis (MS), but it was when she "choked on a pill and stopped breathing" nine years ago that she decided to get active. Zoe hadn't quite considered the possibility that something other than MS could kill her.

For someone not athletic as a youngster, Zoe set high standards for herself. She walked into the Achilles Track Club—on her signature crutches, nonetheless—and announced that she was going to do a marathon.

Zoe started by walking five blocks in each direction. At first, the MS tired her quickly. After two to three months, Zoe was doing three miles at a stretch on crutches. The exhausting effects of a disease like MS made Zoe adapt the way she trained. "Some days I can do more and some days I can't," she explains.

Zoe's crutches help her get around in day-to-day life, and they also help her with her balance. She tried to do the walks without her crutches, but was less successful. Zoe urges everyone who needs them to use body appliances.

To accomplish her goal of completing a marathon, Zoe also weight trains three times a week. In her marathons, she says, "I finish on upper body strength."

Zoe has completed the New York City Marathon eight times, fighting her body's pain and exhaustion the whole way. Her most recent marathon was an all-time high record of almost thirty hours. "For the entire week before the marathon, I visualize crossing the finish line. Mental is 99% of it," she says.

Zoe also did other activities, but mainly to improve her marathoning. For her unstable gait and to regain hip motion, she took an Afro-Brazilian dance class. "It put a swing back in my step," she says, smiling. Zoe didn't worry about the specific steps of the dances, because those are difficult for her. "Improvising—I was able to do that." Zoe also does aerobics several times a week, just focusing on staying in motion throughout the routine.

Regularly playing pinball improved Zoe's hand-eye coordination. It's also a "good stress-

paralysis, spasticity, hyperflexia, tremor and tingling, uncoordinated gait, incontinence, mood swings, depression are all common symptoms. These symptoms wax and wane.

ExRx:

Prevention: There is no evidence that exercise can prevent MS, but it may make your body hardier against the triggering mechanisms, which are fatigue, respiratory infections, and a complicated pregnancy. It also helps you to manage or avoid stress, and to learn new ways to move. Muscle-strengthening exercises will at least maximize your muscle function, if not slow down the progress of muscle weakening. Walking at a buster," as she calls it. For abdominal muscles, Zoe does easy crunches, because she does not have the mobility to do sit-ups. Music has also helped her train. "I wear a walkman. If I can sing, I am training at an appropriate rate."

On the track on which Zoe trains, she "makes up crazy stuff that works" to keep herself motivated, such as keeping poker chips in her pockets and guessing what color they are before pulling them out. She stresses the importance of a safe and comfortable place to train. The first thing Zoe does when she finishes a marathon and she can finally walk again (it takes her a few days) is go to the track she always walks and put in an Olympic victory lap.

Zoe's pain and numbness, which accompany multiple sclerosis, have lessened since she became an athlete, but have not entirely disappeared. She says, "It's what you choose to focus on.

"In every marathon, there's a point where you hit the wall. I've broken that eight times," she says. Zoe also thinks that "marathon" is a metaphor. "It's encouraged people to get on with their lives." Zoe has a strong team backing her. "I have a real pit crew. I see us as a medieval traveling band," she says.

Zoe gets a couple of hundred letters a year. A teacher in Tennessee saw a piece about her on TV and came to the finish line to support her. A woman in Missouri wrote to tell her how inspirational it was to watch Zoe cross that line on TV.

Zoe's incredible feats—all eight marathons—led to her creation of a seminar called "Turtle Power: Life Lessons Learned in Last Place." She gives the talk to a wide range of audiences, from major corporations to schools.

She holds two world records for being the first woman with MS to complete a full marathon and for making the longest women's marathon at twenty-nine hours, fifteen minutes. "I have a great deal of endurance." She subsequently broke her marathon record by completing the New York City Marathon in twenty-seven hours, fifteen minutes.

Zoe doesn't mind that her times are so high. "I start with time goals, and they're nice to have. I'll take what I get with an attitude of gratitude."

slow to moderate pace is good for avoiding flare-ups and falls.

MUSCULAR DYSTROPHY (MD)

This is a group of hereditary diseases including Duchenne's MD, Becker's MD, and facioscapulo humeral MD, all of which primarily affect muscle cells.

Symptoms:
Gradual loss of muscle power, strength, and endurance. These contribute to a distorted gait in later stages.

ExRx:
Concentrate on muscular endurance and strengthening exercises but stop to rest if

DAVE Q

DIAGNOSIS: STROKE/MULTIPLE SCLEROSIS

In 1993, at the age of forty, former computer software engineer and now full-time social-change activist, Dave Q, began to experience weakness in his legs. During July 1994, he suffered a small stroke, followed by MS symptoms. By June 1995, he was in a wheelchair.

During that time, he began researching the disease and, one cool morning in June, he biked for one block. After a week, he managed the fifteen-minute ride to the local swimming pool. "Once I started swimming," he writes, "the rest was easy." Within one month, he was biking forty miles a day and had made what he calls his "99% recovery."

Exercise was just one part of Dave's recovery program. "I received no useful information from the two neurologists I saw, other than the original diagnosis of MS." Instead, he created his own. "I used a plan of exercises, diet, sunlight, stress reduction, and spiritual growth designed from reading 10,000 abstracts on Medline," he reports. (Medline is the computerized database of published medical articles.)

Now Dave bikes for transportation, not just exercise. He bikes an average of forty miles a day, and when he gets the chance, he swims and runs in about four feet of water for about a half-hour.

Dave also publishes a free newsletter entitled "Recovery" that he distributes via e-mail. He has also posted a site on the World Wide Web (http://www.netvoyage.net/~dave q) devoted to telling the story of his and others' recovery from MS.

Dave believes that an important part of his amazing recovery is that he created his own recovery program based on his own research. "Dozens have sent me stories indicating I've been a part of their recovery," he writes, "although the only ones as dramatic and complete as mine produced their recovery on their own."

Dave doesn't claim that recovery is easy. "Expect to make massive changes in your life," he writes. "Admit you caused your illness, and only you can cure it. Take any action to increase your overall health, however improbable it might seem, on the theory that the body will heal itself if given the proper tools."

excessive fatigue or muscular cramping occurs. MD patients can conquer a physical challenge as part of building up their self-esteem.

MYASTHENIA GRAVIS

Sporadic weakness and abnormal fatigue of skeletal muscles worsened by exercise and repeated movements. Also affects face, lips, tongue, throat, and neck.

Symptoms:
Symptoms wax and wane. Muscles can be strong in the morning, then weaken in the course of the day and after exercise. First signs are uncoordinated gait, numbness, tingling, and visual impairment.

ExRx:
Avoid strenuous exercise and activities that cause accidental injury. Frequent rest, shallow breathing, small movements, rather than large ones can all help. Organize your activity and rest periods around high and low energy peaks. Exercise that distributes the work load over many muscle groups at once is a better choice than those that stress only one muscle group at a time.

PARKINSON'S DISEASE

Progressive muscle rigidity and involuntary tremors. Affects slightly more men (usually over age 50) than women.

Symptoms:
Often starts with finger tremor (pill-roll tremor), then muscle rigidity, tremors, walking difficulty, drooling, loss of posture control, difficulty in eating, swallowing and speaking, and lack of coordination. Tremors increase during periods of stress or anxiety, but decrease during sleep and purposeful movement.

ExRx:
Hand-eye coordination exercise, standing balancing exercise, walking techniques, facial, posture, breathing, balance, and eating exercise. Parkinson's patients benefit most from slow motion, ROMs, and circulatory exercises (see illustration of Parkinson's Rehab Exercise, p. 268.) which helps them to gain movement control and avoid falls. Use seated arm and leg cycling to maintain and improve aerobic endurance capacity. Use short bouts of exercise, for example, walking twenty to thirty yards or cycling one to seven minutes following brief rest and up to sixty minutes a session, three to six times per week. Practice strengthening and stretching exercises of arms, shoulders, legs, and hips using light weights three sessions per week. Slowly increase duration of each approximately every four weeks.

The gradual loss of balance and muscle control that characterizes Parkinson's disease is helped by balancing, posture, and ROM exercises, in addition to low-impact, continuous motion exercises such as walking in place. These will help the patient become stronger, more flexible, and more coordinated in handling such everyday movements as personal care, eating, sitting, and standing. Depending on the progress of the disease, patients can practice the MuSkel Rx preventive program for slight tremors (one to two years), the therapeutic program for moderate tremors (three to five years), and the rehab program, under a care giver's supervision, for severe tremors.

PERIPHERAL NERVE DEGENERATION

Degeneration of nerves at extremities caused by severe infection and alcoholism. Usually occuring between ages thirty and fifty with a slow onset.

Symptoms:
Muscle weakness, tenderness, and painful to touch; also sensory loss and diminished deep tendon reflexes. This is usually compensated by muscle overuse. There are also pains of varying intensities.

ExRx:
Use rehabilitation exercises for habit retraining. Counteract physical symptoms of muscle weakness with strength exercises, and offset the sensory loss with balance exercise.

BILL SANDGRUND

DIAGNOSIS: PARKINSON'S DISEASE

Bill Sandgrund, eighty, was diagnosed for Parkinson's disease seven years ago. His posture had become disturbingly stooped and the entire stride of his walk seemed to have changed. In order to identify these symptoms, Mr. Sandgrund decided to go to a neurologist and take a number of tests. The tests pointed to Parkinson's. He remembers his initial reaction to the news as painful, "You go into a kind of depression—the more you hear, the worse it feels."

But in spite of his depression, Mr. Sandgrund tried to find out every possible piece of information both about the disease and its treatment. He was prescribed to take to kinds of medication: sinemet and eldepryl; both of them help to increase the dopamine in the basal ganglia. Believing that even such an incurable condition as Parkinson's could be controlled, Mr. Sandgrund's doctor suggested he exercise systematically. Exercise cannot cure Parkinson's, but it can slow down its development. "Knowing I had Parkinson's was helpful," says Mr. Sandgrund. "I realized that I could do something to directly slow it down."

Mr. Sandgrund agrees with his physical therapist that although many people who don't have Parkinson's think of it mainly as of the tremor disease, tremor is not the greatest danger. In reality, a far more dangerous result of Parkinson's disease is that it makes the person who has it very rigid and stiff. The rigidity of the internal muscles can cause constipation and vulnerability to pneumonia and other lung diseases. The rigidity of the external muscles results in difficulty in the simplest everyday physical activities, such as getting up, getting dressed, and taking a shower.

Unfortunately, medications alone are not enough to prevent the growing rigidity. It is, therefore, crucial that the people diagnosed with Parkinson's disease exercise their muscles. "Fortunately," Mr. Sandgrund tells us, "I was always a very athletic man, an exercise person; I am eighty, and I have been playing ball till six months ago when my coordination got worse." In addition to this type of general exercise, Mr. Sandgrund is a practitioner of the Feldenkrais Method.

Dr. Dolphin, one of the major practitioners and advocates of this method, notes that among the hardest things about Parkinson's is the initialization of a movement. Feldenkrais Method allows a patient with Parkinson's to battle this condition because this method is built on the idea of unity of body and mind. It carefully explores the smallest and simplest parts of each movement through a series of commands given by the instructor.

Mr. Sandgrund says that Feldenkrais Method allows him to become aware of the muscle work that goes on in his body. "You are not exerting your body, but at the same time your muscles are in motion." Most of the exercises are quite simple. You can be sitting on your chair, pressing your heels hard into the floor. This immediately starts the tension in the muscles of your thighs. Keep pressing and releasing slowly, letting your mind go into each region of the tension, exploring a feeling, trying to understand how to initiate it on your own. Repeat this exercise several times with both heels and then try it with left or right heel, respectively. Do it about a dozen times. But the important thing is to think about what you do and how you do it. "Do it slowly: give your mind a chance to pick up your body's movements," instructs Mr. Sandgrund.

Here is another exercise can be done either sitting or standing. Your hands are touching, arms in a lotus position. Slowly, at a 30- to 40-degree angle, you begin lifting them until they meet again above your head. Next, slowly lift your head to look at how the fingers touch. Then start bringing your arms down again. "Do it slowly, feel each muscle. As you are doing it, your mind concentrates on the motion," says Mr. Sandgrund.

"For example, I have just noticed that while my toes are on the ground, my heel is up. This is typical for Parkinson's. I don't notice it until it becomes a bit painful. But even though I am not aware of my heel coming up, I can bring it down," Mr. Sandgrund tells me. This is an issue of voluntary muscles acting involuntarily. And that's why the Feldenkrais Method is so important: "It teaches you to exercise a muscle control."

And although the change in a patient's actual condition might be minimal, the Method develops awareness and enables the patient to initiate a movement. This, in turn, prevents muscle rigidity.

Another value of the Feldenkrais Method concerns the process of adjustment to Parkinson's: "Adjustment is very hard for anyone: young and old," says Mr. Sandgrund. "The Feldenkrais Method helps you to adjust; its prime function is to adjust to the new, disturbing condition."

Mr. Sandgrund says that medication makes up 60% of his treatment while the remaining 40% is exercise. He practices the Feldenkrais Method five days a week and goes to the YMHA gym twice a week. "My objection is to taking too many pills. My doctor agrees and says to 'take as low dosage of pills as possible'." Mr. Sandgrund continues to battle the disease with astonishing and inspiring determination and advises other Parkinson's sufferers to consult a physical therapist, to read Feldenkrais's *Awareness Through Movement,* and to exercise as much as they possibly can.

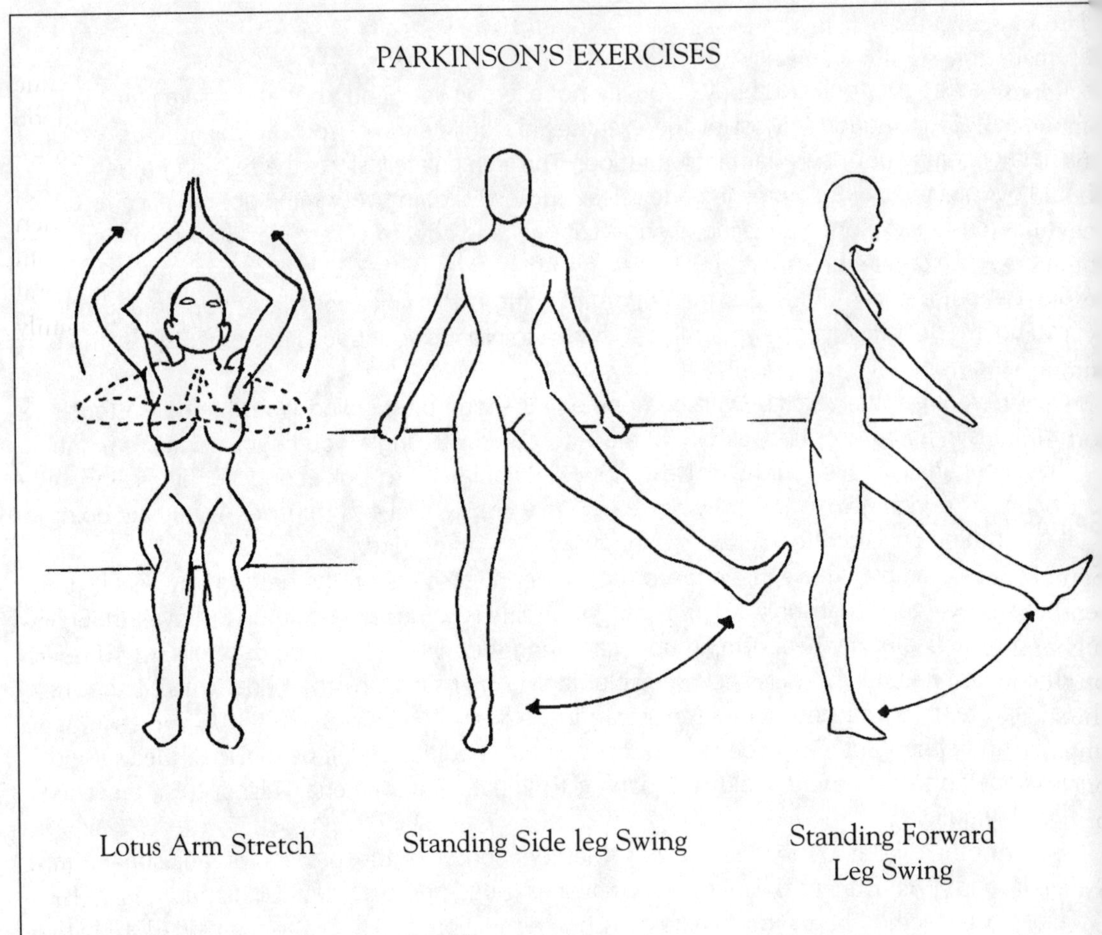

POLIO AND POST-POLIO SYNDROME

This is a severe viral disease that attacks the motor neurons causing paralysis and atrophy of certain muscles. Post-polio syndrome (PPS) is a later recurrence of the symptoms that causes additional muscle weakness.

Symptoms:
Fatigue, weakness, and pain.

ExRx:
For maximum cardiovascular benefits, use four-limb ergometry: arm crank, bicycle pedals, and water exercise. Practice strengthening exercises in the seated or lying down positions as needed. Fasten one or more limbs to ergometer pedals or cranks. If necessary, minimize the use of the painful limb, letting other limbs get as much exercise as possible. Support your joints with braces or splints where the surrounding muscles have been weakened. Practice intermittent exercise to minimize damage to joints and muscles. Do aerobic and strengthening exercises on alternating days. Do five sessions a week of stretching exercises, which will help prevent contractures and alle-

iate muscular tension in the lower back and hips caused by walking with an impaired gait. Water exercise in warm water is especially recommended for PPS, as are gentle stretching and low-intensity aerobic exercise. Beginners should do aerobic exercises at 40 to 70% of maximum heart-training rate in two- to four-minute intervals of up to twenty minutes per session. Intermediates should build up gradually to twenty-five-minute sessions with five-minute intervals, three sessions per week. If you already exercise regularly, do thirty- to forty-minute sessions without rest.

SPINAL CORD SEVERANCE INJURIES

Spinal cord injuries can impair the motor and sensory functions of the trunk or limbs. The higher the placement of the spinal cord injury on the lower back up to the neck, the greater the degree of damage done by the injury, impairing arms, legs, trunk, and pelvic organs. Patients are often wheelchair-bound or need crutches.

Symptoms:
Loss of arm and/or leg muscular control and muscle weakness, for example bladder functions and loss of organ control.

ExRx:
Prevent overusing muscles and joints of the upper body by varying exercises from week to week. Alternate arm cranking, swimming, wheelchair propulsion, and walking with crutches or braces. Strengthen and stretch the upper body muscle groups on alternate days as follows: day 1—upper back and back of shoulders; day 2—chest and front shoulders. Develop arm muscle endurance to achieve aerobic heart-training rate of 50 to 80% of maximum heart-training rate.

STROKE (CEREBROVASCULAR ACCIDENT)

Predisposed risks include: transient ischemic attacks, hardening of the arteries, high blood pressure, irregular heartbeat, electrocardiogram changes, rheumatic heart disease, diabetes, gout, decreased blood pressure when rising or standing, enlarged heart, high serum triglyceride levels, lack of exercise, use of oral contraceptives, cigarette smoking, and family history of stroke.

Symptoms:
Headache, neck or nape of neck rigidity, and paralysis.

ExRx:
The best prevention against strokes is accomplished by maintaining better arterial health through lifelong aerobic exercise. Rehabilitation is achieved through a variety of exercises, including posture and balance exercises, massage of paralyzed limbs, ROMs, strengthening nonaffected body areas to make them supporters of the damaged limbs, exercising the unaffected side (left vs. right or vice versa), walking, and speech pathology. Doctors and therapists will also add a variety of specific assisted and/or unassisted exercise prescriptions for stroke rehabilitations.

Preventing a stroke is the job of Cardio Rx; providing therapy and rehabilitation from the damage caused by a stroke is the job of the Age Rx program and the MuSkel Rx program. Stroke prevention not only includes exercise but also involves managing the risk factors that can lead to the disease, including high blood pressure, diabetes, and poor arterial system health. Therapeutic exercise for a post-stroke patient incorporates strengthening, stretching, and ROM exercises that will bring feeling, function, and coordination back to

EVELYN KATZ

DIAGNOSIS: SPINAL STENOSIS

Evelyn Katz's spinal stenosis caused problems that reached further than the compressed nerves in her spine. Evelyn's condition caused five falls in a six-month period. She received severe bruising in these falls. Once, she landed on her eye. Another time, she broke her arm, and another, her nose. All these injuries caused traumatic arthritis.

Evelyn, an economist and financial advisor, began using a walker out of fear of falling. Her ankles became weak, and she soon had to take taxis for her eight-minute walk to work. Her difficulty in getting around also forced her to drop some extracurricular classes she had been taking. Stenosis was also damaging nerves in her left knee.

Any change in her body caused pain. "Getting up was the worst," she says. The only relief she got was when sitting down. Evelyn also had balance problems. When she first came in for therapy, she was unable to balance on one foot.

Evelyn had never been an athlete, but she had led an active life before the stenosis and the subsequent falls, participating in such activities as walking and swimming. Evelyn began seeing Evelyn Ordman of Joint Effort Physical Therapy. She went to Joint Effort for four months, twice a week. Ordman prescribed a series of exercises for Evelyn to do twice a day. One of the main focuses was pelvic tilt exercises, which are, today, somewhat obsolete as a single movement exercise.

The pelvic tilt exercises were a huge factor in her recovery, "They helped my back," Evelyn says. One pelvic tilt that Evelyn practiced is done as follows: lie on your back with bent knees. Tighten your abdominal muscles, squeeze your buttocks muscles, flatten your back to the ground, and hold for five seconds. Exercises such as this strengthen the abdominals. An

numb and paralyzed limbs. Rehabilitative exercise will involve a care giver or occupational therapist who will guide the patients through the exercises to help them recover what function they can, and to show them how to exercise the unaffected areas. (Also see head injury, p. 261.)

NECK AND HEAD DISEASES, DISORDERS, AND INJURIES RX

The head and neck area are perhaps the most vulnerable of all body areas to injuries and disorders that affect both balance and mobility. The exercises that help this body area are posture, balancing, breathing, stretching, and strengthening exercises. The symptoms that predominate this area range from such extreme symptoms as paralysis, dizziness, nausea, and headaches to those that are more moderate like clumsiness and lack of coordination and control.

CONCUSSION

Blow to head, less serious than brain contusions (bruises) and lacerations (tears).

upright pelvic tilt exercise begins by standing in a normal, correct posture, then bending the knees slightly, while tightening the abdominal muscles, squeezing the buttocks muscles, and flattening the back by rolling out the small of the back. This takes pressure off of irritated nerve roots.

Evelyn's therapy also included leg lifts, often done with a Theraband (an exercise band made of rubber strips or tubing; the thicker the band the greater the resistance offered) for added resistance. Sit-ups and ankle exercises done with a Theraband wrapped around the leg of a chair were two more of her main activities.

For strength and balance, Evelyn began walking again. The treadmill was not only a cardio workout, but it improved her balance. Also, for the balance problem, Evelyn did such exercises as holding on to a bar, standing on one foot, letting go of the bar, then switching feet. Evelyn also began using an exercise bike that had arm cranks.

Evelyn was given simple exercises with weights when arthritis in her right elbow joint began causing her pain. With a light weight (e.g. one to two pounds), Evelyn lifts and straightens her arms repeatedly.

After six weeks of therapy, Evelyn had gone from using a walker for any movement whatsoever to the occasional use of a cane. Now, she says she uses the cane rarely.

Having gained some weight during her illness, Evelyn has joined a health club and exercises three to four times a week. She walks generally three to four miles to keep up the strength in her legs and ankles. She also bikes, but her health club doesn't have a bike with an arm rotator, which helped her so much at Joint Effort Physical Therapy. She also plans to begin swimming again soon.

Evelyn is not cured of spinal stenosis, but she is cured of the disabling back pain she once had. Of her recovery, she says, "My doctor was impressed. Everyone was."

Symptoms:
Brief loss of consciousness, trouble recalling, irritability, sluggishness, dizziness, nausea, anxiety, headache, and fatigue.

ExRx:
Relaxation for twenty-four hours, gradually resuming activities. Slow-motion exercises and ROMs—start in prone position and graduate to seated and standing positions. Rehab head and neck area very carefully, with any rehab exercise program monitored by a doctor.

HERNIATED DISK (ACUTE CERVICAL DISK DISEASE)

Spinal disk breaks up and fragments impinge on nerves. Caused by contact injury or degeneration with age. There is danger of permanent arm weakness if there is too much nerve impingement. This injury should first be evaluated by a physician.

Symptoms:
Arm and neck pain on one or both sides, slow reflexes, pins and needles, numbness.

ExRx:
Depends on severity, therapy ranges from medication and muscle relaxants to soft collar, cervical traction, and surgery. Stretching and strengthening, proper posture techniques, and avoiding contact sports are good preventive actions. (To rehab lower back, see pp. 284–285, 289–293; to rehab neck, use head and neck Rx exercises, pp 278–280.)

BRIAN PHILLIPS

DIAGNOSIS: BROKEN NECK

You *can* come back from the dead. Just ask Brian Phillips.

Brian, a college student, dove into a pool six years ago and broke his neck, but that was the least of his troubles. At the time, he also drowned and was legally dead. His lungs were filled with water, and he had no pulse. Luckily for him, his girlfriend knew CPR and revived him.

Brian is a C6 quadriplegic. (See illustration, p. 274) After his accident, he had no movement from the neck down, but soon he began to regain some residual movement. For the first month, he couldn't do anything for himself. He says that he was somewhat depressed, but he considers himself "fortunate to be a very motivated person."

During this time period, while still in his hospital bed, his surgeon came to see him. At the time, breathing was just about the only thing Brian could do on his own. The surgeon said, "The way you are right now is the way you're going to be for the rest of your life."

Brian spent four years in outpatient rehab. The beginning of the rehab consisted of daily stretching and ROM exercises. Weight lifting was another essential element. Brian was very dedicated and spent three to four days per week, three to four hours per day on this rehab routine, although he adds, "Some days are better than others. Some days the spasms that I have are so bad, I can't range without help." He is very loyal to his routine mainly in case "they ever come up with a cure." Brian wants to be in top shape to take full advantage of a such an occurrence, if it should ever happen.

Brian has had a lot of success with his mobility. He can now ambulate with a walker, which is different than functionally walking, but it means he goes on walks every day from ten minutes up to an hour. "I can do just about everything everyone else can do," he says. Luckily, at the moment of his accident, the damage to his spine was not all permanent, some of the injury was swelling and bruising. Standing is one of Brian's favorite things. He says it's "good for you."

Brian was a runner and played soccer prior to the accident. After the accident, Brian became interested in wheelchair racing. He has been in five races already and says he does one every two weeks in the summertime. "There's a lot of technique to it," he states.

Brian says that many people find it hard to dig up the strength to try to do things for themselves. "[It's] easy to let someone else do things for you." Brian prefers the hard way.

NECK SPRAIN (WHIPLASH)

Overstretching or tearing of ligaments that link spinal vertebrae.

Symptoms:
Pain on one side of neck, muscle spasm, and neck stiffness.

ExRx:
Rehab with neck and head exercises, pp. 278–279.

NERVE STRETCH SYNDROME

Forceful sideways bending resulting in stinging or burning sensation at back of neck or shoulder. Usually caused by impact forces in such sports as football and wrestling. Permanent nerve damage can result.

Symptoms:
Burning and/or stinging.

ExRx:
Neck muscle exercises, and padded neck protection. Over-the-counter anti-inflammatories and ice packs are also effective.

SPINAL INJURIES

Neck or head injury, resulting in contusions and compression of spine.

Symptoms:
Muscle spasm, radiated pain, numbness, tingling, quadriplegia (paralysis of limbs), dysreflexia, excessive nervous system activity long after spinal cord injury, irregular urination and bowel movements, skin itching or burning.

ExRx:
After ten to twelve weeks of stabilizing the fracture, begin posture training in the prone position and progress to seated, then to standing. Also begin back-strengthening exercises; a back brace or corset may also be necessary to support the back while walking or exercising.

NECK AND HEAD INJURY EXERCISES

NECK INJURY PREVENTION

Do at least one set of neck stretching and strengthening exercises (e.g. forward and side to side rotation) prior to your workout. If you practice a sport in which your neck is under constant stress (e.g. football, sailing, driving) do two or more sets a day to increase strength and flexibility.

NECK INJURY THERAPY

With diseases or injuries that do not require surgery or neck immobilization, neck ROM exercises should start as soon as pain and swelling go down (usually twenty-four to forty-eight hours after being injured). Neck therapy and rehab promotes blood flow to the area which, in turn, speeds the healing process. It also relieves stiffness and prevents muscle atrophy and tightening.

NECK INJURY REHABILITATION

With surgery or immobilization, neck ROMs can start as early as five days after surgery. Remove neck braces for exercise. Especially after a severe injury, your therapist may at first use passive-assisted exercise, moving your neck through all allowable ranges of motion. Later, your therapist will go to active-assisted exercises helping you use your own strength to move your neck.

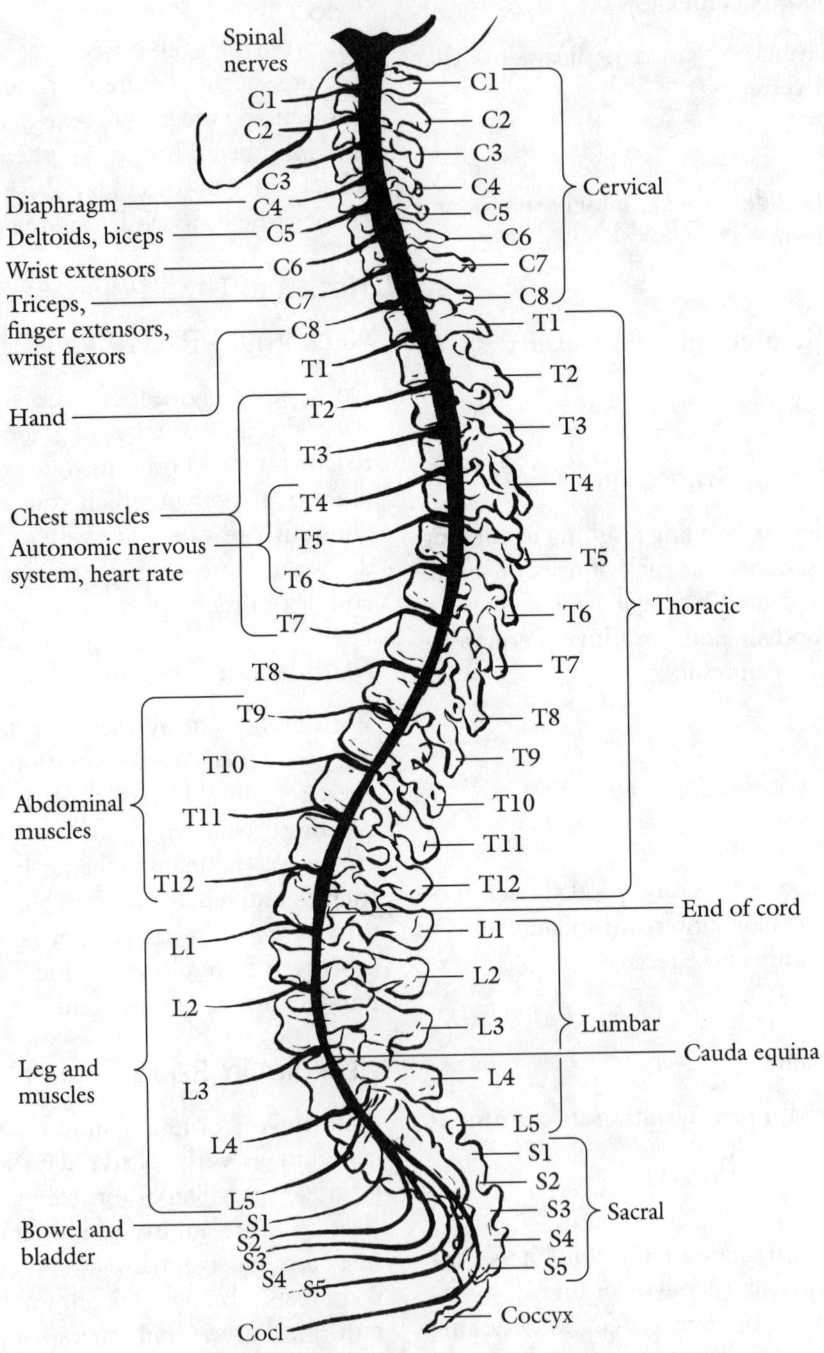

Spinal Column

GENERAL REHABILITATION GUIDELINES AND PROCEDURES

PHASE I: FOR ACUTE INJURIES

1. After surgery, the physical therapist will use either active or passive-assisted exercise. Passive will consist of four to six major range of moving the injured body area in the four ranges of motion: flexion, extension, supination, and pronation.

2. After you are able to move the injured area unassisted, the physical therapist will supervise unassisted ROMs and then isometric exercises on the muscles that are connected to the injured body area.

PHASE II: FOR MODERATE TO SEVERE INJURIES

1. When you are able to move the injured body area and you can do isometric exercises with your own strength and without undue pain, begin Phase II exercises.

2. Phase II exercises (bend/extend, flexion) are those that let you bend and strengthen the body area through the full range of its motion.

PHASE III: FOR MILD INJURIES

These involve dynamic exercises to strengthen muscles as well as stretch them through a full range of motion. They also involve regaining balance and motor-sensory pronation. After this phase is completed, you may begin the three levels of preventive and conditioning exercises in Part Two.

WEIGHT-LOADING EXERCISES

The amount of weight that you add depends on your own body weight and on your muscle strength and size. Here are the general guidelines. In general, do not use any weights until your doctor or physical therapist says that it is okay. Weight-loading exercises can then be added in Phase II and III of the rehab schedule.

WEIGHT LOAD/REPETITION SCHEDULE

	LOAD	REPETITIONS
Phase I	No weight	determined by MD or PT
Phase II	See schedule	1–5
Phase III	See schedule	6–12

WEIGHT-LOADING SCHEDULE

USE FOR PHASES II AND III

TYPE OF WEIGHT	AMOUNT OF WEIGHT SMALL FRAME	MEDIUM FRAME	LARGE FRAME
Hand-held	0–¼ lbs.	¼–½ lbs.	½–1 lbs.
Ankle	0–½ lbs.	½–1 lbs.	1–5 lbs.

NECK AND HEAD REHAB EXERCISES

Use Phase I Neck and Head Rehab exercises for severe injuries or for rehabilitation after surgery. Practice Phase II Neck and Head Rehab exer-

AMY SCARAMUZZINO

DIAGNOSIS: PARALYSIS

Amy Scaramuzzino, now thirty-one, suffered a T5 and T6 paralysis (paralysis of the body measured from the thoracic vertebrae T5 and T6; see figure 13.2) during a car accident in December of 1991. At the time of the accident, she was driving drunk and not wearing a seatbelt. Amy had surgery three days after the accident. Harrington rods were put in her back, and her spine was fused from T2 to T7. She spent four months as an inpatient—the first two of which she spent in a hard, shoulder-to-pelvis cast. Amy began a twice-a-day physical therapy regimen, and she also worked once a day with an occupational therapist. After such a trauma, Amy's upper body strength was slim to none. Amy had no sensation in her limbs, except for that of hot and cold.

As a paraplegic, Amy still had use of her arms. She began working on her upper body (mainly her hand grip and arms) by weight lifting. She worked her way up the weight scale little by little. Amy also began using the arm pedaling machine, which simulates a bicycle. Another part of her workout involved wearing weights on her arms while doing exercises. Playing catch was another exercise prescription her physical therapist gave her.

Floor exercises on a mat taught her how to roll over and crawl. Her therapist would also add resistance by holding her ankles as Amy tried to crawl away. Balance problems also came along with Amy's injury. To work on that, Amy sat on a large rubber ball and tried not to fall off. "It was very difficult," she explains. This balance exercise also helped her regain some trunk and abdominal muscles that were missing because of the location of the spinal injury—her neck area. A standing frame helped with spasticity in Amy's legs and lower back. "Plus, it felt great to stand," Amy says.

The outpatient program was similar to the inpatient program. Amy continued to lift weights and use the arm pedaling machine, but she also began to practice the kind of activities she needed to be independent. One of the most important and most difficult was learning the floor-to-chair transfer. In case of an emergency, Amy also wanted to learn how to go down stairs in her wheelchair, since she lives on the third floor of her building. She explains that the stairs process is achieved by going backward, lowering yourself down step-by-step, and that it takes a lot of upper body strength.

cises for moderate to mild injuries or for severe injuries or postsurgery, when you can do Phase I exercises without pain or assistance. Start Phase III Neck and Head Therapeutic exercises when you can do Phase II without pain or difficulty. Start at Phase III for mild neck injury rehab.

PHASE I SEVERE NECK AND HEAD INJURIES (POSTSURGERY THERAPIST-ASSISTED ROMS)

Within the limits of your injury, you will work on the four directions of motion of your neck:

One of the side effects of Amy's surgery was, in fact, caused by a medical mistake. The Harrington rods put into her body were too long, and actually protruded from her skin. This caused a lot of pain and emotional depression. Therefore, in February of 1993, Amy had the rods surgically removed, and so began another recovery. Although this did not entirely regress Amy's rehabilitation, it was several leaps backward.

During outpatient rehab from this second surgery, Amy went to a different rehab center, which lacked the free weights and the standing frame. It did, however, have a set of parallel bars. Amy was placed in "Frankenstein" leg braces and put between the parallel bars to stand. To everyone's amazement, Amy began to move. She hopped up and down the parallel bars in her braces. Amy was switched to a walker, then a wheeled walker. She spent a year building her endurance at walking. She often walked "the circle," that is, the corridors at the rehab clinic. She sometimes walked outside but had difficulty because of the uneven ground. At home and in front of her house, she walked with her walker and full leg braces. She even walks around the CBS parking lot, which is near her home.

Now that Amy has experience ambulating, she has taken up other exercise activities. She bought a "sit-ski" and has taken up water skiing. She goes canoeing and camping in the summertime and has recently taken to indoor rock climbing. She also bird-watches twice a week. Amy says that it takes a lot of energy, because she has to walk all over the place following her "prey."

Amy was an athlete before the accident turned her into a paraplegic. She went to college on a basketball scholarship, where she also swam and lifted weights. Recreationally, between college and her accident, she played tennis and cycled. She describes herself as a very active young adult. "I had a motorcycle," she states.

Amy also spent ten years studying ballet, to which she attributes the fact that her muscles have not atrophied. Five years after losing the use of them, Amy still has muscles and tone in her legs.

Her sports background helps her these days. "I know how to push myself. I can take risks," she explains. These risks include going down the stairs in a wheelchair or rock climbing.

Today she says she is very independent and "as long as I'm independent, I'm happy. I'm really around."

forward flexion, lateral flexion (side bending), and rotation (turning your head, not circling). Severe injuries require active-assisted exercises; less severe, passive-assisted. Backward flexion is rarely used; if utilized, it should be done very gently with hand support.

PHASE II MODERATE NECK AND HEAD INJURIES ROMs

Head Tilts

- Sit or stand up straight; align your head properly over your shoulders

- Slowly tilt your head left, then back to center
- Slowly tilt your head right, then back to center
- Slowly tuck your chin into your neck
- Slowly tilt your head forward, then back to center
- Repeat five times, building up to fifteen; practice one to three sets, three times a day

Head Turn

- Sit or stand; align your head properly over your shoulders (your chin should be back with your jaw line, parallel to the ground)
- Slowly, turn your head toward your left shoulder; hold
- Return your head to the center position
- Turn your head toward your right shoulder blade; hold
- Return your head to the center position; be sure not to let your head tilt down, back, or sideways as your turn it
- Repeat these turns five times building up to fifteen; do one to three sets daily

Phase III Neck and Head Injuries Exercises

Supine Head Lift

- Lie on your back with proper prone alignment, arms resting by your sides
- Slowly lift your head and bend it forward until your chin touches your chest or you can see your feet; don't raise your shoulders or arms, keep them loose and relaxed; hold
- Slowly lower your head back down to the floor
- Repeat five times building up to fifteen; do one set a day building up to three

Prone Head Lift

- Lie face down
- Slowly lift your head up while looking down; hold
- Lower your head back down
- Repeat five times building up to fifteen; do one set a day building up to three

Side (Lateral) Head Lift

- Lie down on one side with your floor-side arm stretched out; bend your arm and cushion your head with your hand
- Place your other arm on the floor in front of your chest for balance
- Slowly lift your head up off your arm; hold
- Slowly lower your head back down
- Repeat five times, building up to between eight and fifteen repetitions
- Change sides and repeat
- Do one set a day, building up to three

Side (Lateral) Head Turn

- Lie on your left side, head resting on your outstretched left arm (i.e. the same position as the start of side (lateral) head lift, above)

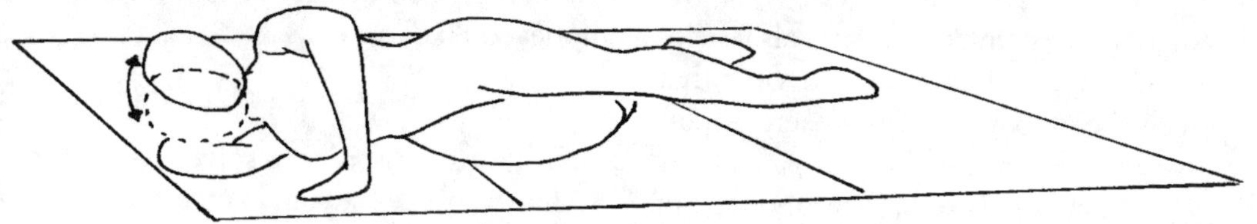

Side (Lateral) Head Lift

- Slowly raise your head so your right ear is moving toward your right shoulder
- Slowly turn your head to look at the ceiling; hold
- Slowly turn your head back down to look at the floor
- Repeat five times, building up to fifteen
- Change sides and repeat
- Do one set a day building up to three

PREVENTION AND CONDITIONING NECK AND HEAD EXERCISE

When your neck strength is at least 95% of its preinjury strength, move on to Prevention or Conditioning Exercises Level I in Part Two. Additionally, to prevent a neck injury or the recurrence of one, practice Levels I through III of the following neck prevention exercises:

Head and Neck Exercises, pp. 183–188

Face and jaw exercises, pp. 171–172

EAR DISEASES, DISORDERS, AND INJURIES RX

The ears help your body control its position and balance, especially during movement. Thus, similar to nervous system disorders, balancing exercises help restore balance and reduce the symptoms of dizziness and vertigo associated with ear disorders.

Earaches, dizziness, and hearing loss are the most common exercise-treatable symptoms. If the symptoms are too severe, medical treatment and bed rest must precede any exercise program. As part of therapy and rehabilitation, you should begin doing posture, balance, and ROM exercises. For severe symptoms, start with relaxation training exercises, pp. 244–248).

The ears, mouth, nose, and throat is a system of organs, muscles, and openings in the head and neck area, which share many of the same physical illness symptoms. Because the mouth, ears, and nose have openings, they are entryways for viruses and bacteria that enter the mucous membranes and cause them to become inflamed and swollen. Infections can spread through the three areas. Additionally, a disorder in one of these body areas usually affects the others. For example, dripping sinuses in the nasal area are associated with headaches, sore throats, and earaches. Exercise improves the circulation of blood and fluids working on the symptoms caused by the inflammation from infection and also helps reduce the amount of bacteria and virus that can attack these body areas. For exercise purposes, we include the ears here as part of the sensory and nervous system. The disorders of the nose and mouth, which involve breathing symptoms, are covered in Chapter Sixteen, Cardio Rx.

Hearing Losses and Deafness

Hearing loss is a condition that makes hearing and understanding speech difficult; deafness is a condition of being unable to hear. The causes include aging, hereditary factors, head trauma, and such diseases as encephalitis, measles, meningitis, Meniere's disease, mumps, and scarlet fever.

Symptoms:
A person with hearing loss or deafness may exhibit poor balance, along with depth perception and spatial-orientation difficulties. Also associated with these symptoms are hyperactivity and restlessness, which can contribute to low physical fitness, low self-image, and low self-confidence.

ExRx:
Posture and balancing exercises for special symptoms, along with a regular total exercise program to improve overall fitness.

Infectious Myringitis

Inflammation of the eardrum; middle ear infection.

Symptoms:

Severe ear pain, tenderness of mastoid, which is the bone behind the ear that is filled with a honeycomb of air cells.

ExRx:
Self-limiting disorder, resolves itself in three to fourteen days. Avoid exercises or activities during earaches. Practice proper posture holding of head, neck, and jaw. Also, use head lifting and turning exercise to rehab after pain subsides.

Meniere's Disease

Endolymph fluid pressure increases, causing pressure and symptoms. Dysfunction of labyrinth of inner ear, with hearing being affected. Onset at ages thirty to sixty, men slightly more than women. Multiple attacks cause residual hearing loss. Sudden violent attacks last for ten minutes to several hours.

Symptoms:
Fullness or blocked feeling in inner ear, dizziness, severe vertigo, hearing loss, ringing in ears (tinnitus).

ExRx:
Prescribed drugs, and eventually surgery. Relaxation and balancing exercises can help relieve symptoms.

Middle Ear Infection

A catch-all description of various types of infections, which are often preceded by upper respiratory infections. A history of air travel or scuba diving is often associated with this type of infection.

Symptoms:
Acute—dizziness, nausea; chronic—thickening and scarring of ear drum.

ExRx:
Antibiotics, decongestants, don't blow your nose, don't get your ears wet when in water. Choose exercise position (upright or prone) that reduces dizziness and earache during rehab period.

MOTION SICKNESS

Loss of equilibrium caused by irregular movements or motion (e.g. rocking of boat, plane, train, automobile).

Symptoms:
Nausea and vomiting, headache, dizziness, fatigue, and sweating.

ExRx:
Balancing exercises (see especially head balancing exercises), stretching exercises, head down stretches and relaxation exercises; learning to properly position body can help relieve symptoms.

AGE RX: LIST OF ADDITIONAL EAR DISEASES, DISORDERS, AND INJURIES BENEFITED BY HEAD AND NECK REHAB EXERCISES

- earaches and pains
- ear injuries
- inflammation of the mastoid
- labyrinthitis
- otosclerosis
- perforated eardrum
- swimmer's ear

SINUS INFECTION

Infection of the four pairs of air pockets that drain into the nose; caused by viruses, colds, or persistent bacterial infection.

Symptoms:
Stuffy, runny nose, facial pain, headache, and sore throat.

ExRx:
Mouth breathing until nose breathing becomes easier; regular aerobic exercise helps clear sinuses over the short term and may prevent recurrences by keeping fluids and blood flowing through the nasal area. (See also Cardio Rx for sinusitis, p. 420.)

EYE DISEASES, DISORDERS, AND INJURIES

Your eyes contain both muscles and blood vessels that respond to exercise prescriptions. The most common medical risks predisposing you to eye diseases and disorders are close-up eye work, high blood pressure, diabetes, age-related degeneration, and traumatic injuries. The most common symptoms are fatigue, blurred vision, and eye muscle and headache pain. Exercise can help many symptoms, especially eye fatigue and headache.

The best exercises to help slow down or prevent loss of vision are those that involve less strain on blood vessels such as easy, lifting exercises and those that promote continuous blood circulation to the head and neck area. To help prevent traumatic injury use protective glasses during ball playing and other sports (e.g. hiking) where sticks or protrusions may poke your eyes. If you have lost some or all of your vision, posture and balancing exercises can help improve your neuromotor control. You can also practice stationary forms of aerobic exercise such as stationary cycling and standing water exercises.

Eye exercises, as well as balancing exercises, can help strengthen weakened eye muscles.

Eye diseases and disorders that involve blurring or loss of vision include bulging eyes, cataracts, chalazion, crossed eyes, drooping eyelid, eye strain, extraocular motor nerve palsies, glaucoma, optic atrophy, detached retina, and vascular retinopathies.

Eye diseases and disorders that involve eye pain include corneal abrasion, corneal ulcer, glaucoma, inflammation of the cornea, conjunctivitis, hordeolum (stye), and uveitis.

Eye injuries that involve both pain and vision difficulties include black eye, corneal abrasion, detached retina, hyphema, and particles in the eye.

Age-Related Macular Degeneration

Atrophy of the disk near the center of the retina, resulting from hardening of the arteries of the retina. This causes 12 to 17% of blindness, especially among the elderly.

Symptoms:
Blank spot in the center of vision.

ExRx:
Low-vision optical aids, and laser photo coagulation surgery. Because this condition involves the arteries, exercise may slow down the artery hardening process and, therefore, the disease itself.

Eye Strain

Overuse of three different sets of eye muscles: ciliary (focusing), eye movement muscles (point and turn eyes), and eyelid muscles (blinking and squinting). Affects 75% of those who work in front of computer screens; also caused by intense close-up work, e.g. editors, proofreaders, accountants. The ciliar[y] muscles can hold one position causing fatigu[e] and stress.

Symptoms:
Blurry or double vision.

ExRx:
Use well-lighted work space, free from glare[.] Practice blinking exercises.

Glaucoma

Caused by a fluid in front of the eye (calle[d] "aqueous humor") that doesn't drain properly[,] resulting in high internal pressure (intraocular hypertension) causing optic nerve damag[e] and vision loss. This is the leading cause o[f] blindness. Affects 2% of the population ove[r] age forty, and accounts for 12% of new blindness. African Americans have the highes[t] rates of glaucoma. With early treatment[,] prognosis is good.

Symptoms:
Chronic—progresses gradually with mildl[y] aching eyes, leads to eye inflammation, pain[,] pressure, and nausea.

ExRx:
Drug therapy and laser surgery. Studies show that vigorous cardio exercise such as cycling helps reduce intraocular hypertension, providing a therapeutic effect similar to drug[s] prescribed for this purpose.

Vascular Retinopathies

Poor blood supply or blockage through retina[l] arteries and veins; causes include high bloo[d] pressure, diabetes, glaucoma, and atherosclerosis. Onset mostly in the elderly; withou[t] treatment, 50% have complete vision loss within five years. There are five types of retinopathy: (1) sickle cell, (2) central vein occlusion, (3) central artery occlusion, (4) diabetic, and (5) hypertensive.

Symptoms:
Poor vision.

ExRx:
Posture and balancing exercises help compensate for imbalances caused by loss of vision. Preventive treatment should be accompanied by a cardio exercise therapy program aimed at controlling high blood pressure. For the nonproliferative diabetic (i.e. diabetics who do not have a lot of peripheral circulatory problems in their legs), controlling blood sugar levels may delay onset or reduce severity later. Hypertensives can control blood pressure with medications, exercise, and diet. Central retinal artery occlusion may benefit from medications and eyeball massage.

AGE RX: LIST OF ADDITIONAL EYE DISEASES, DISORDERS, AND INJURIES BENEFITED BY EYE EXERCISES AND NECK REHAB EXERCISES

- cataract
- chalazion
- extraocular motor nerve palsies
- inflammation of the cornea
- motor nerve palsy

EYE EXERCISES

Blinking Exercise

This exercise stimulates the flow of fresh blood into eye muscles as well as increasing the lubrication of dry eyeballs. Repeat blinks by slowly opening and closing your eyelids, squeezing the lids together as you close them; hold that closed position for one to two seconds.

Focusing Exercise

Place your left hand one foot in front of your left eye and your right hand extended out three feet from your right eye. Look out a window at an object, for example a tree or a lamppost, which is more than fifty feet away. The outside object should be seen between your outstretched hands. Now, alternate looking at close and extended hands and the far-off object. Hold each focus for one to two seconds. Practice changing from near to farther to faraway eye focus, for five to twelve repetitions.

Pointing Exercise

With your upper body erect and your head centered over your shoulders, look straight ahead. Imagine you are looking at a giant clock whose circumference or face outlines your field of vision. You see the center of the clock when you look straight ahead. Without moving your head, turn your eyes upward and point them at the 12, 3, 6, and 9 o'clock positions, remaining one to two seconds in each spot.

LOWER BACK INJURIES RX

A majority of Americans (60 to 80%) have lower back pain at some time during their lives; 1 to 5% are disabled by it.

Protecting your back from injury and degeneration should be one of your top health priorities because as soon as your back goes, you can become further disabled from back pain. Inactivity caused by back pain can lead to the breakdown of other body areas and systems. You must exercise your back and abdominal muscles, and practice good posture and body mechanics when standing, walking, lifting, sitting, lying down, and especially when exercising and playing sports.

Paradoxically, however, you can also damage your back by overexercising it. Overuse back injuries can be caused by repetitive forward and backward bending and aggravated by anatomical abnormalities and muscle imbalances. For example, strong quadriceps and weak hamstrings can cause runners to experience lower back stress and pain unless they can balance out their exercise program. Many nonathletes have weak abdominal muscles that can also cause the pelvis to tilt out of proper alignment.

Preventing Lower Back Injuries with Posture Training

Posture refers not only to how you hold your body in the three static positions of sitting, standing, and lying down, but also to how you adapt these correct positions to everyday movements and situations. The following three sections will help you to achieve better posture in your common daily activities.

Standing, Walking, and Lifting Postures

1. Avoid standing still for long periods. If you must, alternate by leaning on one foot, then the other, while slightly bending your knees. You can also walk in place or do heel-toe rolls (see p. 177) to keep the blood circulating through your legs as you pump with your calf muscle. When standing and working, put one foot up on a stool or riser to take the pressure off your lower back.

2. Whenever you're standing or walking, keep your lower back as flat as possible. Squeeze your buttocks and pull in (brace) your stomach muscles. Hold your shoulders slightly back. Chest breathing enables you to hold this position for many minutes, even through all the hours you have to spend standing in movie and checkout lines every day.

3. Keep your knees slightly bent when standing and leaning over something—locked knees cut off blood circulation. Slightly bent knees allow your blood to better circulate to and from your lower legs.

4. Avoid bending over to pick up things. Instead, sink or squat straight down and keep your back straight. Keep the object close to your body as you lift it. Pivot on your feet to turn your whole body instead of twisting your body to turn while carrying a heavy object. If you have a bad knee, bend your healthy knee and brace yourself with one hand. (i.e. sink down with your weight over your healthy knee only.)

5. When starting to walk or turn, move your feet first, then turn your body in the direction of travel. To avoid tripping or falling, look at the terrain in front of you.

6. When walking, standing, or running let your arms hang loosely by your sides, with your elbows slightly bent. Keep your hands in front of your body—rather than

behind—and lean slightly forward to avoid arching your back.

SITTING AND DRIVING

1. Do not sit or drive for prolonged periods without a lower back support and without occasionally getting up and walking around or stretching your muscles.
2. Sit with your lower back flat or slightly convex (bent forward, meaning extended with a curve in the neutral position). Your shoulders should be slightly pulled back and not hunched over. Keep your knees higher than your hips by using a foot stool or pulling the car seat closer to the steering wheel.
3. Center your head, with your ears aligned over your shoulder joints. Keep your chin tucked back into your neck and chin line parallel to the ground.
4. Sit with your knees bent and your feet about hip-width to shoulder-width apart. Sitting for long periods with your legs crossed puts extra strain on your hip joints; sitting with your legs straightened puts strain on your lower back.
5. Sit in hard-backed rather than soft-backed chairs. Change your position from time to time when sitting for prolonged periods. For example, sit with your back against the chair, then sit forward with your back erect for some time. Avoid leaning forward more than a 5- to 15-degree angle. When working at a desk, pull the chair up so that you don't have to lean over too far. Stand up and walk around if you catch yourself slouching. Also, too much twisting and turning can strain your lower back. When you feel yourself jutting out or slouching too far forward or too far back, correct this bad posture by becoming more erect, putting your shoulders back, and tucking in your chin, buttocks, and abdomen.
6. For driving, add a flat back rest to support your lower back and keep the seat upright—no lounging.

LYING DOWN POSTURES

1. Exercise in the prone position (lying down), and sleep on flat, firm mats and mattresses. If you wake up with a sore neck, hip, or back, do not sleep on your stomach or put a pillow under your ankles because it makes you overarch your back for long periods of time. Sleep, instead, on your side with your knees bent and in front of your hips, and your arms in front of your body. To keep the pressure off your hips and lower back, place a small pillow between your knees to keep your legs hip-width apart. For the same purpose, if you are lying on your back, place the pillow under your knees.
2. Avoid overtwisting or turning your body from the prone position. Instead, bring your knees forward and roll over. Likewise, use your arms and stomach muscles to brace yourself as you draw your knees in and swing your legs over the side of the mat or bed when getting up.

ACUTE LOWER BACK INJURIES

These injuries are caused by falls, collisions, or sudden twists. Exercise therapy or rehabilitation cannot start until the patient has been stabilized and then only with permission of the treating physician.

Back Contusions

A bruise or muscle bleeding caused by direct impact from collision or fall.

Symptoms:
Local pain, tenderness, swelling.

ExRx:
Prevent this type of injury by not playing contact sports and avoiding falls or reducing their severity with a wider stance or foot placement. For mild injuries, practice Therapeutic exercise for a two-week period. For moderate injuries, start at Phase II Rehab with a recovery usually in four weeks. For severe injuries, recovery is usually in six weeks. Start Phase I Rehab, recovery in six weeks.

Back Muscle Strain or Back Ligament Sprain

An overstretching or tearing of the back muscles or ligaments caused by twisting, overbending, strenuous lifting, or any sport or activity that causes quick or powerful trunk rotations and lifts.

Symptoms:
Sudden, sharp pain, and later, tenderness, swelling, continuing severe pain and muscle spasm.

ExRx:
Prevent this type of injury by strengthening your back as well as your abdominal muscles. For severe injuries, start with Phase I Rehab within three weeks or with doctor's approval as soon as pain subsides. For moderate injuries, start with Phase II Rehab for one to two weeks. For mild injuries, practice Phase III, Therapeutic back exercises for three to five days.

Overuse Lower Back Injuries

Disk Disease

Disks slip and disk shells crack causing them to herniate or rupture. The pulpy center leaks out slowly or in a spurt putting pressure in the surrounding nerve roots. This usually occurs in people over the age of twenty; results from degeneration and compression of back vertebrae caused by pounding or lifting.

Symptoms:
Radiating pain, tingling, and numbness from lower back through buttocks to the toes. Legs may also give way from muscle weakness.

ExRx:
Slow down the degeneration with back-strengthening exercises and overall exercise. Walking is the best overall lower back exercise. Cardiovascular exercises also nourish the back area. When pain subsides, start back rehab exercise at Phase II or III. Postsurgery rehab exercises begin at Phase I and can continue up to three months or longer.

Mechanical Lower Back Pain (Backache)

No specific injury, but back pain caused by a combination of factors: poor posture, muscle strain or weakness, or previous injury, among

DOMINICK PERROTO

DIAGNOSIS: DEGENERATIVE DISKS

Disk degeneration usually hits after age forty, but some experience this back disorder prematurely. For example, in November of 1993, Dominick Perotto, a thirty-seven-year-old Federal Express employee, bent down one day at work and felt a pain in his back. As most people would, he thought he had merely pulled a muscle. That night, he went home, took a hot shower, and laid down in bed. He couldn't stand up again for over a week.

To move around his house, Dominick had to literally roll out of bed onto the floor and crawl on his hands and knees, pausing often for rest breaks, and holding on to the wall for stability. Unable to work and barely able to walk, he could only do so by sliding his feet across the ground. "I was in pretty bad shape," he explains. When, after a few weeks, he could drive his car to his doctor's office, Dominick was given a CAT scan, which showed bulging disks, then an MRI, which showed he had two herniated disks. His doctors were discussing surgery, but then decided he did not need it. He was told to go into physical therapy. Dominick told them, "I'll do anything it takes to get me back in shape."

Right away, physical therapist Elaine Rosen put heat packs on Dominick's lower back and started him on an exercise routine. The routine consisted of Dominick starting on the treadmill for two minutes, then going straight to the bike for two minutes, and next switching to a pull-down machine for his lateral muscles. After using those machines, Dominick's exercise routine continued with such exercises as sitting on a beach ball-type object, then picking up one leg at a time and trying to balance. Another balance exercise he performed was standing on a round disc, which he compares to a garbage can lid with ball bearings underneath. The trick was to find and keep his balance on the unstable ball bearings, especially when Elaine gave him a push from one direction or another. The final element of this workout was the lifting of light, dumbbell weights for upper body and back strength.

As Dominick progressed, the length of time he spent on the treadmill and bike, his repetitions of the balancing exercises, and the size of the weights all increased. It took Dominick only eight weeks to go from a man who had to crawl to go the bathroom, to someone who today says, "I feel like I never had a problem."

In his younger years, Dominick played softball and basketball. "I was never overweight," he says. A lack of mobility for a "very active" person was difficult to endure, he explained. "I was like a caged animal."

Dominick praises Elaine Rosen's thoroughness. "She taught me how to dress myself, how to put my socks on." He says she taught him the proper ways to bend safely, and how to sit, with his legs in front of him and not crossed, so as not to reinjure his back.

He counts as highly important the exercises Elaine prescribed for him at home. He diligently practices them every morning. They consist of leg lifts, crunches, and upper body raises, done while lying flat on your stomach with arms extended above your head. Dominick hasn't had to take a day off because of his back in the two years since he went into therapy. "I think before every move," he says.

others. Back pain prevents back movement, which further weakens the back in a vicious circle.

Symptoms:
General pain and stiffness, restricted motion, and muscle spasm.

ExRx:
Rest and ice, then Phase III Therapeutic Back exercises.

Spondylolysis (Stress Fracture of the Vertebrae)/Spondylolisthesis (Stress Fracture with Slippage of the Vertebrae)

Caused by repetitive bending of the back. If not treated, this can lead to complete fracture and dislocation. Pain onset can be gradual or sudden from bending backward and can be aggravated by swayback.

Symptoms:
General lower back pain or stiffness on sides of back, difficulty bending, and sometimes tingling or numbness radiating down to toes.

ExRx:
If genetically disposed (thin bones) or already injured, avoid frequent back arching sports and dance moves (e.g. gymnastics, weight lifting, football, butterfly stroke) and such arching exercises as sit-ups. Prevent with abdominal, back-strengthening, and stretching exercise. Treat curvature of the spine with abdominal curls and back stretches, however, surgical spinal fusion may be necessary in severe cases. Mild cases need one week of rest, moderate one to three months, and severe may require six months or more.

Lower Back Rx Exercises

Before you perform any stretching and strengthening exercises, be sure to warm up your back muscles by walking. Because the upper back muscles are large, they can be exercised more vigorously. Lower back muscles are smaller and the area they hold together is subject to more physical stress from constantly supporting the weight of your torso as it rests, bends over, and turns side to side. More time spent sitting and lounging gradually weakens your lower back muscles so that they are more apt to become strained from isolated movements. After your lower back has been hurt or injured, even moving the rest of your body becomes difficult, further weakening your muscles and reducing your level of activity. A back exercise program strengthens your lower back muscles when you use them to hold and raise yourself into various positions. Additionally, anyone who has been inactive for longer than three months should reintroduce back exercises at a therapeutic level because of the potential for injuring an unexercised back with too much exercise.

After your back has been injured, you should begin to rehabilitate it as soon as the pain and swelling subsides. Practice assisted (Phase I) or unassisted (Phase II) ROM and isometric exercises, depending on the severity of your injury. After surgery, you usually start with Phase I Rehab within three to five days in the case of a slipped disk. In general, when your doctor approves, injured backs should be rehabilitated and not allowed to deteriorate further.

AGE RX: LIST OF ADDITIONAL MUSCLE AND JOINT DISORDERS BENEFITED BY MUSCLE STRENGTHENING EXERCISES

- Down syndrome
- Ehlers-Danlos syndrome
- osteomyelitis
- Paget's disease
- surgery

STRETCHING HOLDS

Beginner: three to five seconds
Intermediate: six to fifteen seconds
Advanced: fifteen to thirty seconds

STRENGTHENING REPETITIONS (ONE TO THREE SETS)

Beginner: two to five reps
Intermediate: six to twelve reps
Advanced: thirteen to twenty reps

Phase I Lower Back Rehab Exercises (With a Physical Therapist)

Begin these exercises after the pain subsides from a serious injury or surgery: assisted or passive-assisted back ROM and back isometric exercises.

Phase II Lower Back Rehab Exercises (at Home)

This level of exercise begins when you can exercise your injured (or postsurgical) back unassisted. Your goal is to increase the range of motion of your spine and the strength and flexibility of your back muscles.

Supine, Flat Back, and Pelvic Tilt (Lower Back Strengthening)

- Lie on your back, on the floor or on a firm mattress with your knees bent, feet flat, heels near your buttocks
- Brace your abdominal muscles and flatten your lower back against the floor (see the neutral spine position, p. 157); release and flatten again, five to ten times
- Next, raise your pelvis two to four inches and hold for three to five seconds; press your toes down to fully flatten out your feet; repeat five to ten times

Supine Lower Back Stretch

- Lie on your back with legs extended and knees slightly bent
- Grasp one knee with both hands and pull it slowly toward your chest while keeping your other leg extended; hold for three to five seconds
- Release your leg and slowly return it to the start position
- Now, repeat the stretch on your other leg; hold
- Repeat five to ten times on each leg

Phase III Therapeutic Lower Back Exercises (at Home)

Lower Back Stretch

Please note: You can stretch your lower back from the standing position or from the seated position. (Avoid the yoga "plow" stretch, i.e. bringing both feet over your head because this puts too much pressure on your neck.)

- Lie on your back; relax your jaw and neck
- Extend your arms out to your side at shoulder height
- Extend one leg out, knee slightly bent
- Bend the other leg and cross it over your extended leg and pull it down to the floor; try to keep both shoulders flat on the floor
- Hold for three to five seconds, building up to thirty to sixty seconds
- Repeat on the other side

Supine Lower Back Stretch

- Lie on your back with your knees bent and heels placed near your buttocks
- Extend your arms out at shoulder level and rest them on the floor
- Bring your knees together; hold them there as you roll both of them over to touch one side to the floor
- At the same time, turn your head (and upper body) to the other side; feel the stretch in your lower back; do not be alarmed if you feel or hear cracking sounds
- Hold for three to five seconds and return to the starting position
- Next, roll both legs, knees bent, to the opposite side as you again turn your head away from the direction of the roll; hold for three to five seconds

Seated Lower Back Stretch

- Sit on the floor with your knees bent sideways in front of you, legs splayed, lower legs crossed but not touching, one foot forward a little
- Bend over toward the forward foot and opposite knee
- Let your head hang down and place your arms in front of your legs on the floor; hold three to five seconds, then return to the starting position
- Change sides; place your other foot in front; repeat the stretch by bending over toward your other knee

Standing Hip Stretch

- Place and extend one leg on a sturdy bench or chair; keep your knee bent
- Keep your standing foot pointing forward, knee slightly bent
- Slowly lean forward feeling the stretch in the muscle in front of your hip
- Hold for three to five seconds building up to thirty to sixty seconds; repeat on the other side

Seated Hamstring Stretch

- Sit with one leg extended straight out, the other leg bent inward, knees slightly bent, the foot sole touching the opposite thigh

- Slowly bend forward as far as you can while keeping your back straight
- Hold the bent position; relax; change sides

Standing Trunk Stretch

- Stand with your feet shoulder-width apart
- Place your hands on your hips; straighten one leg and lean your trunk to the opposite side and bend that knee; hold; straighten up
- Change sides

Please note: You can also raise your arms straight up over your head when using this stretch.

Supine Abdominal Curls

Also see alternate abdominal exercises in the Prevention Ex.

- Lie on your back, knees bent, and feet apart and flat
- Cross your arms in front of you and rest them on your chest; rest your chin on your neck
- Raise your shoulders up off the floor, from three inches to the midpoint toward your knees
- Hold for a moment and slowly lower yourself down
- Avoid doing straight-leg sit-ups because they strain the lower back and work the hip flexors more than the abdominal muscles.

Side Curls

- From the supine position, curl up and across your body, touching your elbow to the opposite knee
- Alternate side curls
- Finally, increase the resistance of your curls further by placing your forefeet on the wall in front of you

Standing Lower Back Stretch (For Backache and Spasm)

- Stand in front of an open doorway, about a foot back
- Grasp the door frames with your hands, thumbs down, at shoulder level
- Bend your knees and sit back; hollow out your chest and stomach
- Tuck your buttocks under and hold the stretch

SPECIAL LOWER BACK INJURY PREVENTION EXERCISES FOR AFTER REHAB AND THERAPY

After you are pain-free, begin the following back injury prevention exercises to strengthen the abdominals and lower back and to stretch the hip, hamstrings, and lower back.

Lower Back Stretching

Lie down on the floor and rest your lower legs on a chair seat above you.

Pulling Knee to Chest Stretch (Beginner)

This exercise can be done standing, seated, or prone.

Hollowing Back (Intermediate)

This exercise can be done standing (Door Frame Pull, p. 291) and seated (Forward Cross-Legged Stretch, p. 206, and Advanced Cross-Legged Stretch, p. 207). Crossing one leg over the other adds more resistance to the lower back stretch in standing, seated, and prone positions.

Alternative Lower Back Exercises

Please note: Abdominal strengthening exercises and hip stretches should also be used to strengthen the back. See exercises pp. 202–215.

Abdominal Isometrics

- Hold in your stomach for six to eight seconds when you are standing, seated, or lying down; breathe normally; release
- Repeat three to five times

Abdominal Hollowing (All Fours)

- Get down on all fours; your elbows should be slightly bent
- Slowly pull in your stomach muscles as you use them to make your back concave
- Hold for six to eight seconds, then slowly flatten your back without arching it
- Repeat three to five times

Leg–Arm Raises on All Fours

- Get down on all fours
- Extend one arm and opposite leg so that they are level with your torso; hold
- Lower your arm and leg back to the ground
- Change sides; repeat

Abdominal Curl-Downs

- Sit up on a floor, knees bent
- Rest your arms across your chest and slowly sit back into the recumbent position
- Slowly roll backward, moving your feet toward your buttocks to keep your abdominal muscles working; hold
- Slowly curl up to the recumbent position; repeat curls

Please note: Osteoporosis patients *should not* curl up but should remain with back flat to floor.

Side Abdominal Lifts

- Lie on your side; rest your head on your bent arm and bend your lower leg for body support
- Raise your upper arm and extend it over your head and reach for the floor
- Lift your upper leg high without turning your knee upward
- Now, lift your arm straight up in the air at a 45-degree angle and hold as you lift your head toward the raised arm.
- Next, lower your head down to the rest position; hold
- Lower your arm back down; hold
- Lower your leg back down

- Repeat this sequence several times
- Change sides and repeat sequence several times

HAMSTRING STRETCH

lso see Hamstring Stretches, pp. 237–244.

upine Straightened Knee to Chest Iamstring Stretch (Beginner to ntermediate)

- Lie down on your back
- Bend your leg and grasp your knee from behind, straightening it as you pull your leg toward your chest; also, brace your stomach muscles
- As you straighten your leg, slide your hands up to your calves and pull the leg from behind there; hold for several seconds and then lower
- Repeat with the other leg

ease note: You can also perform this stretch om the recumbent position with one leg nt in front of you and with the outside igh resting on the floor.

odified Hurdler's Stretch (Intermediate)

- Sit bent forward with one leg straight out and the other bent at the knee with the sole of the foot touching the thigh of your straightened leg
- Slowly bend forward; hold
- Change sides

Standing Hamstring Stretch (Advanced)

- Place your feet straight forward, parallel, and hip-width apart; bend your knees slightly
- Now, bend over and touch the floor in front of you
- From this position, slowly straighten out one leg and hold the stretch; avoid bending over with both legs straightened out

LOWER BACK EXTENSOR STRENGTHENERS

Prone Back Extension (Beginner)

- Lie on your stomach with hands by your sides or extended forward for more resistance
- Keep your neck and chin in the neutral position (see illustration, p. 157) as you raise your shoulders off the ground
- Repeat three to twelve times

Standing Lower Back Strengthener (Intermediate/Advanced)

- Stand or sit with your feet shoulder-width apart and your knees bent; clasp your hands behind your neck with your elbows extending outward
- Slowly bend forward at the waist between a 15- and 45-degree angle and straighten up again
- Repeat five to fifteen times
- Stand again with your feet shoulder-width apart and knees bent; clasp your hands behind your neck, elbows outward
- Keep your hips neutral or anchored in the forward position

- Rotate your upper torso to one side and try to look over your shoulder
- Return to the forward position, then execute the rotation to the other side
- Repeat the rotation five to twelve times for each side

Hip Stretches

Beginner, p. 202

Intermediate, p. 204

Advanced, p. 205

Abdominal Strengtheners

Easiest: Isometric Stomach Hold, p. 292

Beginner: Lying Pelvic Tilt, p. 203 or Abdominal Curl Up, p. 291

Intermediate: Seated Curl Down, p. 292

Advanced: Standing Bent-Knee Across Chest Pull, p. 206

CHAPTER 14

MuSkel Rx

Exercise Solutions for Muscles, Bones, Joints, and Skin

THE MUSCULOSKELETAL SYSTEM

MuSkel Rx prescriptions are designed for the rehabilitation of muscles, bones, skin, and joints caused by diseases, disorders, and sports injuries or accidents. The body areas covered are: arms, ankles, feet, legs, and upper torso.

The prescriptions in this chapter use mostly body area exercises, rather than system-wide exercise techniques. Such system-wide MuSkel diseases and disorders as muscular dystrophy, osteoarthritis, scoliosis, and osteoporosis are the exceptions; many other diseases and disorders will only require special exercises for the specific body areas affected. In these cases, find the specific muscle, bone, skin, or joint disease, disorder, or injury for which you have been diagnosed, and then use those specific suggested body area exercises. The basic musculoskeletal exercise prescription is based in low-impact and low-ballistic motion exercise.

The exercises are organized by body areas that surround major joints and therapy and rehab is usually specific to that particular injured body area and joint. For total body conditioning, continue practicing the MuSkel preventive conditioning exercises in Part Two, Chapter Nine for those body areas that are still healthy.

The major portion of this chapter is broken down into eleven areas, which are: (1) muscle, bone, and joint diseases and disorders, (2) cancer care and MuSkel Rx, (3) bone injuries, (4) skin diseases, disorders, and injuries, (5) foot injuries, (6) ankle injuries, (7) lower leg injuries, (8) knee injuries, (9) thigh injuries, (10) shoulder and upper arm injuries, and (11) elbow injuries. Each of these eleven areas is followed by an alphabetic listing of the diseases, disorders, or injuries found under that category. Symptoms are then described for each disease, disorder, or injury, which is followed by an ExRx for that specific ailment. You will note that some of the more common, more rehabilitative disorders and injuries have many exercises associated with them, while other diseases (e.g. multiple sclerosis, cancer) will have only a few exercises associated with them. If you feel you want more exercise than what is given with any ExRx, consult Parts I and II of this book and practice those preventive exercises that are associated with the body system or area that you are rehabilitating. Remember: Always start at a lower level and work your way up to your own personal optimum level. Do not turn your rehabilitative exercise therapy into a competition with anyone—including yourself. That is the surest, fastest way to injury, pain, and setbacks on the road to recovery.

Some of the injuries covered in the eleven areas are caused by overuse. Overuse injuries are more easily prevented by safer exercise techniques and also more directly affected by therapeutic and rehabilitative exercise. Rehab usually begins directly after the injury. There are various levels of injury, ranging from moderate to severe, the most common being bruises, sprains, and strains. A bruise is an injury that usually causes a rupture of small blood vessels, which in turn causes discoloration without a break in the surrounding or overlying skin; a sprain is a partial or complete tear of the ligaments surrounding a joint; a strain is an injury to the muscle or tendon. Sprains and strains may heal without surgery; most bruises require a minimum amount of therapy. For most of these types of injuries, doctors and physical therapists will use the following protocol: Rest, ice, compression, and elevation (RICE) and medical attention for more severe injuries; medications will include acetaminophen, ibuprofen, or aspirin for mild to moderate injuries; for severe injuries, doctors will prescribe bed rest with analgesics and anti-inflammatory drugs.

WARNING: Although many over-the-counter and prescription pain relievers are prescribed for reduction of pain in sore muscles, bones, joints, and skin, do not take any pain relievers before exercising as they tend to mask pain, which can cause further injury resulting from overexercising or overusing an injured body area or part. Take the medication as directed, after exercise and when you are more stationary. Awareness of an injury is key to healing it!

Levels and Types of Rehab Exercise

Practice passive- and active-assisted ROMs only with your medically approved physical therapist, or on your doctor's advice. Otherwise, rehab by starting out at the appropriate phase for your injury. Then progress from less strenuous exercises (Phase I) to most strenuous exercises (Phase III).

After completing the phases of rehab, proceed to the three levels (I–III) of conditioning exercises.

I Passive-assisted ROM
Active-assisted ROM
Isometric strengthening

II Gentle ROM
Gentle stretching and strengthening
Lower body cardiovascular

III Dynamic ROM (Dynamic means against more resistance or dynamic stretching and strengthening)

TABLE 14.1
THE BASIC MUSCULOSKELETAL REHAB PROGRAM

Injuries	*Rehab*
Postsurgery/prolonged splinting	Start within 5 days–3 weeks
Short splint, no surgery	Start within 24–48 hours; allow for joint movement
Severity of Injury	*Exercise Level*
Mild	III (at home)
Moderate (some acute/chronic)	II (at home)*
Severe (postsurgery, acute, chronic)	I (physical therapist)**

*Ice, heat, and continuous passive machines.
**Ice, heat, deep massage, electrical stimulation, and joint manipulation.

JOINT PAIN SCALE

For many joint and muscle disorders, expect some pain and fatigue when exercising. Pain may be local to a body area or may be widespread. Using the scale below, rate your joint pain and take the recommended action. If joint and/or muscle pain persists for more than two hours after exercising, it is an indication that you have overexercised the joint area. The next time you exercise, you should choose a lower level of exercise to avoid further injury to joints and muscles.

PAIN LEVEL	EXERCISE ACTION
1—None	Continue
2—Little pain	Take stretch breaks
3—Moderate/ average pain	Take rests, breaks, or postpone
4—More than average pain	Postpone
5—Severe pain	Stop

TABLE 14.2
STRENGTHENING SCHEDULE

	Phase I	*Phase II*	*Phase III*
% of max reps	20–40	40–50	50–60
reps	light resistance	medium resistance	heavy resistance
Sets	1–2	2–3	3
Repetition	1–3	3–6	6–8
lbs per arm	0–2	2–5	5–15
lbs per leg	0–2	2–5	5–15
Perceived exertion (1–5 scale)	1	2	3
Time per phase (weeks)	2–4	2–4	4–6

WATER-BASED MUSKEL EXRX

Water exercise is an effective and useful way to strengthen injured joints and muscles by providing a low-impact method for working out aerobically. For joint pain and injury, use the Table 14.3, p. 299, to choose the appropriate water depth, temperature, and resistance rate to match your exertion level. Exercise in deeper and warmer water (82 to 88 degrees Fahrenheit). Choose depths appropriate to the level of needed buoyancy or reduction in body weight by 80 to 90% in water that is chin deep, 50% reduction in water that is waist deep, 20 to 30% for water level that is calf to knee deep. Also, choose the appropriate water depth to increase the rate of resistance for strengthening exercise and reduce the pace needed for aerobic exercise.

The water's buoyancy also lets you practice fuller and slower ROM exercises without losing your balance. For example, in water, you can achieve fuller ankle motions when doing heel and toe raises without losing your balance as you would outside the water.

Additionally, water adds twelve times the resistance to the same strength exercise done on land. For example, water reduces the body weight impact on weight-bearing joints making it possible to perform walking, skipping, jogging, and jumping moves that were too painful on hips, knees, and ankles when done on land. In place of impact, you add the resistance of water. It can raise your heart rate using only one-third to one-half the speed of movement needed on land. (See Water-Supported exercises, page 220).

Follow Table 14.3 to gauge the amount and speed of your water exercises. Use the buoyancy section to reduce the impact that exercises have on your back and joints. For example, chin-deep water reduces the impact of walking in place from your normal, land-based body weight to 10% of your body weight. Use the resistance section to add or subtract moving-body areas to control your

TABLE 14.3
WATER DEPTH, BUOYANCY, AND TEMPERATURE

Buoyancy (reduction of impact to the body in percentages):

Ankle-deep	Calf-deep	Knee-deep	Hip-deep	Chest-deep	Chin-deep
10%	20%	30%	50%	75%	90%

Resistance (increase strength/decrease aerobic pace):

Legs only	Mid-torso	Arms and upper body
2× (two times)	3×–12×	3×–12×

Pace reduction (of your land-based exercise routine):

Ankle-deep	Calf-deep	Knee-deep	Hip-deep	Chest-deep	Chin-deep
1/8	1/4	1/3	1/2	3/4	9/10

Water temperature and exertion level:

Warm-up/Posture	ROM	Low-intensity	Moderate-intensity	High-intensity
93–86°F	92–89°F	88–82°F	81–79°F	78°F and lower

heart rate and to add more resistance to both ROMs and strength exercises. For example, using "legs only" doubles the exercise value of any movement; however, using arms, legs, and mid-torso will multiply the effect up to twelve times (12×). Use the pace reduction section to slow down the rate of your leg or arm repetitions based on the water's depth. For example, ankle-deep water should reduce your pace by one-eighth, while chest-deep water will reduce the pace by three-quarters. Finally, use the water temperature section to determine what temperature level the water should be for your specific purposes. Generally, the higher the water temperature, the greater the ability to move weak, sore, or injured joints and muscles. Learn to use the therapeutic effect of water exercise by choosing pools with the right depth and temperature.

Isometric Strengthening Exercises

These are a form of muscular strength-training exercises involving little or no joint movement. Practice these for rehab of severe joint pain or after joint has been immobilized for long periods of time.

Weeks 1–2: Hold the starting position of any strengthening exercise by contracting the muscle and hold it contracted for one to three seconds.

Weeks 3–4: Hold the midpoint position by contracting the muscle and by holding a weight, pushing your arm, leg, head, or torso against your or a care giver's hand. Hold for three to eight seconds.

Weeks 5–6: Hold the final position. (Also see Chapter Seventeen, Psyche-Immune Rx, for isometric progressive muscular relaxation exercise that use isometric exercise for small, tense muscle groups.)

MUSCLE, BONE, AND JOINT DISEASES AND DISORDERS RX

ACHILLES TENDON SHORTENING (CONTRACTURE)

A shortening of the heel tendon. Predisposed risks: family history and genetics, poor posture, wearing high heels, landing on the balls of the feet instead of the heels while jogging and improper stretching prior to exercise.

Symptoms:
Sharp, spasmodic pain and strain, and restricted ankle movement.

ExRx:
Achilles tendon stretch (see illustration below), heel-toe press-downs when walking (p. 177); after surgery, dangling the foot of

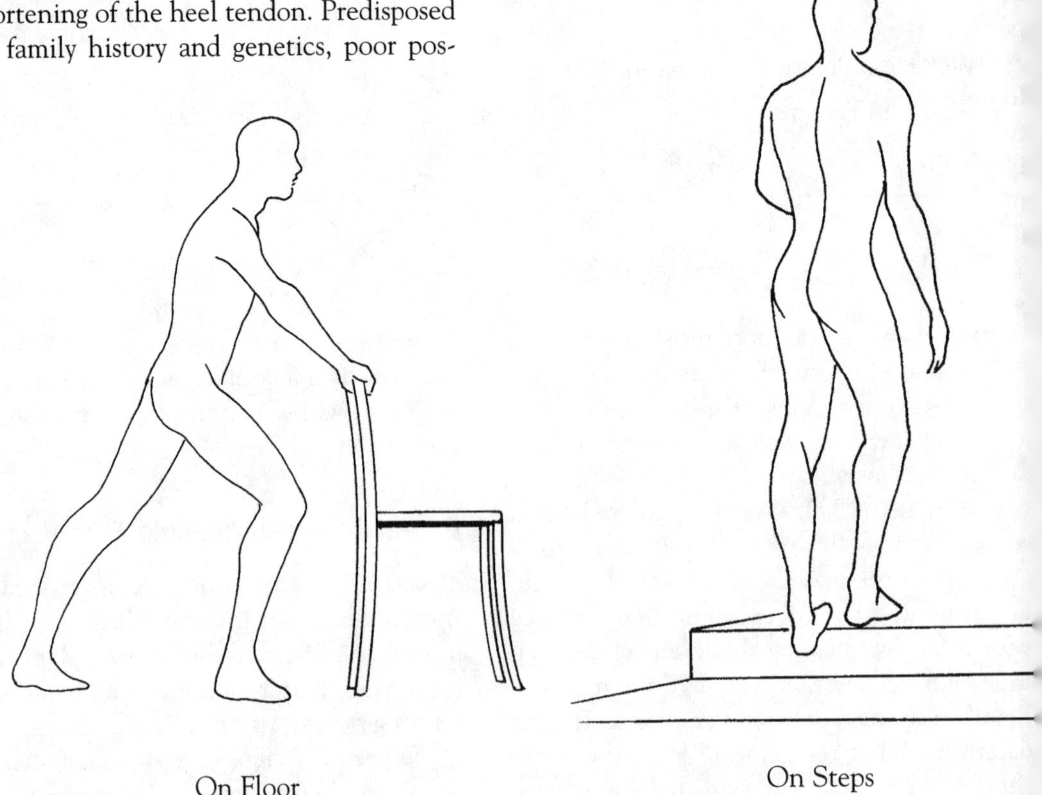

On Floor

On Steps

ACHILLES TENDON STRETCH

the bed (five to fifteen minutes as a warm-up) gradually increases the blood flow to the area; gradual, partial weight bearing on the area with aid of crutches. Heel-lifts can also accommodate the strained tendon. Elevate the injured ankle to reduce swelling and blood vessel pressure. Long-term prevention and rehab—calf stretches.

Arthritic Diseases

Arthritic diseases are those that attack the joints causing inflammation, and tissue and bone dysfunction. They are still incurable and require control of symptoms to maintain normal function. There are hundreds of arthritic diseases that affect over forty million people (about one in four individuals). Arthritic diseases are classified as chronic or long-term diseases. The goal is not a cure but to manage and control symptoms and improve your functioning ability. Some of the major types of arthritic diseases include the following:

- ankylosing spondylitis, which affects the hips, knees, spine, shoulder; symptoms include pain and joint fusion; classified as inflammatory and systemwide
- psoriatric arthritis, which affects the hips, knees, spine, shoulder; symptoms include pain and joint fusion; classified as inflammatory and systemwide
- fibromyalgia, which causes many tender points and muscle pain; classified as systemwide
- gout, which affects ankles, big toes, knees, and waist; symptoms include acute joint inflammation
- lupus, which affects elbows, feet, hands, and knees; major symptom is fatigue; classified as inflammatory and systemwide
- rheumatoid arthritis, which affects cervical spine, feet, hands, wrists, and knees; symptoms include morning stiffness, chronic pain, joint deformity; classified as inflammatory and systemwide

ExRx:
Overall, proper, regular exercise can help break the chronic pain cycle caused by arthritis and related diseases by keeping joints lubricated and by strengthening and stretching muscles around the joints. Exercise can also help you overcome the depression associated with chronic disease and pain by fortifying you physically and mentally to cope more effectively including diverting you from preoccupation with your disease.

Set exercise goals joint by joint depending on degree of pain and inflammation. If hip movement causes more knee pain, avoid stair climbing and jogging. Avoid overstretching, overbending, and overextending the inflamed joint area. Also reduce weight load on your joints by not carrying, lifting, or pushing heavy objects. Practice low-impact and low-duration activities and exercise as needed over a number of shorter sessions. Make sure you get intervals of rest and exercise. Control the pace of your activity with time rather than distance or repetition goals.

For all joint and muscle disorders: Practice slow and gentle exercise, ROM/stretching/strengthening, balance and posture corrections, seated exercise, water exercise, and stationary cycling. Do passive-assisted and isometric strength exercises for severe joint pain with help of a care giver, doctor, or physical therapist.

For pain relief: Practice extended relaxation exercises during cool-downs, tension relaxation, meditation, and deep breathing. Isometric strengthening exercises can help some joint pain by building up muscles' cushioning effect on joints. For isometric strengthening exercises, see pages 299 and 348.

Down Syndrome

A genetic disorder that typically results in mental retardation, abnormal facial features, and other physical abnormalities. Onset is prenatal. Life expectancy is improved with better treatment, including physical exercise.

Symptoms:
Poor muscle tone; dry, sensitive, inelastic skin; short stature, arms, and legs; impaired reflexes, posture, coordination, and balance.

ExRx:
Infant stimulation classes can be prescribed by a doctor. Provide physical stimulation and a balanced diet. Make sure the child gets plenty of exercise and environmental stimulation. Set realistic exercise goals and start with MuSkel Rx therapeutic exercises and build up to MuSkel preventive exercises.

JENNIFER VIVOLO

DIAGNOSIS: EHLERS-DANLOS SYNDROME

Jennifer Vivolo's problems were only just beginning when her left shoulder popped out of its socket at a high school swim meet in November of 1991. During the course of the next two months, her shoulder continued to dislocate with only the slightest applied force. Then, in February of the following year, she underwent arthroscopic surgery to repair the damaged joint, which helped for a while, but a few months later, her shoulder deteriorated again. It would pop out of its socket if she so much as lifted her purse, and the pain was excruciating. So, in December of 1992, just over a year since her original injury, Jennifer underwent a second operation on her left shoulder, but to no avail. Then, two months later, she began experiencing the same symptoms in her right shoulder.

Her doctors discovered that the root of Jennifer's joint problems was that her connective tissue was too elastic. Her ligaments and tendons would not contract after being stretched, rather, they would stretch out and remain stretched—more like silly putty than a rubber band.

Meanwhile, over the course of the next two years, Jennifer's other joints—her wrists, elbows, knees—all started going bad. Her shoulders deteriorated to the point where she couldn't lift her arm, and she began developing nerve problems in her neck that caused further pain and even made her hand turn blue from lack of blood circulation. In January of 1995, she had reconstructive surgery on her right shoulder, and her shoulders have been "okay" since that time.

Next, Jennifer went to see a geneticist and a neurologist. They diagnosed her as having

Ehlers-Danlos Syndrome

A group of genetic disorders of collagen and connective tissue.

Symptoms:
Abnormally stretchy, thin skin that bruises easily. The more serious symptoms include hyperextensibility of both skin and joints; profuse bleeding from wounds, which are slow to heal and leave thin scars. The joints are prone to recurrent dislocation.

ExRx:
To rehab, start with isometric and light stretching for about two to six weeks or until muscles become strong enough to convert to low-weight (e.g. one to ten pounds), high-repetition exercises. Build up reps to the twenty-five to fifty reps, one to three sets range every other day. Then, phase in regular strength-training and aerobic exercise program.

Fibromyalgia (Fibrositis)

A newly recognized rheumatic disease condition characterized by chronic muscle tissue and tendon pain common in chronic fatigue syndrome (see p. 449). Patients are usually between ages twenty and fifty.

---

a 99% chance of having Ehlers-Danlos syndrome, an inherited condition that causes hyperextensibility of connective tissue. The symptoms could indeed be surgically corrected, but there would be no point as the relief would only prove to be temporary.

So, Jennifer began seeing a physical therapist. The goal of her therapy was to strengthen her muscles so that they would provide the tension necessary to hold her joints in place instead of the stretchy connective tissue. Unfortunately, because her joints would dislocate, this made it impossible for Jennifer to practice lifting weights, which are the best exercise for strengthening.

So, she started with isometric exercises. When her muscles became strong enough to compensate for the connective tissue hyperelasticity, Jennifer began doing low-weight, high-repetition weight training. On biceps curls, for example, she did fifty reps of three to five pounds.

The results were dramatic. Jennifer's joints became more stable, her nerve problem corrected itself, and though the painful episodes did not disappear, they did decrease in frequency and severity. Exercises for her pectorals cured her rounded shoulders, and rowing exercises corrected her protruding scapula.

After six months of working with her physical therapist, Jennifer began working out on her own. Today, she works out daily, lifting weights and doing 200 to 250 crunches. In addition to these exercises, she bikes, uses a cross-country ski machine, or rows fifteen to thirty minutes, five days a week, and pacewalks two miles, two to three times a week.

Though not cured of Ehlers-Danlos, Jennifer leads a normal graduate student's life today. She acknowledges, "I still have a long way to go. I know that consistent exercise is a permanent fixture in my life. . . . Muscle is holding my body together."

Symptoms:
Muscle pain and tender points that can lead to poor posture (rounded shoulders and sway back) and fear of movement. Stiffness, sleeplessness, and overall fatigue that becomes worse during periods of inactivity. Also, causes anxiety and depression.

ExRx:
Practice longer, slower warm-up exercises and ROM exercises, preferably in warm water (see Water Supported Exercises p. 220). Make sure that posture is correct before starting and while doing the exercises. Do not exercise any area in which the perceived pain is higher than 3 on the Joint Pain Scale (see p. 297). Practice strengthening exercises at end of exercise sessions and after aerobic and cool-down exercises are complete. Do two or more sets of slower stretching exercises for all major muscle groups. Also use frequent stretch breaks whenever you feel pain or tightness.

HAMMER TOE

Occurs on all toes except the big toe. Often causes formation of corn on top of the toe (hard, calloused skin) and/or bunion (a misaligned joint protrusion of the great toe). Predisposed risks: wearing narrow-toed high heels.

Symptoms:
Big toe swelling, and painful walking. Swelling, redness, callus, and pain.

ExRx:
Wear wide-toed shoes, correct distorted walking technique, and do exercises to strengthen the arches. Keep the affected foot elevated above heart level between activity periods. Arch exercise: with heel at the edge of a step, point and raise up your toe and forefoot. A podiatric evaluation is recommended.

HEMOPHILIA

An inherited (genetic) bleeding disorder in which certain blood clotting factors are deficient or nonfunctioning. Onset at birth; affects mostly males. Bleeding in joints and muscles diminishes physical strength and mobility. As with arthritic conditions, hemophiliacs need an exercise program that strengthens and stretches muscles while protecting joints from injury. Also, high-impact activities that can cause bleeding episodes must be avoided.

Symptoms:
Abnormal bleeding, painful joints, reddened skin, severe bleeding after minor injuries, and large hematomas (collections of trapped blood). Also, swelling, extreme tenderness, possible deformity of joints, and bleeding near peripheral nerves.

ExRx:
Because hemophilia attacks the muscles and joints, you should do MuSkel Rx therapeutic or rehab exercises to help avoid or reduce physical disability. Progress from isometric strengthening exercises (see Chapter Seventeen, Psyche-Immune Rx) to regular strength training. To make your muscles contract, a therapist may use an exercise technique called proprioceptive neuromuscular facilitation (PNF) biofeedback accompanied by electrical stimulation. Prolonged low-intensity stretching and/or positioning (with lightweight splints and braces) works on shortened muscles. Progress very slowly from simple to more strenuous exercises. Chronic pain may require surgery. Joints sup-

›orted by well-developed muscles are better ıble to withstand the trauma of daily living. Children with better muscle development have ewer episodes of spontaneous bleeding. Also, xercise helps create a more positive emotional tate. Start regular exercise early and continue t through adulthood. Recommended sports are hose with the least injuries, such as golf and wimming, but higher-risk activities such as ›aseball, basketball, gymnastics may be necesary to maintain a child's interest, if there is ›roper preparation. Avoid high-impact sports uch as boxing, football, hockey, skateboarding, ınd wrestling.

Herniated Disk

Protruding disk in spine. Onset occurs at any ıge, in either gender. Results from a bad fall, train, or age degeneration. If untreated, back nuscles can weaken, causing faulty mobility ›f spine.

Symptoms:
Severe pain, tingling, numbness, weakness, ınd muscle spasms in lower back and neck hat may radiate to arms, legs, hands, and feet.

ExRx:
Practice low-risk, low-impact exercises. After surgery, do leg- and back-strengthening exercises, posture training, and long walks. Use a firm mattress or bed board. Any nonjarring exercise or activity is recommended. Rehab neck, middle, or lower spine with that specific body area Rx. **WARNING:** Any change in bladder or bowel habits, muscle weakness, numbness or extreme pain may be signs of a serious injury and should be evaluated by a physician.

Hip Fractures

Affects 250,000 people per year. Immediate cause is usually a fall; with osteoporosis, a spontaneous fracture often causes the fall. Affects 17% of all white women over age fifty (lean women have greatest risk because of low bone mass), and 6% of all men. Recent studies show that loss of more than 10% of body weight after menopause also increases risk by causing bone loss. (Also see osteoporosis, p. 307.)

Symptoms:
Hip and groin pain.

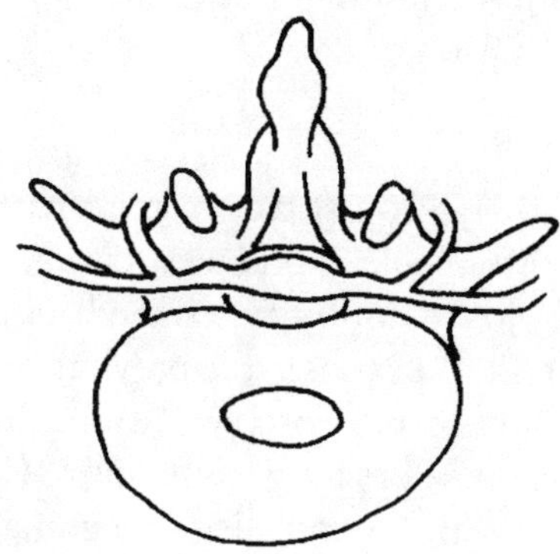

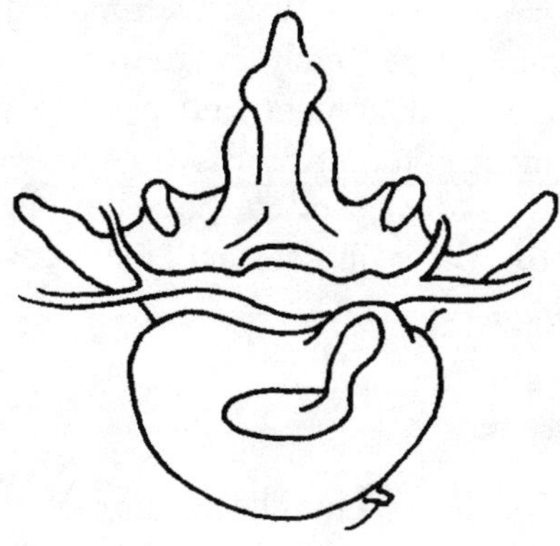

Herniated Disk

ExRx:
After hip replacement surgery, it is important to strengthen hip, buttocks, and thigh muscles and not to engage in activities that make you twist your hip too much and pull out or crack your artificial hip joint (e.g. golf swing, trunk turns, skating, football, horseback riding).

JOINT REPLACEMENT

Surgically replacing damaged and diseased joints is a common treatment for arthritis sufferers and injured athletes. Hip and knee joints are the most common, but ankle, elbow, and shoulders can also be replaced. Often, rheumatoid arthritis sufferers have joint lining (synorium) replaced first.

Symptoms:
Limited range of motion and sensitivity to joint stress.

ExRx:
Practice MuSkel rehab exercises for the replaced joint area. Avoid overbending joints beyond a 70- to 90-degree range. Avoid overloading joint beyond the 40 to 70% of maximum weight range. Practice slower versions of ROMs, stretching, and strengthening exercises on muscles that attach to replaced joint. Maintain proper body posture to promote proper joint alignment and practice proper body mechanics during ROM exercises. Use heat or cold, depending on symptoms, and light to relieve muscle and joint pain and swelling.

KYPHOSIS

Often called "humpback" or "dowager's hump." Convex curvature of the spine. Onset can occur in children ages twelve to sixteen, but this is rare. In adults, caused by aging degeneration, and osteoporosis.

Symptoms:
Back pain, fatigue, tenderness, and stiffness.

ExRx:
With a brace, do gentle pelvic tilts, hamstring stretches, and posture training (shoulders back, buttocks tucked under) to strengthen back and spinal muscles.

MUSCULAR DYSTROPHY

Inherited disorder that involves progressive muscle deterioration. There are two major types: Duchenne's (onset begins at ages three to five, with patient needing a wheelchair by ages nine to twelve; and Becker's (progresses more slowly, onset occurs at ages five to fifteen, sometimes patients can still walk into their forties). Dystrophy of the arms, face and shoulders is slow and less harmful (onset occurs before age ten to early adolescence) Limb–girdle dystrophy is similarly slow and lightly disabling (onset: ages six to ten).

Symptoms:
Loss of muscle control; waddling gait (Duchenne's), falling down, and difficulty climbing stairs.

ExRx:
Physical therapist-assisted exercise with and without orthopedic appliances. Use ROM to promote joint mobility; stretching, and strengthening exercise to prevent muscle atrophy, and to promote activity to prevent constipation. For lung dystrophy (Duchenne's), practice controlled coughing, and deep diaphragmatic breathing. Muscle-strengthening exercises will maintain systems

as long as possible, but will not slow down progress of the disease. Studies show that respiratory (breathing-related) muscle training for Duchenne's muscular dystrophy is useful in the early stages of the disease.

OSTEOARTHRITIS

Also called "degenerative joint disease." Involves a roughening and thinning of the cartilage that cushions the impact between bones, especially on weight-bearing and overused joints. When the disease progresses, the cartilage cracks and wears away, leaving the bone to rub against bone and causing grinding noise, pain, and stiffness in the joint. This is a "wear and tear" form of arthritis that afflicts many older people, but also forms prematurely in injured athletes. Affects sixteen million sufferers, and is widespread after age forty; partly caused by aging and obesity. Predisposed risks are trauma and heredity. Overuse of joints (e.g. sports injuries) may trigger a breakdown of cartilage around bones and new growth around joints, which restricts motion. Areas most affected are hips, knees, ankles, shoulders, hands, and feet.

Symptoms:
Aching joint pain, stiffness, and poor posture.

ExRx:
Prevention—avoid high-impact and ballistic activities that cause injuries to joints and cause further damage. Practice extra warm-ups and ROM, posture training, stretching exercise for improved flexibility, and low-impact exercise to relieve stiffness. Studies show that moderate exercise of joints of osteoarthritic patients will not harm joints and will improve overall fitness, increase longevity, decrease the risk of cardiovascular disease, and improve psychological well-being.

OSTEOPOROSIS

Bones become porous, brittle, and subject to breakage. Four times more apt to occur in women, particularly elderly women.

Symptoms:
Bone cracks and breaks (especially hip fractures), kyphosis, and spinal compression fractures. Causes bone and joint pain.

ExRx:
Weight-bearing, strengthening, and resistance exercises. Walking, biking, gentle exercise, and estrogen therapy will prevent or rehabilitate weakened bones. Avoid twisting moves and prolonged bending. Studies show that moderate weight-bearing exercise helps prevent osteoporosis and bone fractures because it increases bone density and bone strength. Lifetime physical activity slows bone thinning, and studies show that exercising the body's long muscles in the arms, legs, and torso can build new bones, even in older people. Consult a doctor about new drug treatment and calcium supplements. For rehab bone strengthening, gradually increase weight load and resistance levels over a six-week period to at least 70 to 80% of maximum strength effort per body area. Maximum strength effort is how much you can lift with one repetition. For thinning bones, strengthen them by using the physical conditioning exercises for the joint nearest to that bone. For example, use the knee joint rehab to strengthen thin thigh and shin bones. Use the hip joint exercise to strengthen hip bones and hip joints. Use the

LYNN SHERMAN

DIAGNOSIS: OSTEOARTHRITIS

Runner Lynn Sherman, fifty-nine, is used to pain. In addition to the arthritis in her knees, she must bear the many minor pains that go along with competitive athletics. Since she began running eighteen years ago, Lynn has been running through shin splints (stress fractures in the shin bone that result from running on hard pavement), heel spurs (small calcium deposits on the bottom of the heel that irritate the flesh of the heel) and, of course, sore muscles and joints.

Lynn got what most would consider a late start in competitive sports. Starting to run at age 41, Lynn had been a downhill skier. Seven years later, in 1985, Lynn ran her first marathon and has since competed in five others.

Although Lynn was participating in activities that benefited her health, her tendency to ignore pain (the body's warning sign), coupled with the arthritis, was exacting a toll on her joints.

Two and a half years ago, at the Philadelphia half-marathon, after experiencing knee discomfort in training, Lynn felt a "sharp, shooting pain" in her left knee. This time, she knew that what she was feeling was not the result of mere overexertion. But Lynn simply slowed her pace a bit and kept running. For the next two and a half years, she continued to compete, often placing in her age group. During that time, the cartilage in her left knee continued to deteriorate. Then, the pain became unbearable, and when Lynn became unable to run, she went to see an orthopedist.

An MRI revealed that Lynn had torn cartilage and arthritis in both knees. She would require arthroscopic surgery, a very common outpatient procedure in which three incisions are made near the knee to get inside and "clean up" the affected tissues. She had it done on the left knee since it was more painful than the right.

A week after the surgery, Lynn began going to one-hour physical therapy sessions, three times a week for fourteen weeks, to build up strength in the surrounding muscles and connective tissues. During each session, she spends about ten minutes on an exercise bicycle, stair-climbing, treadmill, and weight training—all under her physical therapist's supervision. In addition, she receives fifteen minutes of electric muscle stimulation and fifteen minutes of ultrasound therapy in the area around her knee.

Three weeks after surgery, Lynn has no doubts that she will run again, she hopes competitively, though she knows she mustn't push herself quite as hard as she did in the past. She says she will start to jog, taking it real slow. "The important thing is to go slow and cut down on your mileage when you're recovering from something like this. I plan to maybe jog [to] a pole, walk [to] a pole, alternate like that and keep building up," she explains.

With modern surgical techniques and a positive attitude, Lynn Sherman proves that what many would consider a career-ending injury can be treated as a minor setback.

upper and lower back exercises to strengthen your upper and lower spine. Weight machines offer greater degree of control of weights than free weights, particularly when the weight needed exceeds ten pounds.

Scoliosis

Lateral curvature of the spine. The chest-level curve is more common than the lower back curve.

Symptoms:
Hunchback, swayback (abnormal sagging of spine), backache, fatigue; in severe cases, difficulty in breathing.

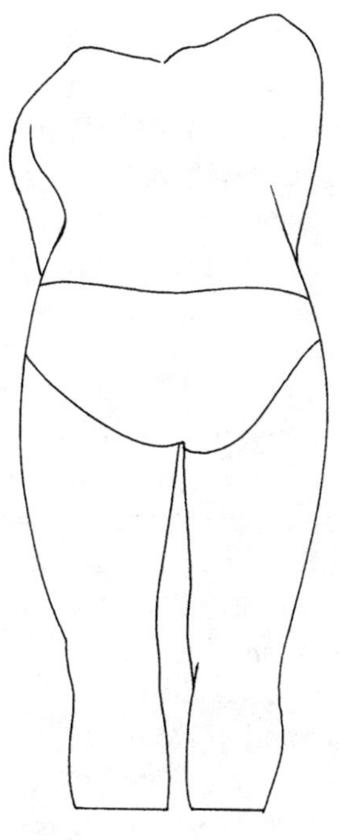

Scoliosis

ExRx:
Posture training, back and abdominal stretching and strengthening. For back curve of less than 25 degrees, do sit-ups, pelvic tilts, spine stretching, push-ups, breathing exercises, and heel lifts in shoes. Back curve of more than 40 degrees requires surgery (spinal fusion), with an exercise program that starts seven to ten days before surgery. Studies show that rehabilitation exercises not only reduce the magnitude of the curvature and counter-curve progression, but also reduce scoliosis-induced pain.

TMD or Bruxism

Temporomandibular joint disorder, sometimes called **TMJ.** This disorder is apparently triggered by stress-induced clenching of teeth at night.

Symptoms:
Jaw and earaches. Pain in the jaw joint and the muscles surrounding it. Pain can spread to other muscles and joints in a cycle of painful muscle spasms.

ExRx:
Various treatments, including relaxation training. Avoid aerobic and such weight-lifting exercises as cycling, jogging, skating, and snorkeling, which may cause you to clench your teeth. Practice jaw stretching and ROM strengthening exercises supervised by a dentist or physical therapist. Studies show that isokinetic exercises reduce joint clicking in a six-month period in young adults. Posture exercises that concentrate on the head and upper body alignment also help, including squaring shoulders, neck and upper back stretches. One special exercise technique involves properly positioning your

KELLY KANE

DIAGNOSIS: SCOLIOSIS

Kelly Kane was fourteen years old when she was diagnosed with scoliosis—the worst case her doctor had ever seen. Kelly's right hip had grown a few millimeters more than her left, so her spine compensated first by turning to the left, then curving to the right in an S-curve. Her back muscles also attempted to account for the difference in hip length by becoming stronger on the left side and atrophying on the right.

Kelly visited many doctors and each of them recommended a different remedy, but they all agreed that Kelly's spine would collapse and leave her immobilized by the time she was thirty if nothing was done. She couldn't wear a Milwaukee Brace (a common treatment for scoliosis) because of the S-curve in her spine. Her chiropractor was unsuccessful in an attempt to realign her spine. The remaining suggestions—to break her back and put in a steel brace, to break her back and put her in traction for two months, or to remove four of her vertebrae—did not appeal to Kelly.

Then she was introduced to dance therapy, a system of slow movements and stretches similar to yoga, which applies the principle "if you stretch something, it will straighten." Kelly began stretching her muscles, especially those of her lower back and hamstrings, every day and noticed a difference in her posture immediately. She continued dance therapy for about six years.

Today, at age thirty-two, Kelly exercises at least five days a week on her stairmaster and treadmill for a total of forty-five minutes, in addition to lifting weights. She also does inline skating for two hours, two to three times a week, and skis as much as possible during the winter. Although her spine will never be perfectly straight, so much for not being able to walk by age thirty!

tongue. Center your tongue in your mouth by saying the letter "N" with your teeth slightly apart. Breathe through your nose with your tongue in this position. Hold your tongue in this position any time you are not eating or talking.

CANCER CARE AND MUSKEL RX

Exercise can be therapy for physical symptoms and can also rehabilitate the physical damage caused by cancer and cancer treatment: after cancer surgery, MuSkel Rx rehabilitates different body areas (e.g. shoulder and chest for mastectomy); immune and cardio systems also can become weakened after radiation and chemotherapy. Exercise before, during, and after cancer treatments helps them go better and makes you feel more comfortable. You may also need to apply special exercise techniques with pouches and other prosthetic devices.

The care and rehabilitation of cancer patients often involves reconditioning parts of the musculoskeletal system that have been affected by surgery, chemotherapy, or radiation treatments. But the cancer patient should also exercise to maintain the good health of the cardio system. This makes the body more stress-hardy. Exercise will also elevate the cancer patient's mood, and help manage the aches and pains associated with treatment. Certain cancer treatments leave the patient too weak to do vigorous exercise, however, and for these patients, slow, intermittent, or moderate exercise is recommended to maintain the health of the circulatory system.

It's very important to strengthen the muscle groups that surround the cancerous area, so they can support any weakening caused by surgery or radiation. Also, muscles may be damaged, removed, or shortened by removal of tumors. For example, if the neck is the site of surgery, the arms and shoulders, in addition to the neck muscles should be strengthened. **Caution:** Check with your oncologist for details.

Bone Tumor

Caused by spreading of another cancer (secondary tumors) in 95% of cases. Occurs mostly in males thirty-five to sixty.

Symptoms:
Intense pain, mobility impairment in the late stages.

ExRx:
Surgery, amputation, chemotherapy, exercising with stump; keep the stump elevated to promote healing. Avoid placing a pillow under hip, knee, back, or between thighs, or lying with your knees flexed.

Multiple Myeloma

Infiltrates bones; 10,000 cases per year, mostly men over age forty. Prognosis poor; early diagnosis has a three- to five-year survival rate.

Symptoms:
Severe constant back pain that increases with exercise, arthritic symptoms, vertebral compression.

ExRx:
Chemotherapy, local radiation, and analgesics for pain. Don't exercise vigorously, but keep moving slowly; practice relaxation training, do low-impact, low-exertion exercises such as slow walking and deep breathing.

Spinal Tumor

The spine is a cord of nervous tissue that goes directly to the brain. Left untreated, a spinal tumor leads to paralysis. There is, however, a possible complete restoration of function if the tumor is surgically removed.

Symptoms:
Pain on spine and through trunk, spastic muscle weakness, decreased muscle tone, exaggerated reflexes, urine retention, accompanied by some loss of bowel and bladder control.

ExRx:
Postsurgery: posture training, back stretching, balancing exercise.

MuSkel Injuries Rx

There are two types of MuSkel injuries: acute and overuse. Acute injuries are caused by a single event (e.g. sprains, strains, bruises, and breaks). Overuse injuries are caused by repetitive trauma to body tissues. The risk factors for sports overuse injuries include fatigue; lack of conditioning, strength, flexibility, and preparation; incorrect technique and body mechanics; muscle imbalances; abrupt increases in the amount, intensity, and frequency of activity; improper equipment; weather, air temperature, and pollution; terrain (including surfaces); inappropriate footwear and clothing; poor coaching; and anatomical abnormalities, diseases, and disabilities (e.g. diabetes, obesity, high cholesterol, cigarette smoking, angina, heartbeat irregularities, and prior history of heart disease or heart attack).

The following are lists of acute injuries (an injury that causes pain with or without physical activity) and overuse injuries (a mild overuse injury causes pain only after physical activity; a moderate overuse injury causes pain before and after physical activity):

Acute

- acute compartment syndrome—swelling within muscle encasements caused by massive bleeding in muscles
- bruises/contusions—bleeding in the muscle fiber
- dislocations/subluxations—the ball of the joint is either forced out of the socket, or the ends of bone that meet at the joint are forced apart (i.e. separation)
- fractures—crack, break, or complete shattering of the bone
- hemobursa—bursa sac filled with blood.
- sprain—stretch, tear, or complete rupture of muscle or tendon (first, second, and third degree)
- strains—stretch, tear, or complete rupture of ligaments (first, second, and third degree)

Overuse

- bursitis (p. 313)
- cartilage wear and tear (p. 307)
- osteochrondritis dissecans (p. 320)
- overuse compartment syndrome (p. 322)
- stress fractures (p. 313)

For acute injuries, practice Rehab Rx (see pp. 325 to 326). For overuse injuries, practice basic rehab Rx, in addition to rest, ice, compression, and elevation (RICE).

BONE INJURIES RX

AMPUTATION

Loss or severance of an arm, leg, finger, or toe.

Symptoms:
Depression, limb pain, postural imbalance, and lower back pain (caused by hip-hiking).

ExRx:
Implantation of a prosthetic device. Begin stretching and strengthening exercises for healthy and/or injured limbs, alike. After surgery, rehab the injured side by practicing balancing and ROM exercises wearing the prosthetic device. If possible, remove any prosthetic device during strengthening exercises using only the stump until the muscles are strengthened. The prosthetic device can then be used to add resistance to strength training.

Amputated limbs should be exercised to maintain postural alignment, enhance funcon, and prevent painful and restrictive movement and muscle contractures. Practice posture exercises and strengthening exercises for muscles, which help relieve postural imbalances.

Depending on ambulation ability, aerobic exercise may have to be done with special devices or a wheelchair. Practice the standard aerobic exercises on all nonamputated limbs, but make sure to prevent excessive strain on unimpaired leg or arm. Avoid hopping, consider doing seated exercise without prosthesis during peak exertions.

ARM, ANKLE, AND LEG FRACTURES

Break, crack, or shattering of bone tissue with or without skin penetration. Muscles, nerves, and soft tissue are also damaged; an open fracture can cause a major blood loss. Stress fractures are caused by weak bone conditions (e.g. osteoporosis), and overuse.

Symptoms:
Pain, weakness, swelling, and tenderness.

ExRx:
Immobilize, then rehab with MuSkel Rx. Do easy stretching and strengthening exercises for affected body parts. Exercise while still in your cast, gradually strengthening and stretching the affected muscles; later, concentrate on rebuilding muscles around or near broken bone. Continue with circulatory and aerobic exercises.

If surgery is necessary, practice seated and prone exercises during the six-month recovery period. Patient can remain fit while working around a leg or ankle break by doing upper body exercises. Some stationary cycles allow one leg and both arms to be worked. Begin water program when out of cast.

BURSITIS

Inflammation of bursa sacs between the connective tissues and bones.

Symptoms:
Warmth, swelling, and painful restricted movement.

ExRx:
Rest and ice within twenty-four to forty-eight hours; thereafter, heat before exercise, ice afterward; correct any repetitive or incorrect movement problem(s). Practice slow warm-ups and stretching exercises. Over-the-counter anti-inflammatories can be helpful.

DISLOCATIONS AND SUBLUXATIONS

Displaced joint surfaces in the shoulders, elbows, wrists, fingers, toes, hips, knees, ankles, and feet.

Symptoms:
Impaired joint mobility, painful movement, swelling, and muscle spasm.

ExRx:
After immobilization, begin with slow ROMs, stretching and strengthening damaged muscles and ligaments. Use prone or seated exercise positions, if necessary.

SPRAINS AND STRAINS

A sprain is a tear in the supporting ligaments surrounding a joint; a strain is a stretch, tear, or rupture of a muscle or tendon.

Symptoms:
Local pain, clumsy joint movement, and immobility. An acute sprain or strain can

cause sharp, brief pain, stiffness, soreness, and swelling. Knee sprains are more likely to recur.

ExRx:
Build up muscles around the sprained or strained area (e.g. for knee sprains, strengthen quadriceps and hamstrings); for ankles, strengthen calf and shin muscles. Reduce your body weight to reduce risk of injury; don't restart sports until joint is completely pain-free.

TENDINITIS

Inflammation of the tendons that connect muscles to bones. Can be in commonly injured muscles of shoulders, hip, Achilles tendons, or hamstrings, or any muscle–tendon unit. Caused by impact or overuse.

Symptoms:
Pain, tenderness, and restricted range of motion.

ExRx:
Rest and avoid repeated injuries and muscle joint overuse. Ice painful area for thirty minutes at a time, several times a day. Practice gentle stretching and begin Rehab Level I or II (depending on the extent of the injury), moving on to strengthening exercise for the affected area.

WHIPLASH

Sharp extension or compression of neck muscles and vertebrae usually caused by rear-end auto crash or in a sports tackle (e.g. football, rugby).

Symptoms:
Moderate to severe pain in back and neck headache, or numbness.

ExRx:
Strengthen neck and back muscles; also d age and MuSkel Rehab exercises.

SKIN DISEASES, DISORDERS, AND INJURIES RX

Skin health is just as important as muscle bone, and joint health. As the body's larges (by area) organ, the skin is more vulnerabl to sports- and exercise-related injuries thar any other injuries, ranging from cuts an rashes to frostbite and sunburn. Skin als plays a large role in foot injuries and othe disease-related problems such as diabetes.

Exercise can harden the skin and make i tougher and more resistant to repeated use an abuse. During exercise, the improved bloo flow to the skin makes it healthier while th increased flow of water through sweat gland helps to clean out excess oil and unclog tissues

Stretching, strengthening, and ROM exercises promote the healing of bruised burned, or wounded skin also by increasing the blood flow to the damaged area Stretching can make "tight" skin more flexi ble (e.g. skin scarred from burns or othe wounds). Improving skin flexibility can als improve overall mobility because tight o scarred skin restricts the normal range o motion and makes movement painful.

Itching is a major symptom of skin disorders, but scratching may spread infection o scar the skin. Exercise helps relieve mild t moderate itching symptoms by distracting you from the source of this mild pain, and by desensitizing your body through the increase flow of beta endorphins.

Special care should be taken by adults and children when exercising outdoors or for prolonged periods in chlorinated water. Exercise often dulls the sensations of too much sun exposure or can distract you from the realization that you are out in the sun too long. It is especially important to protect and even cover skin before and during exercise. Insect repellent, sunscreen (or sunblock for very sensitive skin), and cold weather protection cream properly and consistently applied, as well as washing the skin afterward, can help to prevent or reduce skin problems such as frostbite, impetigo, insect bites, jock itch, jogger's nipple, prickly heat, melanoma, skin allergies, sunburn, and other skin conditions. After you have a skin rash or skin inflammation, however, exercise the affected body area with easy, slow movements.

Abrasion

Scraping off of outer skin, usually caused by falling or sliding on pavement or carpet.

Symptoms:
Burning and tingling.

ExRx:
Easy stretching and strengthening exercises on affected body areas until skin has sufficiently healed.

Burns

Injury from chemicals, fire, or abrasion to various layers of the skin's surface. Severe burns (third degree) lead to scarring and hardening of skin and underlying bone and muscle.

Symptoms:
Pain, itching; also skin can contract and shrink over joints.

ExRx:
After healing process begins, exercise joints and muscles near burned area with warm-ups on a stationary cycle. Gentle stretching, ROMs, and moderate exercise can help reduce swelling and scar tissue formation, and can also promote healing of skin grafts. Strengthening exercises can counteract muscle deterioration from inactivity and from the body's natural tendency to draw from healthy muscle tissue to help heal the skin.

Cuts

Lacerations of face, hands, fingers, legs and feet are most common in sports.

Symptoms:
Pain, bruising, bleeding, swelling, and headache.

ExRx:
To prevent cuts, wear protective helmets, goggles, or face masks. For therapy, apply pressure to wound and bandage. For rehab, do not stress any area that hasn't completely healed or where there are still stitches in place.

Decubitus Ulcers (Pressure Sores)

Occurs on skin areas that are most exposed to friction. Constant pressure on skin and blood vessels leads to ulcers, dead tissue (necrosis), and bacterial infection. Prevalent in wheelchair and bedridden patients. Malnutrition is also an aggravating factor. Most common sites are buttocks, hips, elbows, knees, shoulder blades, and spine.

Symptoms:
Red skin, open sores, swelling, and sensitivity over compressed area(s).

ExRx:
Confined person should be repositioned frequently (at least every two hours), keep knees and elbows slightly bent, use pressure relief pads, massage around affected area, wash and clean skin, and change sheets and clothing often. Practice prone ROMs, stretching and strengthening exercises of all body areas, but especially those areas sore from extensive bed contact.

DERMATITIS

A variety of inflammations of the skin. One common type is "contact dermatitis," which is an allergic or irritated reaction to substances and surfaces that touch the skin. Also caused by such plants as poison ivy, poison oak, and poison sumac. Hands, face, and feet are the most probable sources of contact, but the irritation can be spread by contact to other locations. Dermatitis tends to flare up with increased sweating, psychological stress, and extremes in temperature and humidity.

Symptoms:
Itching, scratching, swelling, crusting, and scaling.

ExRx:
To prevent, find the source of the irritation and avoid it; after becoming inflamed, reduce contact with such surfaces and substances as exercise equipment (e.g. do freehanded exercise until condition clears up); keep skin dry and clean; and avoid tight-fitting and sweat-drenched clothing. Avoid such further irritants as scratchy clothing (e.g. wool); practice nonsweat-producing moderate exercise, which avoids spreading and stimulating inflammation. Keep dry and cool during aerobic exercise by exercising indoors in an air-conditioned room in summer. Apply topical antihistamines and steroids to promote rapid healing.

MUSKEL RX: LIST OF ADDITIONAL SKIN AND BONE DISEASES, DISORDERS, AND INJURIES BENEFITED BY ROMS, STRETCHING, AND STRENGTHENING EXERCISES

- acne
- bleeding
- boils
- calluses
- chafing
- corns
- folliculitis
- frostbite
- jock itch
- jogger's nipple
- melanoma
- open wounds
- penetrating chest wounds
- photosensitivity
- sunburn

PSORIASIS

A chronic, recurring flare-up of overgrown skin with red patches and dry, thick scales; often precedes arthritic symptoms. Affects 2% of the population, mostly whites, both male and female. Flare-up may be aggravated by emotional stress, cold climates, hormonal changes, pregnancy, and infections. There is no permanent cure.

Symptoms:
Itching, redness, flaking; sometimes lesions on back, buttocks, chest, elbows, knees, scalp, and face.

ExRx:
Practice relaxation exercise to relieve itching pain. Practice ROM exercises around affected body areas to improve blood flow to areas of itching.

FOOT INJURIES RX

Feet absorb the brunt of the impact when your body moves. They are similar to the wheels of your car: the arches are the shock absorbers; and the ankles are the tire rims and axles. The muscles are used for propulsion and braking as well as positioning, rotation of the foot and leg, stability, and locking or unlocking of joints.

Of course, sports can produce more foot disorders than everyday living. The repetitive movements place greater stress on the foot and ankle, and aggravate any anatomical abnormalities you may have such as flat feet, high arches, or sensitive areas on skin and bone. The most common problems are stress fractures, bursitis, tendinitis and heel pain. Impact and overuse injuries can also aggravate such foot problems as warts, ingrown toe nails, and pinched nerves.

PLANTAR FASCITIS

An inflammation of the thick, fibrous tissue that runs the length of the long arch on the sole of the foot. Bone spurs can develop where the tissue attaches to the heel. Caused by overstretching and pounding from repetitive jumping and running. Can be aggravated by flat feet or high arches. Obesity is often a factor.

Symptoms:
Pain and tenderness on the inner side of the foot in front of fleshy part of heel, limping. Pain upon first steps when arising.

ExRx:
To prevent, reduce running to less than fifteen miles per week. Insert heel wedge in shoe to lessen stretching of plantar fascia. Therapy for inflammation includes rest and ice, such non-weight-bearing exercises as stationary cycling and swimming. A chronic condition requires surgery to sever plantar fascitis from heel bone and let it grow back again. Custom orthotics are paramount in treatment. After surgery or a severe attack, start Phase I Rehab foot exercises, then practice such low-impact stepping moves as walking in water and soft cycling (see Cardio Ex, pp. 217–222).

RETROCALCANEAL BURSITIS

Inflammation of the bursa sac just above where the Achilles' tendon attaches to the heel bone. In women, caused by high-heeled shoes or low-heeled flats. Faulty biomechanics or incorrect body movements can be corrected with posture training, proper body alignment, and foot placement techniques.

Symptoms:
Pain, swelling, irritation, redness, the soft bump on the back of the heel can become harder.

ExRx:
During the rehab period, avoid sports activities that require shoes. Swimming or stationary cycling is usually okay. Using a flotation device and nonweight-bearing running in deep water is also an option. For therapy use ice massage, cease pain-causing activity for two to three days; if severe, may have to cease painful activity for four to twelve weeks. Wear longer shoes with softer heel contours. For rehab: If bursa is noticeably hardened, seek medical attention. Most of the time,

changes in activities help to work around heel pain. After surgery (i.e. when bursa is removed), depending on patient's build and tendon involvement, start ROM exercises; after four weeks, begin swimming and physical therapy.

Stress Fractures of the Foot (See Stress Fractures of the Tibia and Fibula, p. 323)

MUSKEL RX:ADDITIONAL FOOT INJURIES, CONDITIONS, AND DISORDERS BENEFITED BY STRENGTHENING AND ROM EXERCISES

- athlete's foot
- black nails
- blister
- bunions
- callus
- corn
- fungal infections
- ingrown toenail
- Morton's neuroma
- tendinitis
- trauma (micro or macro)
- wart

Ankle Injuries Rx

Lateral movements, such as the side-to-side steps of racquet and court sports, offer a higher risk of acute ankle injury. With these sports it is important to strengthen and stretch the tendons around the ankle to give it greater range of motion and more strength. Your ankle should be able to bend upward 15 degrees, and you should be able to do a number of heel raises (based on your age and fitness level) for minimum flexibility and strength. Modern medicine emphasizes early mobilization within forty-eight hours of a sprain. Fractures commonly require six weeks of immobilization, with ROM, strengthening, stretching, and proprioception (see lower leg exercises, pp. 224–229) exercises. (Mobilization is difficult to measure with a fracture; it depends on type of fracture and the location.)

If you are in a splint, some of the exercises you can still practice include: stationary cycling, swimming, running in water with a flotation device, upper extremity exercises, and passive-assisted exercises with the aid of physical trainer. Short splinting allows for ankle flexion upward or downward movement of foot without inversion or eversion.

Overuse injuries to the ankle are caused by almost all running and jumping sports, but especially those that involve frequent stop-and-start movements (e.g. football, lacrosse). Overuse injuries in everyday life can result from walking in worn-out shoes that provide little foot and ankle support.

Ankle injuries are rehabilitated with such lower leg exercises as ankle ROMs and calf stretching and strengthening exercises.

Acute Ankle Injuries

Ankle Fractures

Can occur as a crack, break, or shattering of a bone. Left untreated it can lead to deformity, arthritis, and recurring ankle sprains.

Symptoms:

Same as ankle sprain (e.g. pain, swelling,

RANDI C.

DIAGNOSIS: ANKLE FRACTURE

Randi C., 40, was in a car accident in May of 1993, which fractured her foot. A plate, nine pins, and a screw were put in her right ankle. Randi was in a cast for three months. When it came off, the ankle had locked and she was in excruciating pain. Randi said, "I couldn't even stand."

Randi began going to physical therapy three to four hours per day, three to four times per week. In a whirlpool bath, her ankle was twisted, manipulated, and massaged by the skilled hands of her therapist who had to break up all the scar tissue that had built up around the hardware inside her ankle. Randi was thankful for her high pain tolerance, because that experience was extremely painful. She used a walker for three months, and then went to a cane. By about March of 1994, the plates and hardware were taken out. She had to build up her strength again. "I devoted my life to getting better," she explains.

Randi was a modern dancer before the accident. She attributes some of her recovery to that experience. "I knew how to work through pain. I had a sense of my own body," she says. She also touts the importance of working out and staying in shape. "[It's] important to strengthen muscles, because you never know."

Randi swims three to four times per week for three to four hours per day, which she worked up to throughout her rehabilitation. She also uses the treadmill. "I walk perfectly normal now," she says. And instead of the excruciating pain she suffered for months, she is now entirely pain-free.

Although the exercise—before, during, and after the injury—was a huge factor in her recovery, she also says it was "due to hard-working therapists." After she had healed, Randi became pregnant, and her ankle was fine throughout. Her therapists did such an excellent job on her ankle, when she got sciatica during her pregnancy, she went back and her therapist got the baby off of her sciatic nerve!

bruising). Sometimes sharper at the moment of injury and then continuing over the area, which is followed by numbness.

ExRx:
Immediate medical attention, x-ray, and possibly surgery. Phase I Rehab ankle Rx begins at two to eight weeks after injury, depending on severity of injury; rehab continues for four months.

Ankle Sprain

The most common injury involving stretching or tearing of the ligaments that hold the ankle bones together. Inattentive care can lead to recurrence.

Symptoms:
First-degree injury (mild)—some pain, tenderness, swelling, no bruising, and little loss

of function; second-degree injury (moderate)—popping or snapping sound, ligament tears, swelling, tenderness, bruising, and difficulty walking; third-degree injury (severe)—joint slips out of place, severe tenderness, and extreme difficulty walking.

ExRx:
Rest and ice for first-degree sprains. For second- and third-degree sprains, seek medical attention. Recovery is four to six weeks for second degree and six to twelve weeks for third degree. If a fracture is ruled out, doctor should place you on a rehab exercise program. You may need to wear a removable splint for three to six weeks. **Remove it when doing rehab exercises for the injured area.** Start Phase I Lower Leg Rehab exercises within twenty-four hours for first degree, twenty-four to forty-eight hours for second degree, and one to three weeks for third degree. It's important to rehab your ankle to avoid chronic instability and recurrence of injury.

Overuse Ankle Injuries

Osteochrondritis Dissecans (Loose Bodies in the Joint)

Damage caused by repetitive twists and turns of the ankle. Friction causes bone ends (e.g. tibia and talus) to rub together, creating a small crater and loose pieces of bone "floating" around it.

Symptoms:
Pain and swelling during exercise; stiffening of ankle afterward.

ExRx:
Immobilization for four to eight weeks to allow ankle to repair itself. Surgery may be recommended to pin back fragment or remove it if fragment falls into joint; if no surgery, Phase I ankle and lower leg therapeutic exercises with recovery in six weeks or more. With surgery, (removal, drilling, or pinning down of fragment) eight to twelve weeks of recovery.

Peroneal Tendinitis

Inflammation of tendons positioned behind outer ankle. Caused by overtraining and aggravated by bowlegs or high arches, which can make you run on the outside of your feet; can also be caused by running on hard surfaces or in worn-out shoes.

Symptoms:
Tenderness and pain, which can radiate up the outer leg.

ExRx:
Prevent a recurrence by reducing running mileage and using orthotics. Practice such low-impact exercises as swimming, bicycling, and walking. These exercises put less stress on anatomical abnormalities. For treatment, stop running, rest and ice, and about two to three days thereafter, begin therapeutic exercises for lower leg when pain subsides. Recovery takes four to six weeks.

Peroneal Tendon Subluxation

Caused when tendons behind outer ankle bone slip forward and out of their natural grooves. Occurs in skaters and skiers because they spend too much time balancing on the inner edges of their feet.

Symptoms:
Pain when turning foot up or down.

ExRx:
Surgery is usually recommended to deepen groove or reposition ankle bone so it juts out further. Begin Phase I Ankle Rehab exercises three weeks after surgery and continue for twelve to sixteen weeks.

Posterior Tibial Tendinitis

An inflammation of the tendons that go down the back of the tibia; caused by overtraining with running, especially on hard surfaces, and biomechanical abnormalities such as pronation (i.e. inward bending).

Symptoms:
Pain when running, jumping, and walking, especially when trying for a forceful push-off.

ExRx:
For therapy, rest and ice for two to three days. Thereafter, apply heat. For two weeks, stop activity that caused inflammation. If no surgery, begin therapeutic lower leg exercises for four to six weeks; with surgery, begin ankle rehab exercises within five days after surgery and continue for twelve to fourteen weeks or until condition is eliminated. Orthotics are vital if mechanical problems are present.

Lower Leg Injuries Rx

Acute lower leg injuries include bone fractures, muscle strains, and tendon strains. Overuse injuries are caused by excessive and repetitive sports and exercises. They are aggravated by anatomical abnormalities and improper and inadequate strength and flexibility training.

Prevent lower leg injuries by avoiding contact sports and stretching and strengthening the leg muscles.

Achilles Tendinitis

A series of microtears in tendons caused by repetitive stretching of the tendons by an overpowering calf muscle. Anatomical abnormalities including high arches and pronated feet may predispose you to this condition. Hard roads and worn-out shoes can also play a role. After age twenty-five, degenerative changes begin, which make the calf muscle stronger and the tendon lighter and weaker. Finally, footwear without proper support and cushioning can also be a contributing factor.

Symptoms:
Early on, gradual swelling and redness, and a creaking sensation. Later, tender to the touch, with reccurring pain during and after exercise.

ExRx:
Catch it early to clear it up in one to two weeks. Orthotics, such as leather arch supports or heel wedges will also help relieve pain. Prevent by strengthening and stretching calf and Achilles tendon with in-place, heel-toe exercises, and walking instead of running. Practice Achilles tendon–calf muscle stretch. We recommend extra sets of this stretch for those with a very tight Achilles tendon condition. Do two to three extra sets, at first holding each stretch from three to five seconds, building up to fifteen to thirty seconds, or even a minute.

If surgery is called for, practice lower leg rehab exercises starting one week after the operation. If condition persists and is severe, more surgery may be needed to give the tendon more room and to cut inflamed areas. This suggests that constant inflammation of this or any tendon will permanently damage tissue and that tendinitis is something to be avoided in the long run. You should avoid overly repetitive exercises and sports-training methods (e.g. reduce your weekly running to under fifteen miles). Also, choose two to three activities that distribute the work load over your entire body. Mix high-impact running with low-impact swimming and cycling to give your lower leg tendons a rest. Cease activity early on when telltale signs (i.e. pain, swelling, limitation of motion) appear. Seek medical help when pain or discomfort recurs.

Achilles Tendon Rupture

A stretch, tear, or rupture of the Achilles tendon, which extends down the back of the leg connecting the calf muscle to the heel.

Symptoms:
Snap of the tendon, which feels like being hit in the back of the leg, then intense pain.

ExRx:
In a cast for six weeks, or surgery to reattach and then a cast for six weeks. Begin Phase I Rehab lower leg exercises as soon as cast is removed. Because this is often misdiagnosed, see a sports-oriented podiatrist or orthopedist instead of a general practitioner.

Calf Strain

A massive contraction and tearing of fibers of the calf muscle caused by a quick stop and planting a flat foot followed by a sudden straightening of the knee. Occurs in stop-start and jumping sports such as basketball, squash, tennis, and volleyball.

Symptoms:
First-degree injury (mild), tearing of less than 25% of fibers—mild pain and tenderness, twinges the day after; second-degree injury (moderate)—stabbing pain felt immediately, discoloration beneath the skin, and limping; third-degree injury (severe)—muscle completely torn in two.

ExRx:
Prevent by doing more warm-ups of muscles, especially in cold temperatures. To prevent both excess scar tissue and reduced flexibility, rehabilitate with calf stretching and strength-conditioning exercises. First degree—rest and ice, begin Phase III in one to two days and continue for three to five days; second degree—begin Phase II rehab within eight days and continue two to four weeks; third degree (complete rupture)—begin Phase I Rehab lower leg exercises when the cast comes off.

Compartment Syndrome of the Lower Leg (Anterior Compartment Syndrome)

Excessive muscle pressure caused when muscles become too big for their membranes, compartments, or encasements. Muscles grow larger during exercise by swelling with blood. This condition can also be caused by increased osmotic pressure, which puts pressure on nearby nerves and the blood supply; aggravated by incorrect footwear, hard training surface, and improper running techniques.

Symptoms:
Severe tightness, dull aches, numbness, and tingling in lower leg; may progress to death of muscle unless surgery is performed.

ExRx:
Cease or reduce activity that causes this condition and switch to other activities that put less stress on those restrained muscles. Rest

and ice and extra stretching of the lower leg muscles help.

Medial Tibial Pain Syndrome (Shin Splints)

An inflammation of tissue covering the tibia or shin bone caused by repetitive pounding of the feet on a hard surface; can also be the result of an imbalance between strong posterior muscles and weak anterior muscles.

Symptoms:
Pain, swelling, and tenderness that is felt on the front surface of the lower leg (i.e. the shins) when running and walking or just bending toes down. Sometimes, these symptoms are also a sign of either stress fractures of the lower leg or compartment syndrome.

ExRx:
Avoid running high mileages and high-duration, high-impact, weight-bearing exercises. Practice the bulk of your cardiovascular activities in low-impact mode, for example, walking, using a cross-country ski machine, or cycling. Stretch the calf and Achilles tendon so they do not overpower the weaker shin muscle during lower leg moves. Do strengthening exercises for anterior shin muscles. If shin splints have already occurred, use rest and ice along with exercises that do not aggravate the shins (i.e. movement that bends the toes downward). When cycling, place your heels rather than your forefoot on the pedals. Recovery time is one to two weeks for mild cases, and six months for chronic conditions.

Muscle Cramps

A painful, spasmodic muscular contraction in the lower leg, usually in the calf muscle. Can be caused by overuse, underuse, disease (e.g. intermittent claudication), fatigue, dehydration, lack of nutrients (e.g. calcium or potassium), or by a sudden contraction or twisting of the muscle. There are two types: (1) tonic, and (2) intermittent. (Tonic is type in which the muscle remains in contraction.)

Symptoms:
Sudden, sharp pain or hardness of the muscle, limping, "Charlie horse," or cramping.

ExRx:
An accurate diagnosis helps because intermittent claudication requires exercise, medication, or surgery (bypass), whereas a nutrient deficiency may only require supplements. Stretching and strengthening of the calf muscles, including heel-toe roll, heel and toe lifts, and achilles tendon/calf stretch, all can relieve painful symptoms and prevent recurrence.

Muscle Pressure

This is a general condition resulting from insufficient circulation of blood to muscles in which one muscle overpowers another muscle.

Symptoms:
Muscle tightness, soreness, and warmth.

ExRx:
If not too painful, stretch the affected muscle.

Stress Fractures of the Tibia and Fibula (also of the Foot and Ankle)

Microfractures caused by repetitive impacts usually from airborne or jumping-like movements (e.g. aerobics, marching, running, ballet dancing). Can also be caused by poor technique or faulty mechanics. When your muscle is sore, overworked, or tired, more of the work load is transferred to your bones, which can cause a stress fracture. Muscles also repeatedly bend bones back and forth, which can cause them to crack. Additionally, if your bones are thin, they can fracture more often. In 95% of cases, the stress fracture occurs in the shin or heel.

Symptoms:
Pain and localized tenderness during running and jumping activities. If located in the tibia, pain is felt at the top third of the lower leg. If located in the fibula, pain is felt just above the ankle bone on the outside of the leg.

ExRx:
Prevent by avoiding exercises in which you frequently leave the ground with both feet (e.g. running). Switch to such nonpainful and nonweight-bearing activities as swimming and stationary cycling for a two- to six-week recovery period; ice the affected area. Walking and cross-country skiing will also aggravate stress fractures. Practice Phase III Therapeutic lower leg exercises until pain-free, then go to preventive level. Orthotics may be used if there is a mechanical problem.

GENERAL REHABILITATION GUIDELINES AND PROCEDURES

PHASE I: FOR ACUTE INJURIES

1. After surgery, the physical therapist wil use either active- or passive-assisted exercise. Passive will consist of four to six major range of moving the injured body area in the four ranges of motion: flexion, extension, supination, and pronation.
2. After you are able to move the injured area unassisted, the physical therapis will supervise unassisted ROMs and ther isometric exercises on the muscles tha are connected to the injured body area.

PHASE II: FOR MODERATE TO SEVERE INJURIES

1. When you are able to move the injurec body area and you can do isometric exercises with your own strength and withou undue pain, begin Phase II exercises.
2. Phase II exercises (bend/extend, flexion) are those that let you bend and strengthen the body area through the full range o its motion.

PHASE III: FOR MILD INJURIES

These involve dynamic exercises to strengthen muscles as well as stretch them through a full range of motion. They also involve regaining balance and motor-sensory pronation. After this phase is completed, you may begin the three levels of preventive and conditioning exercises in Part Two.

WEIGHT-LOADING EXERCISES

The amount of weight that you add depends on your own body weight and on your muscle strength and size. (See chart on facing page.) In general, do not use any weights until your doctor or physical therapist says that it is okay. Weight-loading exercises can then be added in Phase II and III of the rehab schedule.

ANKLE AND LOWER LEG INJURY EXERCISES

Rehabilitation (Phases I and II) is needed after surgery, sprains, and fractures, beginning as soon as possible (between five and twenty-one days after the operation). Rehab will promote blood flow for faster healing, prevent atrophy and tightening of the surrounding muscles, and will help relieve pain from joint stiffness. Use isometric, active- or passive-assisted ROM exercises in areas that don't have open surgical wounds. Use Phase III Therapeutic for mild lower leg, ankle, or foot injuries, or after you have done the Rehab series for approximately three weeks (a longer time period may be required for severe injuries). When your injured ankle, foot, or lower leg has returned to between 90 and 95% of its original strength, you may proceed to the prevention level of exercise for this body area (see Part Two).

WEIGHT LOAD/REPETITION SCHEDULE

	LOAD	REPETITIONS
Phase I	No weight	determined by MD or PT
Phase II	See schedule	1–5
Phase III	See schedule	6–12

WEIGHT-LOADING SCHEDULE

USE FOR PHASES II AND III

	AMOUNT OF WEIGHT		
TYPE OF WEIGHT	SMALL FRAME	MEDIUM FRAME	LARGE FRAME
Hand-held	0–¼ lbs.	¼–½ lbs.	½–1 lbs.
Ankle	0–½ lbs.	½–1 lbs.	1–5 lbs.

Phase I Ankle and Lower Leg Rehab Exercises

Ankle ROM I

- Draw the whole alphabet in capital letters with your foot, toes pointed
- Repeat two more times

Ankle and Toe ROM

- In a seated or prone position, flex your foot upward, straightening your toes
- Point your foot downward, bending your toes
- Repeat two more times in each direction

Ankle and Lower Leg ROM

- Rotate your ankle in clockwise and counterclockwise circles, eight to twelve circles in each direction
- Repeat two more times in each direction

Toe ROMs

- Squeeze your toes together, gripping and holding an imaginary pencil
- Release the grip and slowly spread and straighten your toes out and back

Ankle ROM II

- Seated or prone position, slowly turn your foot, soles facing inward, then soles facing outward
- Repeat eight to ten times

Achilles and Calf Stretch

- Stand with your feet shoulder-width apart and parallel to each other

- Step back with one leg, at the same time bending your forward knee
- Place both hands on the forward thigh just above the knee and bend forward; press your back heel against the floor and lean forward
- Hold the stretch, building up from three to ten seconds
- Relax the muscle by stepping forward and slightly straightening out your legs
- Slightly bend both knees for a short time
- Repeat the stretch on the other leg
- Repeat one to three times on each leg

Ankle and Calf Strengthener (Simple Heel Raises)

- Stand with your feet parallel and shoulder-width apart
- Slowly raise your heels and lower them back to the floor, extending your arms forward to keep your balance
- Repeat this exercise, first with your feet parallel and then with your feet turned inward
- Repeat each position one to six times

Phase III Ankle and Lower Leg Rx Therapeutic Exercise

Calf and Achilles Tendon Stretch and Strengthener

- Stand with your feet parallel and hip-width apart on a step with your heels hanging off the back edge
- Extend your arms forward to keep your balance
- Raise and lower heels slowly

Ankle ROM With Resistance

- Place a folded towel or bed blanket on the floor
- In a standing or seated position with one foot in front of the other, firmly plant the forward heel on the floor and lift your big toe and forefoot to scoop the towel back toward you
- Place a soup can or book on the towel to add extra resistance
- Repeat the exercise with each foot three to ten times

Ankle and Foot Proprioception

Please note: Proprioception is your ability to feel your movements without looking. It involves coordination, reflexes, and reaction time.

Balance yourself on a board that is straddling another board or over a tennis ball. (Physical therapist may use a balance board.)

Knee Injuries Rx

The knee is the largest joint in the body and bears the greatest load of activity in sports and exercise. The knee is acted upon by large muscles that subject it to a great deal of stress but also support it.

Before the fitness boom, knee injuries were exclusive to active and retired college and professional athletes. Now, they are among the most common injuries.

With an increase in various forms of arthritis and osteoporosis, a damaged knee will worsen and require greater protection or rehabilitation. Such anatomical differences as high arches, flat feet, turned-in thigh bones, knock-knees, bowlegs, and inequalities in leg length can also aggravate or complicate a damaged or diseased knee. Orthotics or shoe inserts can correct these differences in some circumstances, as can well-constructed athletic shoes. But foot aids often cannot stop the damage done by increased impact forces on the knees that are created when exercising at a high-intensity level.

When you jump, your body leaves the ground, then returns with a shock force that is three to four times your body weight. Shoes and orthotics can only reduce impact forces by 5 to 15%, whereas changing the way you move eliminates 75% of the force! By eliminating jumping and jogging motions and substituting them with walking and sliding motions, you reduce the force from 300 to 400% down to between 50 and 150% of your body weight.

You can prevent many knee injuries by eliminating lateral and jumping movements and keeping your knees slightly bent during physical activities. Strong thigh muscles also help protect your knees from twisting forces. Develop balanced leg muscles by strengthening and stretching front and back leg muscles equally (your quadriceps may require more work, however). Choose sports that complement each other in regard to equal muscle use, for example, running, walking, skating, skiing, bicycling, and swimming. Also, do not increase the intensity or duration of your exercise routine by more than 10% per week.

Practice correct foot position and posture techniques to help condition the body for proper alignment during sports and exercise. This will, in turn, reduce injuries to knee joints by redistributing forces on the knees to other parts of the body.

Warming up, stretching, and cooling down are the most important exercises especially for your knees because they make body tissues more pliable and, thus, more able to withstand fast or intense movements. They reduce the impact of muscle or tendon pulls on the knee joints.

ACUTE KNEE INJURIES

KNEE PLICA

The roughening of the ends of your thigh bone caused by the repetitive snapping of the plica, which are bands of tissue surrounding the knee joint. They can become too tight or too loose from repeated bending of the knee in sports or exercise.

Symptoms:
Pain when walking down stairs, squatting, or kneeling; mild locking of knee when bent too far.

ExRx:
First rest and ice, then practice Phase II Rehab knee exercises as soon as the pain subsides. If surgery is performed, begin with Phase I Rehab. Both recoveries require four to six weeks of rehab.

KNEE SPRAINS

An overstretching, tearing, or rupture of one or more of the seven ligaments of the knee; caused by twisting or impact. Most often damaged are the medial collateral ligament and the anterior cruciate ligament.

Symptoms:
Medial collateral ligament injury—immediate pain, which recedes and then recurs when

HOWARD TUROFF

DIAGNOSIS: DAMAGED KNEES FROM SPORTS AND OVERUSE

Howard Turoff's knees have gone through five surgeries. First, he blew out his right knee in 1973 playing baseball in high school. In 1975, he was less than successfully operated on. His knee bent sideways. If he twisted it, it would give way and collapse. Howard had another surgery in 1983 in which his knee was irrigated. Howard blames his damaged knees on the sports he played in high school—football, baseball, and basketball.

After his second surgery, Howard changed his exercise lifestyle. He began swimming, biking, running, and taking karate lessons. He had his knee irrigated once more in 1989. Then in 1992, after years of training in swimming, biking, and running, Howard competed in the Iron Man Triathlon, completing it in sixteen and a half hours.

Unfortunately, his right knee was popping out of his socket on a regular basis. In 1993, it popped out of its socket, but this time, he couldn't get it to go back in place. Finally, Howard had to have full, reconstructive knee surgery. The twenty-year-old injury had now become arthritic. Even with the surgery and the arthritis, Howard had a relatively easy recovery. "Being fit enabled me to recover faster," he explains.

Howard became busy with biking. His wife's company, La Corsa Tours, Inc. runs bike tours in Italy and France, and Howard leads the tours. He is a big proponent of biking as a healing method. Howard says, "Biking works because it is not fully weight-bearing, and there is no impact." And while there is no way to build up your knees, biking is great for strengthening the muscles that support the knees—the quads and hamstrings.

Karate also helped Howard strengthen those supporting muscles, as well as teaching him how to move in safer ways. Howard has had two falls off of his bike, but neither one was serious because karate taught him how to fall. He also learned to protect his joints by being relaxed, so his body is loose and can take an impact more effectively.

Howard does his two-and-a-half-hour karate workout three times a week. That involves stretching, kicks, punches, push-ups, an abdominal workout, and situational role-playing. When Howard is biking regularly (mainly in the summer) he does long rides over hills. Usually, he rides 150 to 200 miles a week, but when on tour, leading a trip, he covers 500 miles. He bikes long distance, keeping his heart rate in the 130 to 140 beats per minute (bpm) range. When racing, however, it can climb to 165 bpm.

While on the twelfth and last training ride six weeks before a tour trip, Howard severely injured his left knee. Although he had full, reconstructive surgery on that knee, he was back on a bike four days after surgery. His doctor was unsure, at first, whether Howard should lead the upcoming tour. He had just come out of major knee surgery, but Howard is a speedy recoverer. His doctor told him, "You're far ahead of where you ought to be because you rode so much before the surgery and because you got right back on the bike after." His diligence about riding the bike was the key to Howard's successful recovery: He led the bike tour.

trying to move the knee, also stiffness, swelling, and instability. First-degree injury (mild): stretching or a few tears, minor pain, and stiffness. Second-degree injury (moderate): tearing of many fibers, which results in the inability to straighten the leg or place any weight on the foot. Third-degree injury (severe): complete rupture, which causes no immediate pain, but loss of stability and possibly pain later.

An anterior cruciate ligament injury is almost always a complete rupture caused by a violent twist. There is an immediate popping sound and the knee feels as if it is falling apart; becomes very swollen and cannot be walked upon.

ExRx:
Medial collateral ligament—For first-degree sprains, as soon as pain and inflammation abate, practice rehab knee exercises (see pp. 334–338) for six weeks before returning to the preventive level. For second-degree sprains, first three days of rest and ice and splinting, then practice rehabilitative exercises for six to twelve weeks. For third-degree sprains, first three to five days of rest and ice and brace for six weeks, then practice rehab knee exercises for another twelve weeks.

A sprain of the anterior cruciate ligament requires the same treatment as a medial collateral ligament injury, but for three months duration; nine to twelve months if surgery is involved. After three months, some will be able to start light aerobics.

OSGOOD-SCHLATTER DISEASE

An irritation in the area where the tendon from the kneecap attaches to the shin bone from repeated knee bends in running-type sports. Caused by growth spurt of the bone and damage to bone ends that have not fully hardened. Usually found in boys ages ten to fourteen.

Symptoms:
A gradual, mild ache, which worsens over weeks and prevents the child from running and fully bending the knee. Also, child walks with a limp. Condition can persist for up to three years. Also, 10% can develop an enlarged piece of bone at the top of the shin, just below the knee, causing a knee bump and pain throughout life.

ExRx:
To prevent, child should abstain from strenuous running activities during growth spurts. In severe cases, the bone piece may be surgically removed. The knee can be immobilized with a cast until inflammation has subsided. Depending on severity, practice knee therapeutic or rehab exercises after pain has subsided.

OSTEOCHRONDRITIS DISSECANS OF KNEE

Grinding together of knee bones to form a crater and/or loose chips of bone that may fall into the knee. Caused by repetitive impact between the ends of the thigh and main shin bones. Occurs in adults, but also children ages twelve to sixteen are especially at risk because of their softer bones.

Symptoms:
Pain grows gradually worse during dynamic bending. If a bone chip dislodges, knee joint may lock and be very painful to straighten or even to touch.

ExRx:
Adults usually need knee surgery to correct. A child needs injured knee immobilization

AMY MCKHANN

DIAGNOSIS: RUPTURE OF THE ANTERIOR CRUCIATE LIGAMENT

Amy McKhann, a financial advisor, has always been athletic. She had been a professional dancer.

In her thirties, she would go skiing all day, then play tennis afterward. Consequently, Amy overloaded her body. Finally, she ruptured her meniscofemoral ligaments and the anterior cruciate ligament on her right knee. After the necessary surgery, she couldn't walk or put any weight on her right leg.

Therapy began with ice on the injured knee and then putting it in a cradle, which moved the leg up and down. After five or six days, the bleeding in her knee stopped. Amy then began swimming every day. "The swimming was the miracle," she says. She also spent one and a half hours a day riding a bike, or using a ski simulator. Amy found the bike to be the most comfortable exercise: there was no pressure or tension.

Up to this point, Amy's surgeon and her physical therapist had been her healers. Now, she acquired a trainer, Angela Fischetti. At first, Angela worked with Amy just on her upper body, until the rest of Amy's body was strong enough to join in. Leg extensions would have further damaged her knees, so her lower body workout began with stretching the quads, hamstrings, and calves.

Amy did a squat variation, no deeper than a 90-degree angle. She also did back squats, where the machine is on an approximately 45-degree angle. Amy rested back in the unit and slid up and down with her feet up high so the toes didn't bear any of the weight. Another of Amy's squats was done on the Smith press machine; this was done with her toes lifted to put the weight back on her heels.

Amy also worked on the leg press, keeping her feet up high and never bringing the knee into flexion. She kept her toes over the edge of the foot rest, again so as not to put any weight on her knee. Some exercises that she was advised not to do (and, consequently, did not do) were weighted leg lifts and anything with isolation of the quadricep. Amy did modified lunges that were no deeper than 90 degrees. For leg curls, she used the hamstring isolator and the hip abductor/aductor machines.

Angela put Amy on a recumbent bike for less flexion. Amy also did calf work, lifts, and donkey raises, to work the larger calf muscle. Seated calf raises worked the smaller calf muscles. Amy's regimen also included crunch variations. The ski simulator brought her abs, hips, and thighs back up to speed.

Amy is now 100% recovered and is told she has twenty-one-year-old legs. She promises not to try to be WonderWoman anymore. She does everything, just not all at once, and not on the same day. Yoga has played a big role in that fact. "My life was unbalanced before," she explains.

Amy says, "Physically, I could live until 110 or 120!"

DR. ALBERT ROSEN

DIAGNOSIS: PLATEAU FRACTURE OF THE TIBIA; KNEE REPLACEMENT

Bones break at any age, but older bones break more easily.

"August 15, 1987 was not one of the better days in my three score and ten years of existence," says Dr. Albert Rosen. "It was a beautiful day. I decided to combine business and pleasure by biking to the hospital to examine a newborn." Instead, he arrived at the hospital in an ambulance, and never got to see the newborn.

Dr. Rosen eventually learned that, while on the bike path in his country park, an out-of-control car had crashed into the park at a tremendous rate of speed, and hit him. He was thrown onto the hood of the car and his head smashed into the windshield. He was then thrown thirty feet in the air and landed on his head; the car ended up in a duck pond. "Without my helmet I would never have survived the two smashes to my head," he explains. "I sustained several fractures. The most serious was a plateau fracture of the tibia, which is notorious for its poor end result, a cerebral concussion, and numerous lacerations and bruises."

After surgery to repair the fractured tibia, which required bone grafts, he started rehabilitation. "I was determined to regain my usual lifestyle. I went religiously to rehab, spending hours on the stationary bike, and doing straight leg raising with weights," he says. He reached a point when he could lift thirty pounds thirty times with his injured leg and only ten times with his undamaged leg.

Unfortunately, the plateau fracture failed to heal properly, so he underwent a total knee replacement. Right after surgery, he was allowed to bear weight and start walking the stairs in the hospital. He did seven flights up and down in addition to his regular physical therapy. As a result, he was discharged in seven days, instead of the usual fourteen. Back home, he started walking instead of using the elevator, and hiking.

Nine years after the accident, Dr. Rosen still uses the stationary bike every morning for a half hour and still walks. "The secret of my recovery is exercise, exercise, exercise," he says.

for two to three months to allow the knee to heal itself. During this period, you can exercise stiff-legged with a cast.

After the cast comes off, practice Phase I Rehab knee exercises for six weeks and go on to Phase II Rehab and Phase III as you gain the appropriate strength. The whole process may take up to six months in nonoperative treatment. With surgery, the recovery period is eight to twelve weeks.

PATELLAR TENDINITIS (JUMPER'S KNEE)

An inflammation of the tendons of the kneecap.

Symptoms:
Pain felt below the kneecap when seated or straightening out the leg.

ExRx:
Prevent by developing more thigh muscle strength and flexibility. Treat by ceasing jumping and squatting activities (e.g. basketball, weight-lifter's squat) until condition abates (between two and four weeks). Because tendons heal slowly, maintain muscle condition with low-impact, cardiovascular exercise, for example, swimming, bicycling, or walking. Adjust the height of the bicycle seat so your knee does not fully straighten. Sometimes treated by trimming off scar tissue with surgery. Begin knee Rehab Level I within twenty-four hours. Recovery can take several months if condition is severe.

PATELLOFEMORAL PAIN SYNDROME

Damage to the kneecap caused by misalignment of the kneecap combined with repetitive bending and pounding of the knee during running and jumping-type exercises. Misalignment may be caused by an anatomical abnormality (e.g. flat feet) or muscle imbalances (e.g. weakness of inner thigh muscles versus tightness of outer thigh muscles). Can be either chronic or acute.

Symptoms:
Pain in kneecap that intensifies during running sports activities or when walking up stairs. Also, crackling or crunching sensations and sounds.

ExRx:
Prevent by reducing running and jumping activities and by practicing balanced leg development. Treat nonsurgically by stretching outer thighs and strengthening inner thighs with Phase III exercises. Also, can be treated surgically to realign kneecap. After surgery, rehabilitate with Phase II Rehab exercises. Recovery for both injuries is six to twelve weeks. Of extreme importance is the medical evaluation of the feet and the use of orthotics, which can realign the angle of the knee, helping the patella to track properly.

SESAMOIDITIS OF THE KNEE

Inflammation of the sesamoids, the oval-shaped bones that lie within a tendon (your knee cap is the largest sesamoid).

Symptoms:
Knee pain.

ExRx:
Practice parallel foot placement and low-impact versions of stepping exercises to reduce force of ground impact and side-to-side motions on knees.

OVERUSE KNEE INJURIES

BURSITIS IN THE KNEE

Inflammation from repetitive stress to one or more of the seven bursa sacs in the knee, causing fluid to fill up the sacs. Can also be caused by a single blow (hemobursae). Most frequently injured is the bursa over the kneecap (prepatellar) caused by kneeling too much, ballet, trampolining, and wrestling.

Symptoms:
Tenderness and swelling over kneecap, limited range of motion.

ExRx:

First, rest; then, practice such non-knee bending exercises as walking on level ground, which involves much less bending or kneeling of the knee. Practice therapeutic exercises for the injured knee. If knee bursa becomes chronically inflamed, adhesions may form and surgical removal of the bursa may be necessary. If surgery is performed, practice Phase I Rehab exercises. Recovery period for both surgical and nonsurgical healing is ten to fourteen days.

MUSKEL RX: LIST OF ADDITIONAL KNEE AND THIGH INJURIES BENEFITED BY KNEE REHAB EXERCISE

- quadriceps tendinitis
- subluxing kneecap
- thigh bruise
- thigh fracture

Illiotibial Band Friction Syndrome

An inflammation of the thick tendon running from the outside of the pelvis down to the outside of the knee at the top of the large shin bone. Caused by too much running, ballet, aerobic dancing, and so forth.

Symptoms:

Gradual tightness on the outer knee which changes to a burning sensation while running. Pain grows worse going downhill. This syndrome forces you to walk or run with your leg fully straightened to relieve pressure.

ExRx:

Prevent with more warm-up exercises. For recovery, treat by refraining from running or other aggravating activity and substituting with non-knee bending/straightening activity such as swimming. Do illiotibial band (outer thigh) stretches (p. 337) up to six times a day, thirty-second hold per stretch. For mild cases, two or three days of recovery; moderate cases, recovery takes up to two weeks; severe cases, recovery can last up to six months. Also, use shoes with adequate cushioning.

Knee Injury Exercises

Phase I Knee Rehab exercises are used after knee surgery and are done with a physical therapist. Phase II Knee Rehab exercises are used for moderate or severe knee injuries (you may exercise with a knee brace at this phase). If you have been exercising at Phase I, start Phase II when you are able to move your knee by yourself. Phase III Knee Therapeutic exercises are used for mild to moderate knee injuries as well as for mild thigh injuries. You will stretch and strengthen the thigh and groin muscles while continuing to improve knee joint range of motion. Start Phase III when you can do Phase II without pain. (See General Rehabilitation Guidelines and Procedures and Weight-loading Schedule, pp. 324–325.)

Phase I Knee Rehab Exercises

After surgery, do passive-assisted and active-assisted ROMs and isometric exercises (e.g., isometric quadriceps strengthening) that do not interfere with surgical sutures. Continue these until you are able to use your own strength to do the knee exercises.

Phase II Knee Rehab Exercises

Knee ROM with Thigh (Extensor) Muscles (Seated)

- Sit on a mat or the floor

- Place a rolled up towel under your injured knee
- Contract your thigh muscles and raise your foot to straighten your leg; your injured knee should keep contact with the towel
- Hold the raised position for five to ten seconds; rest five seconds
- Repeat one to five times
- Do two to five sets a day

Knee ROM with Hamstring (Flexor) Muscle (Seated)

- Sit back on a table or tall chair, thighs supported, legs dangling
- Position the front of the ankle of your healthy leg behind the heel of your injured leg
- Bend the injured knee backward, gently pushing against the healthy leg; hold for five to ten seconds
- Use the healthy leg to guide the injured one back to the starting position
- Repeat two to five times a day

Knee ROM with Hamstring (Flexor) Muscle (Lying Down)

- Lie face down; place the ankle of your healthy leg behind the heel of your injured leg to help guide it
- Bend your injured leg back toward your buttocks as far it will go; hold for five to ten seconds
- Repeat two to five times a day

Thigh (Extensor) Strengthener

Please note: This exercise is not for people with lower back problems.

- Lie on your back; contract the thigh muscle of your injured leg
- Straighten the knee of your injured leg then raise and lower your leg two to ten times; heel comes three to twelve inches off the ground
- Rest fifteen to thirty seconds between repetitions
- Increase the number of repetitions from between ten and twenty to between twenty and thirty as your leg feels stronger

Hamstring (Flexor) Strengthener

- Sit on a stoop or thick mat with your injured leg bent and healthy leg extended
- Pull the injured leg back until it meets the stoop or mat
- Press against it for five to ten seconds
- Stretch out the injured leg and hold for five seconds
- Repeat the exercise five to ten times, building up to thirty times

PHASE III KNEE THERAPEUTIC EXERCISES

Knee ROM with Hamstring (Flexor) Muscles (Lying Down)

- Lie on your back on a mat placed near a wall; wear socks
- Place your injured leg up against the wall

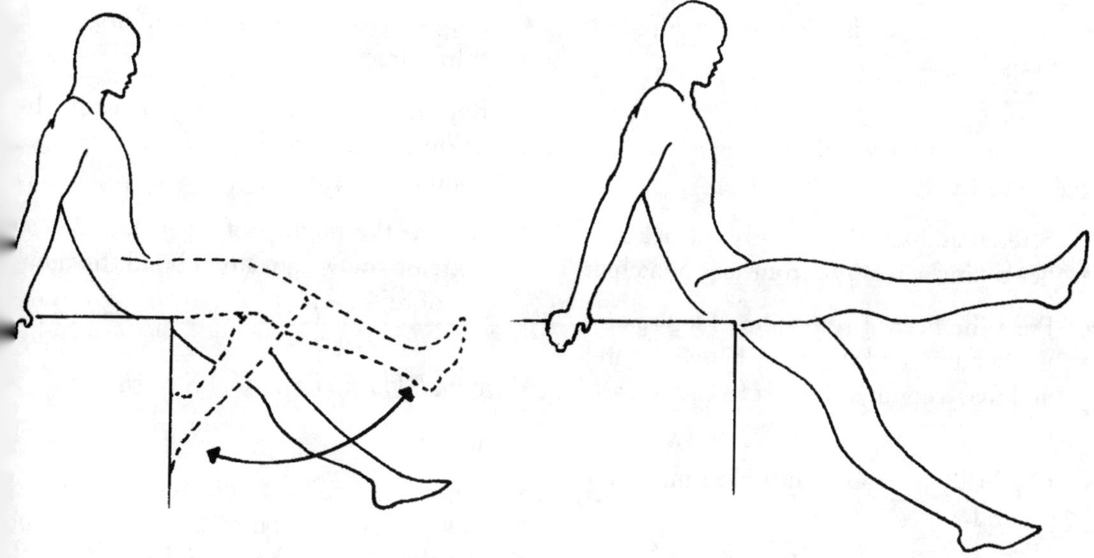

Hamstring (Flexor) Strengthener

- Let your foot slide down the wall as you bend your knee
- Raise your leg again and repeat two to five times

Knee ROM with Hamstring (Flexor) Muscles (Standing)

- Stand and place the foot of your injured leg on a chair (knee bent at a 90-degree angle)
- Slowly lean forward as you bend your injured knee further (can be bent from 45 degrees down to a 15-degree angle)
- Hold five to ten seconds before returning to the starting position
- Repeat two to five times

Knee Strengthener for Thigh (Extensor) Muscle

- Attach an ankle weight (one to five pounds) to your injured leg
- Sit back on a table or tall chair with legs dangling
- Slowly raise, straighten, and lower your leg five to ten times
- Hold one to six seconds in a straightened position; rest five seconds between each repetition
- Repeat the set of exercises two to three

times a day, building up to thirty repetitions

Knee Strengthener for Hamstring (Flexor) Muscle

- Stretch and attach a length of thick rubber tubing across the front legs of a chair
- Press the heel of your injured leg against the tubing; hold the press between three and five seconds, then rest five to ten seconds
- Gradually increase your hold time to ten seconds
- Repeat the exercise three to five times; do two to three sets per day

Knee Strengthener for Thigh (Extensor) Muscles

- Stand with your back against a wall and your feet shoulder-width apart
- Bend your knees as you slowly slide your back down the wall
- Hold the position for ten seconds, then rise up to your starting position and rest for five to fifteen seconds
- Gradually increase your hold time
- Repeat two to five times; do two to three sets per day

Knee Strengthener for Hamstring (Flexor) Muscles

- Attach ankle weights to the injured leg; lie face down
- Slowly raise your lower leg and bend your knee backward, then lower it
- Repeat five to ten times, building up to thirty times
- Repeat the exercise as you increase the ankle weights first by a pound, then two pounds
- Reduce the number of repetitions as you increase the weight, then build the number of reps back up

Knee and Thigh (Extensor) Stretch

- Lie face down
- Grasp the ankle of your injured leg and pull it to your buttocks keeping your thigh pressed to the ground
- Hold the stretch for three to five seconds; build up to between thirty and sixty seconds

Please note: Repeat this stretch at the end of every thigh strengthening exercise.

Knee and Hamstring (Flexor) Stretch

- Lie on your back in a doorway; your injured leg and buttocks should rest on the bottom of the door frame; your healthy leg should stick out of the door opening
- Bend your toes back as you straighten your injured knee
- Hold stretch for three to ten seconds; build up to fifteen to thirty seconds

Knee and Groin Stretch

- Sit on the floor with your knees bent and the soles of your feet pressed together

Hold your ankles and rest your elbows on your knees

Slowly press your knees down with your elbows and hold the stretch for three to ten seconds; build up to fifteen to thirty seconds

Repeat one to three times

Iliotibial Band (Outer Thigh) Stretch

Sit on the floor with your healthy leg extended out in front of you

Raise the injured leg and place the foot of the injured leg on the outside of your healthy knee

Place your healthy side elbow on the outside of the injured knee; brace yourself with your other arm

Gently press the injured knee toward your healthy leg while turning your shoulders in the opposite direction

Hold for three to five seconds, then rest for five to ten seconds

Repeat one to three times

Thigh Injuries Rx

The thigh is the bone in your body with the largest and most powerful muscle group, the quadriceps (also called the *rectus femoris*), on the front side, and the hamstring (another powerful muscle) on the back side. For balanced muscle development, your hamstrings, composed of three muscles, should have 60 to 70% of the strength of the quadriceps, which consists of four muscles.

Overuse thigh injuries are rare because this muscle is strong and well protected. Acute injuries (much more common) are prevented by strengthening and stretching the thigh muscles. When playing sports or practicing vigorous exercise, protect the thigh from impacts and falling-down injuries by wearing protective thigh pads.

Hamstring Strain

A stretch, tear, or rupture of one or more of the three muscles behind the thigh.

Symptoms:
First-degree injury (mild)—slight pull in muscles behind thigh when running, next day soreness. Second-degree injury (moderate)—twinge causes you to stop running, then continued pain, tenderness, and bruising under skin. Third-degree injury (severe)—sharp pain, collapse, walking impossible.

ExRx:
Prevent by muscle warm-ups and reducing running mileage. Treat properly or this injury will recur. First, rest and ice for forty-eight to seventy-two hours. Second-degree and third-degree injuries may need bed rest and crutches until you can walk without a limp. Gentle thigh stretching will minimize scarring from a rupture. For first-degree injuries, practice Phase II Thigh Therapeutic exercises. For second-degree injuries, do Phase III Rehab. For third-degree, do Phases I and II Rehab. Practice cardiovascular activities (e.g. swimming) for the upper body; walking, stationary cycling, and stair climbing for the lower body. None of these exercises will overstress the hamstrings.

Quadriceps Strain

A rupture, stretch, or tear of one or more of the four muscles that together make up the quadriceps.

Symptoms:
Stabbing pain when trying to straighten the knee caused by a violent contraction of the muscle during explosive, stop-and-start running moves.

ExRx:
Prevent by strengthening and stretching thighs, and by doing warm-up and cool-down exercise before and after stop-and-start and running sports play. Treat first with rest and ice immediately, continue for forty-eight to seventy-two hours. Treat mild strain with Phase III Therapeutic knee exercises for three to five days. Rehab moderate strain with Phase II Rehab exercises for two to three weeks. Rehab severe strain with Phases I and II Rehab for up to ten weeks.

THIGH INJURY EXERCISE

Similar to the rehabilitation of any large or important muscle group, the thigh injury rehab should be performed in a comprehensive manner because of the danger of strength and mobility loss that can lead to recurrent injury and permanent disability. Phase I Thigh Rehab exercises are done with a physical therapist after surgery. Phase II Thigh Rehab exercises are used as a starting point for moderate to severe injuries that do not require surgery. Phase III Thigh Therapeutic exercises are used for mild injuries or when you can do Phase II exercises without pain.

PHASE I THIGH REHAB EXERCISES

Thigh Physical Therapy

After surgery, therapist will use active-assisted and passive-assisted ROM exercises and isometrics that do not compromise surgery.

Phase II Thigh Rehab Exercises

Quadriceps Stretch
(see pp. 239–244)

Quadriceps Isometric Strengthener (Lying Down)

- Lie face down
- Grasp the ankle of your injured leg an pull it toward your buttocks
- Keeping your thigh flush to the floor, tr to straighten your leg while resisting wit your hand; hold for up to six seconds
- Repeat this exercise with your other leg

Standing Quadriceps Stretch and Strengthener

- Start with your feet hip-width apart an brace yourself on a wall with the han opposite the side of your injured leg
- Grasp the ankle of your injured leg, hol your hip straight or slightly back
- Stretch your thigh by pulling your ankl toward your buttocks and hold for count of six seconds
- Then strengthen the thigh by pushin against your hand resistance for up to si seconds

Prone Hamstring Strengthener and Stretche in Door Frame

- Lie on your back with your buttocks nea the door frame and let your healthy le stick out into the doorway
- Stretch your thigh by straightening you knee as you bend your toe toward you knee and lean forward

- Hold for five to ten seconds
- Now, strengthen your thigh by pressing your heel against the doorway and hold for another five to ten seconds

Standing Groin Stretch (see p. 206)

Seated Thigh Stretch (see p. 240)

Seated Outer Thigh Strengthener

- Sit on the floor with your healthy leg extended out in front of you
- Place the foot of your injured leg on the outside of your healthy knee
- Place your healthy side elbow on the outside of your injured knee
- Grasp your injured side shoulder with your healthy side hand and your healthy side ankle with your injured side hand for greater resistance
- Now, press your injured side knee against the elbow resistance, brace yourself further by pushing against your shoulder and ankle with your two hands

Phase II Thigh Rehabilitation

Lying Hamstring Strengthener with Ankle Weights

- Attach ankle weights and lie face down
- Curl your ankle so it approaches your buttocks, then curl it back down slowly

Standing Groin and Outer Thigh Strengthener

- Attach ankle weights to your leg; place your hand against a wall for balance
- Pull your outer leg across the front of your body toward the wall, then extend that leg back across and away from your body
- Do each exercise ten to thirty times

Thigh Injury Prevention Exercises (see pp. 237–244)

Shoulder and Upper Arm Injuries Rx

Shoulder injuries account for 10% of all sports injuries. They can be caused by repetitive throwing and pushing as well as batting, overhead and side stroking, and swinging motions as in swimming, golf, and tennis. Shoulder injuries are also among the most difficult of all injuries to rehabilitate because of the many bones, joints, and muscles involved. Shoulder movements are controlled by three major joints and twenty different muscles, which make shoulder injuries difficult to rehabilitate. Three major bones—the collarbone, shoulder blade, and the upper arm bone all meet at the shoulder. These are held together by relatively weak ligaments and surrounded by powerful muscles that cross from the neck and upper torso.

Overuse shoulder injuries are common and can be caused by such low-impact activities as swimming. Acute injuries are usually caused by ballistic or jerking motions such as those associated with swinging a bat.

Acute Shoulder and Upper Arm Injuries

Biceps Strain

A pull or tear of the muscle fibers caused by a sudden, powerful movement such as in throwing or lifting.

Symptoms:
Pain, tenderness, and stiffness.

ExRx:
Rest the arm and begin either Phase II or III Rehab when pain subsides.

Chest Muscle Strain

Pulls or tears of the tendons where the chest muscles attach to the upper arms. Caused by a single, extremely powerful lift, pull, or push as in weight lifting or field sports.

Symptoms:
Acute pain when lifting, extensive bruising, and possible loss of chest muscle definition.

ExRx:
Rest and ice for first-degree strains (mild). For second-degree strains (moderate), rest the injured area; begin Phase II Rehab after three days, then three- to six-week recovery. For third degree strains (severe), begin exercising with Phase I; or with surgery, four weeks of immobilization and then Phase I; severe strains have a six- to twelve-week recovery period. If pain is severe, wear an arm sling for five to ten days. Continue rest and ice for all degrees of injury.

Dislocated Shoulder

The ball at the top of the upper arm bone comes out of the socket in the shoulder blade. Caused by a collision or a fall with an outstretched arm and results in susceptibility to further dislocations, even during daily activities.

Symptoms:
Extreme pain, muscle spasm, and the injured arm goes limp.

ExRx:
Professional must realign shoulder—the sooner the better for fewer complications. Apply ice in the meantime and immobilize the injured arm in a sling. Adults, two to three weeks in a sling; children, six weeks. Very important to begin rehab exercises as soon as pain permits because adults, especially, are at risk of long-term dysfunction and are also more apt to redislocate the injured shoulder. Begin isometrics and ROMs as early as twenty-four to forty-eight hours, if possible. After two to three weeks, you should be able to lift your arm to shoulder height and rotate without pain. Complete recovery time is two to three months.

Separated Shoulder

A stretching or tearing of the ligaments that hold the shoulder bones in place. Most common is acromioclavicular separation caused by a fall or impact to the tip of the shoulder.

Symptoms
First-degree injury (mild)—ligaments are only stretched, there is pain and tenderness on movement, but no bone displacement. Second-degree injury (moderate)—shoulder aches constantly, ligaments are partially torn, and there is significant pain and tenderness. Third-degree injury (severe)—there is extreme pain, ruptured ligaments, bruising, and swelling.

ExRx:
For first-degree—apply ice twenty minutes on, twenty minutes off for seven to ten days while arm is in a sling. For second-degree—apply ice in similar manner to first-degree injury and contact doctor if unable to lift arm overhead. Expect up to ten days of pain and

decreased range of motion. For third-degree—apply ice and seek immediate medical assistance; immobilize the injured arm and secure it with an elastic bandage. This severe injury probably needs surgery.

For a third-degree injury and postsurgical, begin Rehab exercises two weeks after injury. Remove the immobilizer to exercise. Start with Phase I ROM exercises until full mobility returns. Strength training begins six weeks later and lasts about one month before starting preventive shoulder exercises.

Shoulder Subluxation (Shoulder Popping)

The ball of the shoulder joint slips in and out of the socket. Can recur if front lip of the socket is deteriorated. Caused by overarm and side arm throws and strokes.

Symptoms:
Popping in and out accompanied by severe pain for about a minute; numbness and weakness follows.

ExRx:
Isolated movement can be treated with ice and a two-day rest. Heat treatment thereafter. After a week, start ROMs and strengthening exercises. If recurring, surgery may be necessary to tighten up the area with eight weeks to six months of rehabilitation and therapy.

Upper Arm Fractures

A crack, break, or shattering of the humerus bone caused by a direct blow or a fall with the arm outstretched.

Symptoms:
Immediate pain and swelling; the break may be felt through the skin.

ExRx:
Ice over area (twenty minutes on, twenty minutes off) while waiting for immediate medical attention. Immobilize the injured arm in a splint and secure with an elastic bandage. For severe breaks, a realignment of the bone or surgery might be needed. After approximately a ten-day immobilization period, Phase I Rehab exercises can begin with physical therapist-assisted ROM exercises. When you are able to move yourself through ROMs, Phase II Rehab can begin and continue through Phase III for a total of about three to six months after surgery.

Overuse Shoulder and Upper Arm Injuries

Biceps Tendinitis

An inflammation of the tendon that connects the biceps muscle to the shoulder joint; injury is caused by repetitive overarm motions and overtraining for sports (e.g. golf, tennis, rowing, swimming, baseball).

Symptoms:
Onset of pain is gradual in front of shoulder. Hurts when you raise and lower arm and cracks when lifting arm over shoulder.

ExRx:
Catch it early and rehabilitate before pain becomes a more difficult chronic condition. Begin Phase III exercises for a mild condition after one to two days rest. For moderate injuries, begin Phases I and II within one week and continue for about two to three weeks. After surgery, rehab can take up to twelve weeks.

FROZEN SHOULDER

A condition in which the joint capsules stick and can even grow together leading to a severe loss of mobility in as little as two to three weeks. This condition is made worse by inactivity and requires immediate physical therapy to head off disaster. Otherwise, it may take years of rehab to correct. Commonly occurs in injured athletes, diabetics, menopausal women, and smokers.

Symptoms:
Ache in shoulder, extreme pain during overarm movements, and reduced mobility.

ExRx:
Avoid letting shoulder overuse injuries go untreated. Inactivity allows the adhesions to grow stronger, so it is important to begin rehabilitation exercise immediately. Rest and ice, and then begin shoulder ROM exercises, staying within your pain threshold. If the condition does not clear up in four to six months, surgery may be necessary to break the adhesions.

PECTORAL MUSCLE INSERTION INFLAMMATION

Caused by a series of mini-tears in the tendon fibers that attach the chest muscle to the upper arm just below your armpit. Caused by excessive weight lifting and across-the-chest sports moves in tennis, golf, and swimming. When a person is over forty, frequent mini-tears can lead to a rupture.

Symptoms:
Gradual onset of pain just below the armpit where chest muscle attaches to the upper arm; pain increases when you try to move your arm toward and away from your chest against resistance.

ExRx:
Treat early to avoid having a chronic injury; rest and ice. For mild injuries, if you begin gentle ROMs and isometric exercise right away, the condition can clear up in one week. Phase II exercises begin in ten to fourteen days. For moderate injuries, start Phase II in two to three weeks; rehab takes another two to three weeks. For severe injuries or postsurgery, rehab starts at Phase I and can continue for twelve weeks.

ROTATOR CUFF TENDINITIS

Inflammation of one or more of the tendons that holds the ball of the shoulder joint in its socket. Caused by a sudden increase in training or powerful, repetitive, overarm motions. This tendinitis usually affects the tendon of the suprapinous muscle and is part of the shoulder impingement syndrome (see below).

Symptoms:
Gradual onset of pain, weakness, swelling, and tenderness in the front and upper part of the shoulder. Shoulder hurts when arm is extended or raised and lowered.

ExRx:
Catch it early to avoid larger, ongoing problems later. Mild symptoms can be cleared up in three weeks with ice (twenty minutes on, twenty minutes off) three times a day. Modify overarm activity so it does not cause pain or cease arm activity altogether if still painful. For mild to moderate injuries, begin Phase II Rehab right away, and go to Phase III within a week for a six-week recovery period. For severe pain or postsurgery, begin Phase I exer-

cises in about three to five days for a twelve-week recovery period.

Shoulder Bursitis

An inflammation of the bursa sac located between the rotator cuff tendons and the shoulder blade, caused by repetitive overarm motions in sports. After age thirty, it can be precipitated by calcium deposits around the rotator cuff tendons that can penetrate the sac, too.

Symptoms:
Pain in front and upper part of shoulder, tenderness, swelling, loss of motion. (Symptoms are similar to tendinitis and shoulder impingement syndrome.)

ExRx:
Cease the overarm activity, but keep your shoulder otherwise active to avoid a frozen shoulder condition. Medication for pain and swelling. Rest and ice first, and later, heat treatment. May need draining of the bursa sac or surgical treatment. In severe cases, the injured arm may need immobilization, but not for too long. For mild to moderate bursitis, begin Phase II Rehab right away for a recovery of two to three weeks. For severe or postsurgery, begin Phase II within one week; recovery takes about six to eight weeks.

Shoulder Impingement Syndrome (Rotator Cuff)

Chronic shoulder pains caused by repetitive pinching of muscle and bone against soft tissues (i.e. tendons, bursae, ligaments) that surround the shoulder joint. This leads to development of internal scar tissue and degeneration, which, in turn, causes more irritation. It can be caused by frequent and intense overarm motions in such sports as swimming, weight lifting, tennis, and so forth, as well as arthritis caused by an old separated shoulder injury. This syndrome can also be aggravated by muscle imbalances.

Symptoms:
Onset of pain is gradual, but is usually felt early when doing circular arm motions; intensifies with raising and lowering arm straight out in front of your chest as you do when looking at your wristwatch.

ExRx:
Prevent with rotator cuff warm-ups and stretching before any vigorous or strenuous activity. Stop the aggravating motions; apply ice to the injured shoulder twenty minutes on, twenty minutes off, three to four times a day. But avoid totally disengaging shoulder muscles or you may cause "frozen shoulder." Depending on the severity of the injury, start with Phase II or III Rehab. Recovery is within six to eight weeks and is completed within three months. Steroid injections are no substitute for good physical therapy and they can weaken tendons.

Shoulder and Upper Arm Injury Exercises

Phase I Rehab exercises are done after a severe upper arm or shoulder injury or postsurgery. They consist of passive-assisted and active-assisted ROM exercises under the supervision of a physical therapist. Following a severe injury or surgery, begin Phase II when you have completed Phase I for several weeks. For mild to moderate injuries, begin Phase II Rehab (at home) when you are able to move your shoulder by yourself without pain. Start

Phase III Therapeutic exercises (at home) when you can do Phase II exercises without pain or difficulty. (See General Rehabilitation Guidelines and Procedures and Weight-loading Schedule, pp. 324–325.)

MUSKEL RX: LIST OF ADDITIONAL SHOULDER AND ARM INJURIES BENEFITED BY SHOULDER RX REHAB EXERCISES

- biceps bruise (or contusion)
- biceps tear
- collarbone fracture
- separated shoulder II (S-C separation)

Phase I Shoulder and Upper Arm Rehab Exercises (With Physical Therapist)

Phase I consists of six major assisted ROMs: flexion, extension, abduction, adduction, external rotation, and internal rotation.

Phase II Shoulder and Upper Arm Rehab Exercises (At Home)

Pendulum Swings

- Stand behind a sturdy chair with a back
- With your good arm, grasp the chair back for support and lean forward; let your injured arm hang down
- Begin to do full-range swings of your injured arm, swinging only as far as the pain allows; start each swing with five reps and build up to thirty reps

  (1) Rotations: swing your arm clockwise one to five times and counterclockwise one to five times

  (2) Flexion and extension: swing your arm forward 15 to 90 degrees and backward 15 to 90 degrees, one to five times

  (3) Adduction/abduction: swing your arm side to side, out 15 to 90 degrees and back in 15 to 90 degrees
- Repeat the above three pendulum exercises, three times a day, building up to between five and fifteen reps

Lying Arm Raises (Flexion/Extension)

- Lie on the floor, clasp your hands behind your neck, and rest your elbows on the floor
- Alternately, raise each elbow up to your ear and lower it again, five to fifteen times on each side, three times a day

Shoulder Rolls (Internal/External Rotation)

- Sit or stand; place each hand on the top of its shoulder
- Now, trace circles with your elbows, clockwise and counterclockwise, five to fifteen times for each shoulder and in each direction, three times a day

Please note: You can alternate arms or rotate them together—one going clockwise and the other counterclockwise.

Lying Chop (Internal/External Rotations)

- Lie on the floor with your arms stretched out 90 degrees from your body
- Bend your injured arm to a 90-degree

angle with your fingers pointing straight up in the air

- Lower your hand to your hip and hold for five to thirty seconds
- Return to the starting position and lower your hand to your ear and hold there for five to thirty seconds; return to the starting position
- Repeat movement five to fifteen times, three times a day

Phase III Shoulder and Upper Arm Therapeutic Exercises (At Home)

For Phase III, do the same exercises as for Phase I, but now add weights. Do these exercises for mild shoulder injuries or when you can do Phase II exercises without pain or difficulty.

Start with a one-quarter pound weight and increase the weight in increments of one-quarter pound to one pound (see Weight-Load Schedule, p. 325). Add an additional weight at the beginning of each week and increase the repetitions in one to five rep increments until the maximum of thirty is reached. Your goal is to restore your shoulder to 95% of the strength it was before the injury.

After Phases I to III have been completed, begin conditioning and strengthening with the following arm and upper torso exercises:

Shoulder Prevention (Conditioning or Strengthening) Exercises

Lying down strengthening shoulder raises—rotator cuff (internal), pp. 189–190

Biceps curls—rotator cuff (external), pp. 198–199

Seated front raises—deltoid (front), p. 192

Seated overhead raises—deltoid (middle), p. 192

Seated behind the neck—deltoid (back), p. 187

Standing shoulder shrug, upright row—trapezius, p. 191

Standing bent over row—latissimus dorsi, p. 193

Seated chest press, chest cross—pectorals major, pp. 195–196

Seated biceps curl—biceps, p. 199

Standing triceps extension—triceps, p. 195

Underside cuff stretch, p. 189

Front cuff stretch, p. 191

Back cuff stretch, p. 191

Elbow Injuries Rx

Elbow Bursitis

Caused by fluid filling the bursa sac at the elbow point underneath the skin as a result of either a single or repeated blows to the elbow.

Symptoms:
Pain and reddening of the skin, accompanied by an egg-shaped swelling at the elbow point, which can spread to the back of the forearm.

ExRx:
Rest and ice until swelling goes down—avoid heat, which increases the swelling. Start with gentle ROMs as pain and swelling permit and continue throughout to avoid joint stiffness. Then begin Phase I knee rehab exercises.

Elbow Dislocation

This injury is when the head of the radius or ulna bone comes out of its socket. Can be caused when you try to break a fall with your hand while your arm is bent. It also involves damage to surrounding tissue, which increases your recovery time.

Symptoms:
Intense pain, swelling, tenderness, loss of mobility, deformity of the elbow joint.

ExRx:
Phase I Rehab should start within five days to three weeks; Phase II starts when muscle function returns; and Phase III, when you can move your arm fully again, or in about six to eight weeks. Recovery is within six to twelve weeks.

Elbow Fracture

May be a complete break or tiny, hairline cracks or shatterings of the humerus, radius (radial head), or ulna bones. Should be treated as medical emergency because any one of these may involve the danger of losing elbow function unless promptly and properly treated by an orthopedist. Also, 20% of these injuries involve nerve and blood vessel damage, which may require surgery to correct. Humerus fracture occurs in the upper arm bone just above the elbow. The pull of your biceps and triceps muscles will easily pull the ends of the bone apart unless it is surgically reattached. Also, surgery may be necessary to correct twisting of arteries, nerves, and veins above the elbow. Caused by contact sports and falling accidents.

Symptoms:
Extreme pain, tenderness, swelling, and bruising; deformity behind elbow joint.

ExRx:
After surgery, wear a removable splint and sling for three weeks. One week after surgery, begin Phase I exercises; after two to three weeks, go to Phase II with an emphasis on range of motion; six to eight weeks after surgery, go to Phase III to correct stiffness and muscle atrophy. Adults should stay away from contact sports for six months; children, three months.

Elbow Sprain (Hyperextension)

Caused by a violent straightening of the elbow. This can occur when ligaments are stretched or torn.

Symptoms:
Immediate pain, followed by swelling within a half hour; tenderness, stiffness, and difficulty straightening elbow. In severe cases, the elbow joint may also be dislocated.

ExRx:
Rest and ice. Do not underestimate this injury; seek immediate medical attention and physical therapy. Do gentle ROMs within twenty-four to forty-eight hours after surgery. Depending on the degree of the injury, start with Phase I, II, or III exercises. Recovery time for mild to moderate is two to three days; for severe, ten days to two weeks.

Little League Elbow

Damage to the growth of cartilage on the inner side of the elbow in children and adolescents. Caused by the snap of powerful, downward and inward throwing motions. It is very serious and can interrupt a child's growth, creating a long-term disability, because in children, the tendon is attached to growth cartilage (at the ends of growing bone). There is a danger that this cartilage can be pulled off and cannot be reattached without surgery. In adults, this injury causes tears in the tendon where it is attached to the bone.

Symptoms:
Gradual onset of pain over bony knob on inside of elbow joint along with stiffness or inability to straighten arm. Extreme pain when growth cartilage detaches.

ExRx:
Your child must refrain from sports as soon as this elbow pain happens and then taken to an orthopedist who specializes in pediatrics. If it is a mild displacement, the doctor will splint the child's arm for six weeks. After a two-week rest, remove splint regularly to do ROM exercises and begin Phase II exercises building up to Phase III within four to six weeks. Children must wait six to nine weeks before returning to throwing. You can prevent Little League elbow by having Little League coaches supervise and control the total number of throws a child makes in a week, in a game, and in practice. The injury rates go up dramatically with more than 350 weekly throws. Keeping the number of throws under 250 would help avoid overusing the elbow and shoulder areas.

TENNIS ELBOW

An inflammation of the tendon of the forearm extensor muscle where it attaches to the bony knob of the outside elbow. It is one of the most common sports injuries, the "Achilles heel" of tennis. More likely after age forty. It can occur in tennis players who play at least two times a week and use too much wrist action in their strokes. It can also be aggravated by a heavier or more tightly strung racket. In general, the harder the racquet hits the ball, the more stress is transmitted to the elbow. The condition also occurs in golf and other racquet sports. Can also be caused by overused forceful grasp and poor technique.

Symptoms:
Pain over the outer elbow knob increases when you turn your wrist or hand against resistance.

ExRx:
Treat early before scar tissue builds up. Frequent rest and ice of the injured area and use of anti-inflammatory drugs. Recovery in mild cases is two weeks; in severe cases, up to two years.

Prevent by not only strengthening the elbow but also the wrist and the shoulder because all connected areas contribute to overcoming the stress of swinging a racquet and golf club. One technique for preventing overgripping is to learn to make a loosely clenched fist. When you notice that you are gripping too tightly, release the grip on your middle finger and thumb.

MUSKEL RX: LIST OF ADDITIONAL ELBOW INJURIES BENEFITED BY ELBOW REHAB RX EXERCISES

- fracture of the elbow point
- loose bodies in the elbow joint
- nursemaid's elbow
- pitcher's elbow
- radial head fracture
- slippage of the ulnar nerve
- triceps tendon rupture
- upper arm fractures

ELBOW INJURY EXERCISES

Keeping your elbow immobilized for more than three weeks can lead to elbow dysfunction, so it is important to start exercising as soon as possible.

For mild injuries, begin your Phase III ROM exercises as soon as pain and swelling diminish. For moderate injuries, begin Phase II exercises when you are able to move your elbow unassisted and without pain—usually after doing two weeks of Phase I exercises or when you are rehabilitating moderate to severe elbow injuries that did not require surgery. Begin Phase I five days after surgery unless joint is still not fully healed. Remove slings and splints during rehab exercises. Do Phase III, Dynamic Strengthening Exercises, when rehabilitating a mild injury or when you can do Phase II exercises without pain or difficulty.

Phase I Assisted ROMs and Isometrics

Physical therapy exercises should begin after surgery or within three weeks of a serious injury. Work the elbow in four ranges of motion—flexion, extension, supination, and pronation—with the active or passive assistance of a physical therapist.

Phase II ROM Exercises

Elbow Flexion and Extension

- Sit or stand with your injured arm hanging loosely by your side
- Slowly bend and raise your arm until it is bent at an angle that is between 90 and 45 degrees; hold briefly
- Now, straighten out your arm as you lower it back down
- Do ten to thirty repetitions each, three times a day

Elbow Pronation and Supination

- Sit with your forearm resting flat on a table, palm facing down
- Slowly turn your forearm palm up until the back of your hand is touching the table
- Do ten to thirty repetitions each, three times a day

Phase III Dynamic Elbow Strengthening Exercises

Weighted Biceps Curl

- Sit or stand and hold a small weight (see Weight Load Schedule, p. 325) in your hand; your arm should be straightened, elbow slightly bent, hand resting palm up on your thigh
- Bend your arm between 90 and 45 degrees as you curl the weight up toward your shoulder; be sure to keep your elbow pointing straight down; hold
- Slowly lower your arm back down as you straighten your elbow
- Repeat the exercise six times building up to fifteen times; practice one set a day building up to three sets

Triceps Extension

- Sit or stand; hold a small weight
- Raise your arm straight up next to the side of your head
- Slowly lower your weighted hand back behind your head to a 90-degree angle; keep your elbow stationary, pointing straight up

- Now, straighten your arm upward
- Repeat the exercise six times, building up to fifteen times
- Practice this set of exercises once a day, building up to three sets

Towel Turns

- Sit or stand and hold a rolled up towel in front of you
- Slowly twist the towel one side forward and one side backward
- Repeat the exercise six times, building up to fifteen times
- Practice one to three sets a day

Elbow Prevention/Conditioning Exercises

After Phases I to III have been completed, begin conditioning and strengthening with the following elbow and upper arm exercises:

Weighted biceps curls (palms up, in and down), pp. 199 and 348.

Weighted triceps extensions (elbow forward, up and back), page 348.

Weighted wrist curls, rolls (forearm extension), pp. 198 and 236.

Weighted reverse curls, rolls (forearm flexion), pages 198 and 236

CHAPTER 15

Meta Rx

Exercise Solutions for the Digestive and Reproductive Systems and Organs

NUTRITIONAL AND METABOLIC SYSTEM

The Meta Rx program provides therapeutic exercise and rehabilitative prescriptions for digestive, nutritional and metabolic, liver and gallbladder, pregnancy-related, male and female reproductive systems, and kidney and urinary diseases and disorders. Meta Rx covers all the body organs used to help metabolize food and control the body's weight. The body areas included in Meta Rx are lower trunk, hips, groin, peroneal areas, abdominals, and lower back. Not only are the basic metabolic and nutritional diseases and disorders examined, but also related diseases and disorders of the digestive tract, liver, gallbladder, and kidney and urinary systems. The major symptoms of the metabolic diseases and disorders are abdominal and back pain, interior uterine cramping, bladder and anal incontinence, and frequent urination. Pregnancy, and female and male reproductive system diseases and disorders are also included because they involve prescriptions for controlling weight, changes in metabolism, and they share similar lower trunk, pelvic girdle, and peroneal muscle exercises.

The body's main metabolic challenge is maintaining the balance of nutrients. Too much or too little of one nutrient can lead to a disease or disorder. Meta Rx uses exercise to help manage imbalances in the body's ability to absorb, use, and dispose of nutrients from the food and vitamins it ingests. The balancing act keeps the digestive system strong and functioning well.

Moderate aerobic exercise helps the body burn calories and improves blood and fluid flow to the metabolic organs, which provides relief from discomfort while promoting the healing process. Although diet and drugs are the most common prescriptions for metabolic diseases and disorders, exercise plays a leading role in reducing the need for drug therapy by burning off excess fat and helping you control your appetite for food and drink. Overall, if your body composition lacks a proper balance between fat and lean tissue, it indicates that your metabolism is not in balance. Other indicators are the levels of blood fat, calcium, insulin, magnesium, and acid.

The digestive tract runs from the mouth to the rectum, but the metabolic system's function does not end with digestion. Working through the blood stream, it helps put nutrients to use while also removing waste products on the cellular level.

Weight-bearing and muscle-strengthening exercise can help you to absorb nutrients more efficiently. But exercise can also promote nutrient depletion. To offset this possible depletion, make sure that you are managing your diet properly and taking the necessary vitamin and mineral supplements. Table 15.1 lists many vitamin and mineral deficiencies and their symptoms. Please note: If you are experiencing any of the symptoms listed in Table 15.1, consult your physician before deciding to self-medicate (or self-supplement, as the case may be). These symptoms can be the signs of other serious disorders and diseases, in addition to vitamin or mineral deficiencies, which also can be very serious. Please consult your physician.

The major portion of this chapter is broken down into seven areas, which are: (1) nutritional and metabolic diseases and disorders (2) digestive and excretory diseases and disorders, (3) kidney and urinary diseases and disorders (includes male reproductive system diseases and disorders), (4) liver and gallbladder diseases and disorders, (5) hormone and gland diseases and disorders, (6) female reproductive system diseases and disorders, and (7) abdominal, hip, pelvis, and groin injuries. Each of these seven areas is followed by an alphabetic listing of the diseases, disorders, or injuries found under that category. Symptoms are then described for each disease, disorder, or injury, which is followed by an ExRx for that specific ailment. You will note that some of the more common, more rehabilitative disorders and injuries have many exercises associated with them, while other diseases (e.g. prostate cancer, kidney stones) will have only a few exercises associated with them. If you feel you want more exercise than what is given with any ExRx, consult Parts I and II of this book and practice those preventive exercises that are associated with the body system or area that you are rehabilitating. Remember: Always start at a lower level and work your way up to your own personal optimum level. Do not turn your rehabilitative exercise therapy into a competition with anyone—including yourself. That is the surest, fastest way to injury, pain, and setbacks on the road to recovery.

Some of the injuries covered in the abdominal, hip, pelvis, and groin section are caused by overuse. Overuse injuries are more easily prevented by safer exercise techniques and also more directly affected by therapeutic and rehabilitative exercise. Rehab usually begins directly after the injury. There are various levels of injury, ranging from moderate to severe, the most common being bruises, sprains, and strains. A bruise is an injury that usually causes a rupture of small blood vessels, which in turn causes discoloration without a break in the surrounding or overlying skin; a sprain is a partial or complete tear of the ligaments surrounding a joint; a strain is an injury to the muscle or tendon. Sprains and strains may heal without surgery; most bruises require a minimum amount of therapy. For most of these types of injuries, doctors and physical therapists will use the following protocol: Rest, ice, compression, and elevation (RICE) and medical attention for more severe injuries; medications will include acetaminophen, ibuprofen, or aspirin for mild to moderate injuries; for severe injuries, doctors will prescribe bed rest with analgesics and anti-inflammatory drugs.

WARNING: Although many over-the-counter and prescription pain relievers are prescribed for reduction of pain caused by injuries, do not take any pain relievers before exercising as they tend to mask pain, which can cause further injury resulting from overexercising or overusing an injured body area or part. Take the medication as directed, after exercise and when you are more stationar Awareness of an injury is key to healing it!

NUTRITIONAL AND METABOLIC DISEASES AND DISORDERS RX

ANEMIA

This is a shortage of red blood cells. Anemi blood can't transport as much oxygen, whic can cause iron deficiencies, kidney failure chronic inflammation, hormonal disorders and other diseases.

Symptoms:
Early fatigue during exercise and reduced aero bic exercise capacity can lead to dehydration.

ExRx:
Do only moderate-intensity exercise at most Emphasize duration or total cumulative amount of exercise over a high level of inten sity.

TABLE 15.1
VITAMIN, MINERAL, NUTRITIONAL IMBALANCES AND DEFICIENCIES[1]

Deficiency or Imbalance	*Disease, Disorder, and Symptoms*
Galactosemia	Caused by a rare inability to metabolize milk sugar; symptoms in children include: failure to thrive; cataracts; mental retardation
Hyperlipoproteinemia	Characterized by high levels of lipids (blood fats); fatty deposits and nodules in skin, eyelids, hands; obesity; abdominal pains
Iodine (imbalance)	Deficiency: caused by underactive or overworked thyroid gland;[2] symptoms include: fatigue, loss of energy; goiter; weight gain; in babies: mental retardation and stunted growth; Excess: caused by overactive thyroid gland; symptoms include: inability to

	gain weight, toxic goiter; can lead to Graves' disease
Magnesium (imbalance)	Deficiency: caused by intenstinal disorders; severe kidney disease; alcoholism; prolonged usage of diuretic or digitalis drugs; symptoms include: anxiety; tremors; palpitations; depression; increased risk of kidney stones and heart disease; Excess: usually caused by taking too much antacid; symptoms include: nausea; diarrhea; vertigo; vomiting; muscle weakness; severe excess can lead to heart damage or respiratory failure
Phosphate[3] (deficiency)	Caused by kidney disease; long-term use of diuretic drugs; alcoholism; starvation; symptoms include: bone pain; weakness; tremors; seizures; in severe cases: coma and death
Potassium (imbalance)	Deficiency: caused by gastroenteritis or other digestive tract disorders; prolonged usage of diuretic, corticosteroid, or laxative drugs; diabetes; kidney disease; excessive intake of sugar, coffee, or alcohol; profuse sweating; symptoms include: fatigue, drowsiness, vertigo, muscle weakness; in severe cases: irregular heartbeat and muscle paralysis; Excess: caused by excessive intake of potassium supplements; renal failure; Addison's disease; symptoms include: tingling and numbness; paralysis; irregular heart rhythm; in severe cases: heart failure
Protein malnutrition	In children, symptoms include: stunted growth, muscle deterioration; physical inactivity
Sodium (imbalance)	Deficiency: caused by prolonged usage of diuretic drugs; persistent diarrhea or vomiting; excessive sweating; symptoms include: fatigue; weakness; muscle cramping; vertigo; Excess: can be caused by overuse of table salt and intake of processed foods containing excessive amounts of sodium; symptoms include: fluid retention; leg and extremity swelling; hypertension; heart disease; stroke; kidney damage
Vitamin A (imbalance)	Deficiency: caused by cystic fibrosis; bile duct obstruction; long-term usage of lipid-lowering

	drugs; symptoms include: poor night vision and inflamed eyes; dry, rough skin; lack of appetite; diarrhea; chronic infections; weak bones and teeth; corneal ulcers and sometimes blindness; Excess: caused by excessive intake of vitamin A; symptoms include: headache; fatigue; dry, scratchy skin; hair loss; irregular menstruation; bone pain; enlargement of the spleen and liver; can also cause birth defects
Vitamin B_1 (Thiamine deficiency)	Causes include: poor diet; hyperthyroidism; alcoholism; excessive high-intensity level activities (e.g. manual labor, excessive overexercising); symptoms include: fatigue; irritability; sleep disturbances; beriberi; abdominal pain; constipation; depression; memory loss; Wernicke-Korsakoff syndrome (in cases of severe alcoholism)
Vitamin B_2 (Riboflavin deficiency)	Causes include: poor diet, prolonged usage of antipsychotic or antidepressant drugs; oral contraceptives; malabsorption disorders; alcoholism; severe injury or disease; symptoms include: chapped or cracked lips; mouth and lip soreness; poor vision and photophobia
Niacin (Nicotinic acid deficiency)	Causes include: poor diet; malabsorption disorders; alcoholism; leads to pellagra, which causes cracked and sore skin; mouth and tongue inflammation; emotional disturbances
Pantothenic acid (deficiency)	Causes include: poor diet; malabsorption disorders; alcoholism; severe injury or illness; surgery; symptoms include: fatigue, headache, abdominal cramping and pain; muscle cramps; numbness and tingling; chronic respiratory infections; peptic ulcers
Vitamin B_6 (Pyridoxine deficiency)	Causes include: breast-feeding (in infants); poor diet; malabsorption disorders; alcoholism; oral contraceptives; symptoms include: weakness; irritability; depression; skin ailments; mouth and tongue inflammation; cracked, sore lips; anemia; in babies: seizures
Biotin (deficiency)	Causes include: poor diet; long-term usage of antibiotics or sulfa; excessive intake of raw egg whites; symptoms include: fatigue, weakness, lack

	of appetite; hair loss; tongue inflammation; depression, skin disorders
Folic acid (deficiency)	Causes include: not enough intake of leafy, green vegetables; pregnancy and breast-feeding; dialysis; psoriasis; malabsorption disorders; alcoholism; oral contraceptives; prolonged usage of pain relievers, anticonvulsants, corticosteroid drugs, and sulfa; symptoms include: anemia, mouth and tongue sores; in children: poor growth
Vitamin C (imbalance)	Deficiency: caused by lack of fresh fruits and vegetables in the diet; serious burn or injury; oral contraceptives; cigarette smoking; pollution; major surgery; fever; symptoms include: fatigue; weakness; aches and pains; nosebleeds; scurvy; anemia; Excess: caused by large doses of vitamin C; symptoms include: nausea; stomach cramping; diarrhea; kidney stones
Vitamin D (imbalance)	Deficiency: caused by poor diet; lack of sunlight; symptoms include: low levels of calcium in the blood; soft bones; in children: rickets; in adults: osteomalacia; Excess: caused by excessive intake of vitamin D; symptoms include: weakness; excessive thirst; frequent urination; gastrointestinal cramping; calcium deposits in soft tissues, kidneys, blood vessels; stunted growth in children
Vitamin E (imbalance)	Deficiency: caused by poor diet; malabsorption disorders; leads to the destruction of red blood cells; anemia; Excess: caused by prolonged, excessive intake of vitamin E; symptoms include: nausea; abdominal pain and cramping; vomiting; diarrhea; can also cause deficiency of vitamins A, D, and K
Vitamin K (deficiency)	Caused by poor diet; prolonged usage of antibiotics; malabsorption disorders; chronic diarrhea; symptoms include: nosebleeds; blood seepage from wounds; bleeding from the gums, intestines, and urinary tract

[1]See individual listings in text for calcium deficiency, hypoglycemia, and metabolic acidosis.
[2]Common in pregnant and nursing women.
[3]A salt formed from phosphorus, oxygen, and another element, e.g. calcium or sodium.

HEAT STRESS SYNDROME

Too rapid an increase in heat production or too rapid a decrease in heat loss. When heat loss fails to offset heat production, the body retains too much heat. There are three types of overheating: (1) heat cramps; (2) heat exhaustion; and (3) heat stroke. Heat production increases with exercise, drugs, or infection; heat loss decreases with high temperature, humidity, lack of acclimatization, obesity, dehydration, excess clothing, cardiovascular disease, among others.

Symptoms:
Faintness, nausea, weakness.

ExRx:
Drink plenty of fluids and wear lightweight, loose clothing. For heat cramps and heat exhaustion: Stop exercising, rest fully, and begin again by exercising gradually. For heat stroke: Heat sensitivity will persist for several months; stop exercising until the symptoms disappear and then begin exercising again at a slow to moderate pace, stopping if overheating reoccurs, then starting when body heat normalizes.

HYPERLIPIDEMIA

A condition of elevated triglycerides and cholesterol in the blood or plasma. It is related to hypertriglyceridemia (elevated triglycerides) and hypercholesterolemea (high cholesterol).

Symptoms:
Being overweight; high blood pressure.

ExRx:
Practice aerobic exercises at least five days a week at moderate intensities (40 to 70% of maximum heart-training rate). If necessary, exercise more than once a day until you have reached your minimum caloric expenditure goals.

HYPOGLYCEMIA

A condition characterized by abnormally low blood sugar. There are two types: Type I which is a reaction to the intake of refined carbohydrates (i.e. sugar); and Type II, which is caused by fasting or lack of food. Many people with this condition also suffer from diabetes mellitus; hypoglycemia can occur if a diabetic person misses a meal, doesn't eat enough carbohydrates, or overexercises. Some diabetes drugs can also cause hypoglycemia. A hypoglycemic attack can also be the result of drinking an excessive amount of alcohol.

Symptoms:
For both types—fatigue, nervousness, headache, rapid heartbeat, blurry vision, weakness, hunger, nausea, seizure, and in severe cases, coma. The symptoms can be mistaken for drunkenness because the affected person often acts irrational, with uncoordinated movements.

ExRx:
Eat low-fat, complex carbohydrates snacks (e.g. crackers or orange juice) thirty minutes before exercising. Exercise only at a low- to moderate-intensity level. When exercising for sixty minutes or more, eat snacks every thirty minutes while exercising. Do not exercise alone when the blood sugar level is likely to drop (i.e. five or more hours after eating). For Type I, don't exercise within two to four hours after a meal and don't inject insulin into those body areas that will be used during exercise. Eating frequent (five to six times per day), small, low-fat, complex carbo-

hydrate meals is recommended for overall control of this condition. Carry candy with you at all times for emergencies and practice stress reduction and control through relaxation techniques. Avoid caffeine and alcohol because they cause the blood sugar level to drop. A physician may prescribe glycogen injections to help control this condition. If you are overweight, don't eat extra calories to replace those that are burned during exercise; continue with your prescribed diet.

Metabolic Acidosis

Acid-base imbalance: excess acids, coupled with insufficient base compounds, depress the central nervous system, and can lead to dangerous heart rate and rhythm problems, cardiac arrest, and coma. Causes include uncontrolled diabetes mellitus, kidney failure, severe diarrhea, and aspirin overdose.

Symptoms:
Headache, drowsiness, rapid breathing, and stupor.

ExRx:
Drug therapy, mechanical ventilation. Exercising during an attack of acidosis will only make it worse; however, regular, habitual exercise will help prevent it by maximizing your oxygen delivery capacity.

Obesity

A substantial (20% or more; see Table 4.2, Ideal Body Weight in Pounds, p. 67) excess of body fat. Some 30% of obese persons succeed in losing twenty pounds, but only half of these, (i.e. 15%) keep the weight off. Studies show that exercise is critical to effective weight management because reduced calorie intake alone does not reduce your metabolic rate and without exercise, you are more apt to regain the weight after the diet is done. A high fat and high sugar diet and physical inactivity are the primary factors leading to obesity.

Obesity not only increases the risk of certain diseases but also the severity of disease. The distribution of body fat may be more important than total body fat because upper body fat (i.e. abdominal and upper torso) has been related more to increased risk of coronary artery disease, hyperlipidemia, diabetes, and hypertension, as well as hormone and menstrual dysfunction. (See Table 4.3, Waist-to-Hip Ratios and Risk of Disease, p. 69.)

Symptoms:
Inactivity, uncontrollable appetite, food cravings, large weight gain.

ExRx:
Continuous moderate exercise, especially walking, jogging, and bicycling, when done frequently (five to seven times per week), over a long duration (thirty to ninety minutes per session per day), has the most beneficial weight loss/control results (refer to Table 11.1, Cardio Ex Walking/Cycling Schedule, p. 219.) The overall benefits to metabolic health are greater with moderate exercise than with intense exercise. To lose body fat and weight, you must exercise according to an amount equal to the calories of body fat you need to lose. Monitor the calories expended during the exercise you do. Low-impact cardio exercise (especially walking and cycling) produces the most efficient calorie burn rate. Refer to Table 11.1 for the calories burned during walking and cycling at various degrees of intensity. Multiple exercise sessions of shorter duration for those who fatigue easy, as well as single sessions of longer duration at least five

times a week—but preferably daily—are recommended. Exercise either forty to sixty minutes a day or twenty to thirty minutes two to three times daily at 50 to 70% of max heart-training rate. Strength training with weights, stretch cords, or resistance machines can also help to increase or maintain lean body or muscle weight. Prevent overuse joint injuries by doing extra warm-ups, stretching, and cool-down exercises and gradually increasing the intensity and duration of exercise sessions. The best results come from slow to moderate exercise practiced regularly over a lifetime. For severe obesity, psychological counseling, medication, and sometimes surgery may also be necessary. While the debate rages on whether obesity is a discipline or genetic problem, exercise still works to reduce and control the appetite, and weight control is made easier with a regular, habitual exercise program. For calorie burning and appetite suppression, a properly balanced, lower calorie, and lower fat diet eaten slowly can help.

Systems for defining obesity include Table 4.2, Ideal Body Weight (p. 67), body-fat percentage and body mass index. Body mass index is most difficult to measure. Body fat percentage can also be done with a pinch test. Refer to the Body Mass Index table in Chapter Four, page 71, for your percentage and use the percentages in Table 15.2 to see if you are within your ideal ranges.

TABLE 15.2
BODY FAT PERCENTAGE RANGES

Weight	*Women*	*Men*
Minimum Weight	8%	5%
Below Average Weight*	14–23%	5–15%
Above Average Weight	24–32%	16–25%

*This is the ideal range.

Digestive and Excretory Diseases and Disorders Rx

The digestive and excretory system is part of the Meta System and includes the organs used for the ingestion and processing of foods and the separation and release of waste products. Exercise helps by strengthening muscles and organs involved in the process—the stomach, liver, gallbladder, intestines, kidneys, and rectum. After the mouth has finished chewing the food, the stomach takes in and stores the food, slowly breaking it down with acids. From the stomach, the food passes into the intestines. Vitamins, minerals, and water from the food are absorbed into the body through the intestines and are carried to the liver where they are dispersed into the bloodstream; the residue from this process—small amounts of fat, bile, bacteria, and secretions from digestive organs—become feces and pass into the rectum. The liver also manufactures bile and controls the levels of chemicals in the body. The kidneys filter the blood and excrete waste products and excess water. The gallbladder, situated below the liver, stores and concentrates bile, which is used to rid the body of waste products and to break down and absorb fat.

Too much exercise may aggravate a preexisting digestive condition, such as gastroenteritis. Exercise, however, may also alleviate symptoms of many digestive irritants including alcoholism, overeating, tension, sleeplessness, and blood pooling in the lower tract caused by inactivity. Trunk turns and bends and abdominal exercises are most effective for the digestive and excretory system. Exercise also stimulates blood and fluid flow necessary for healthy digestion. Exercise may also stimulate organ and muscle growth and regeneration.

Digestive problems are also linked to your mental and emotional state. For example, when you are nervous, a high level of digestive juices are excreted causing heartburn and stomach cramps. A continuous unrelieved state of stress can lead to a irritable bowel syndrome or hemorrhoidal flare-ups. Therefore, exercises that relax the body can also help the digestive system to relax and function normally. Posture exercises help the body maintain proper space for the organs to function freely.

Anal Pain

Caused by anal fissure, itching, burning, or anal-rectal abscess.

Symptoms:
Pain, excessive sweating in groin area, tenderness, and discomfort when sitting.

ExRx:
Stop or change any activity that causes or irritates the condition. When exercising, use cotton balls between buttocks to absorb moisture; also apply powder to anal area to absorb moisture and to soothe. Choose or switch to an exercise position—standing, seated, or lying down—that provides the greatest comfort to the affected area. Take sitz baths before and after exercise periods.

Colitis

Chronic inflammation of lower intestine. Peak periods are ages fifteen to twenty and fifty-five to sixty. Studies show that regular exercise reduces the risk of colon cancer, perhaps because it stimulates colon peristalsis, thus spreading the flow of fecal matter and thereby reducing exposure to intestinal mucosa and fecal carcinogens. These same processes can help people with colitis.

Symptoms:
Abdominal pain, spastic rectum, constipation, and diarrhea.

ExRx:
Regular exercise helps digestion, and controlled breathing exercises can reduce abdominal pain. Also see the relaxation training exercises, pp. 244–248.

Colon Cancer

This cancer progresses slowly and affects the colon, which is the portion of the large intestine that extends from the cecum to the rectum. Colon cancer is 75% curable. Predisposed risks include diets high in fat, history of digestive tract disease, and polyps.

Symptoms:
Stomach or intestinal pain; diarrhea or constipation that lasts more than ten days.

ExRx:
Prevent by controlling obesity and constipation with high-fiber, low-fat diet, and abdominal and trunk exercises. After a positive diagnosis of colon cancer, a colostomy will be necessary. A colostomy is an operation in which the colon is brought through the abdominal wall and a pouch is attached to the skin to gather feces. A colostomy can be either temporary or permanent depending on the severity of the illness. A colostomy does not prevent exercising, but you should avoid

KRIS LUCIUS

DIAGNOSIS: SEVERE ABDOMINAL WOUND

In his sophomore year in high school, Kris Lucius joined the school's rowing team. "I liked it somewhat," he writes, "but mainly for the traveling. The actual rowing didn't woo me too much." In the spring of his junior year, a teammate dropped out because of illness, and Kris won a spot on the varsity team.

In his first varsity race, his team finished second, and Kris was awarded his first medal. The next evening, Mother's Day, 1994, he was driving home alone on a country road and collided head-on with another car.

Both cars were travelling at about 55 mph. In the other car, the driver's legs were both broken and the driver's wife, in the passenger seat, was killed. Kris's liver was torn open. He underwent emergency surgery for internal bleeding. "There was talk of a colostomy—a pretty scary thought when you are sixteen years old," he explains.

The surgery was successful, and a colostomy wasn't necessary. Kris was bedridden for two weeks and was in a great deal of pain for some time after. "It was nearly impossible for me to stand up after sitting down; my family had to lift me up."

After two months convalescing, Kris returned to the boathouse, where one of his friends, determined to get him back in shape by fall, began rowing with him in a two-man boat. Without medical supervision, the two rowed every weekday, at first for about forty-five minutes, then gradually up to between an hour and an hour and a half. In the beginning, Kris used only his arms and legs, trying not to use his stomach at all, as it was still healing. However, he rowed with increasing pressure, involving his stomach more and more, until he was again rowing with all his muscles.

Kris developed a new love for the sport, and in late October, the week before the prestigious Head of the Charles race in Boston, he again won a seat on the varsity team, replacing the friend who worked so diligently with him during his recovery. At his high school graduation, Kris was awarded the rowing team's highest honor, the "Etes Vous Pret," mainly, he says, for his newfound work ethic. He is now on the University of Wisconsin rowing team.

According to his doctors, Kris made a speedy and complete recovery because he was in good shape at the time of the accident. Kris believes the most important part of his recovery was that he exercised as his body was overcoming the accident.

weight lifting and contact sports (if you are very active, you will drink more fluids and change your colostomy pouch more frequently); for swimming, use a stoma plug, a soft foam plug that fits into your stoma to block drainage for up to twenty-four hours.

CONSTIPATION

Intermittent or infrequent passing of dry, hard feces. Can be caused by lack of high-fiber foods in the diet, low level of fluids in the body, poor bowel-moving habits caused by poor toilet training, or immobility (in elderly persons). In those who have anal fissures or hemorrhoids, the pain experienced when having a bowel movement may also inhibit the passing of feces thus promoting constipation. People with irritable bowel syndrome also experience intermittent constipation, which alternates with diarrhea.

Symptoms:
Bloating, pain in the intestinal area, and inability to have a bowel movement.

ExRx:
Eat more high-fiber foods (e.g. fruits, vegetables, and whole grains) and drink more water. Also see Exercise Guidelines for Constipation and Hemorrhoids, pp. 382–383.

Crohn's Disease

Chronic inflammation of digestive tract (usually in the area where the small intestine joins the large intestine), swelling caused by inflammation. Ulcers and abscesses may also form. Unknown causes, but believed to have a genetic predisposition. It is a chronic disease that may require long-term care and multiple surgeries.

Symptoms:
Diarrhea, abdominal pain, stress, fever, lack of appetite, anemia, and weight loss.

ExRx:
Sulfa drugs and corticosteroid drugs may be prescribed; long-term medical care is frequently required. Surgery may be necessary to remove the most affected areas of the intestine or to remove an abscess. After surgery, begin rehab after two weeks with low-intensity, short duration trunk-bending and stretching exercises; also more rest, relaxation, and deep breathing exercises, pp. 244–247.

Diverticulosis

Bulging pouches push through the intestinal wall usually in the lower portion of the colon. Mainly affects men over forty. Caused by straining, lack of dietary fiber. Fecal matter hardens and bowel tunnel narrows requiring higher abdominal pressure during bowel movement.

Symptoms:
Irritable bowel, alternating constipation and diarrhea.

ExRx:
Practice abdominal exercises to strengthen area in order to withstand greater pressure; eating a high-fiber diet helps to widen the bowel tunnel; trunk exercises help strengthen muscles used in bowel movements; improved circulation resulting from exercise increases the blood supply. Exercise also increases your intake of fluids, which can also help soften the stool, making it easier to pass through affected areas.

Gastroenteritis

Severe upset stomach. Second-most common cause (after common cold) of lost work time. Food poisoning, dysentery, and various diseases (e.g. thyphoid fever, cholera) are all forms of gastroenteritis. Can also be caused by food intolerance, spicy foods, and alcoholism.

Symptoms:
Diarrhea, nausea, and abdominal cramping.

ExRx:
Rest and liquids, relaxation, and breathing exercises done from the prone side-lying (fetal) position (below).

HEARTBURN

Burning sensation in throat and chest. Back flow of stomach acid or upper intestine contents into esophagus; often occurs with obesity and pregnancy.

Symptoms:
Persistent flare-ups can lead to inflammation of throat lining; may also worsen during vigorous physical exercise.

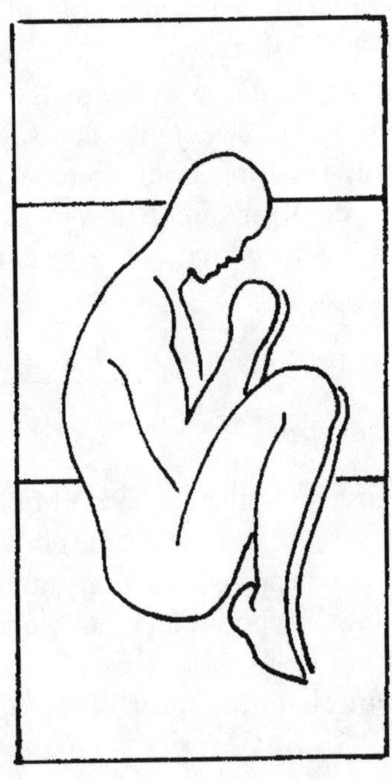

Fetal Position

ExRx:
Mild cases—antacid and diet change; los weight; practice sitting, upright, moderat exercise instead of vigorous. Avoid lying down exercises. Rest and exercise in th upright position or with the head elevated Avoid cigarettes and alcohol, which reduc sphincter control.

HEMORRHOIDS

Enlarged, bleeding veins in the region of th anus. Affects adults ages twenty to fifty an postpartum women. Coexisting condition prolonged sitting and standing; straining c anus and rectum, (e.g. constipation, diarrhe birth crouching); heart failure; liver diseas (e.g. cirrhosis); alcoholism; loss of muscl tone resulting from aging, pregnancy, and rec tal surgery; anal intercourse.

Symptoms:
Painful, intermittent bleeding.

ExRx:
Take sitz baths; spend less time on the toil and do not strain to have a bowel movemen practice circulatory exercises, such as th heel-toe rolls while standing or seated (177), to improve venous health; Kegel exe cise (pp. 204, 380–382) to improve surroun ing muscle tone; and walking.

HERNIA

Organ (e.g. intestine) pokes through a torn weak area in the abdominal wall. Oft requires surgery to repair.

Symptoms:
Bulging of organ; groin pain during standi or exertion.

ExRx:
Postsurgery, rehab with seated exercises including breathing, strengthening, stretching, abdominal, and lower back. Progress to standing exercises.

Hiatal Hernia

A common defect in the diaphragm, in which a portion of the stomach protrudes into chest. Caused by weakening of esophageal muscles resulting from old age, surgery, or genetic predisposition.

Symptoms:
Heartburn and pain in the upper chest; complications can occur if not treated.

ExRx:
Surgery may be necessary, especially when there is a risk of strangulation. Strengthen lower esophageal sphincter muscle by avoiding positions that cause continuous abdominal pressure (e.g. recumbent). Do trunk-bending, stretching, and diaphragmatic breathing exercises.

Irritable Bowel Syndrome (IBS)

Intermittent abdominal or intestinal pain coupled with constipation and/or diarrhea. Causes are unknown, but usually associated with a disturbance of involuntary muscle movement in the colon. The most common disorder of the intestine; twice as common in women than in men. Many physicians believe that stress and anxiety are highly causative factors for IBS.

Symptoms:
Abdominal cramps, bowel movement straining, diarrhea, constipation, and anxiety.

ExRx:
Eliminate or avoid from your diet those foods that you are sensitive to (e.g. caffeine, alcohol, spicy foods). Do relaxation training and deep breathing exercise (pp. 244–247).

Pancreatic Cancer

A malignant tumor of the pancreas, which is located in back of abdomen. Predominant in men ages thirty to seventy, especially in Israel, United States, Sweden, and Canada. Predisposed risks include cigarette smoking, high fat and protein in the diet, and food additives.

Symptoms:
Weight loss, stomach pain, lower back pain, depression, anxiety, and pronounced itching.

ExRx:
Lower back stretching and relaxation training (pp. 244–247). Wear a cotton glove to scratch.

Pancreatitis

Inflammation of the pancreas. It starts with a stomachache and can lead to swelling and tissue damage. In men, linked to alcoholism; in women, linked to diseases of the bile tract.

Symptoms:
Steady stomachache.

ExRx:
Eat less fat; reduce alcohol consumption; see Psyche Rx program (p. 429) for substituting exercise for alcohol.

META RX: LIST OF ADDITIONAL DIGESTIVE AND EXCRETORY DISEASES AND DISORDERS BENEFITED BY META EXERCISES

- abdominal cramps
- appendicitis
- inflammation of the stomach lining
- peptic ulcer
- peritonitis
- rectal polyps
- rectal prolapse
- stomach cancer

KIDNEY AND URINARY DISEASES AND DISORDERS RX

Kidney disease can be slowed down significantly by exercising while following a special, doctor-prescribed diet which will change with the different stages of your disease. These changes include regulating the balance of fluid and salt, restricting protein intake to prevent accumulating wastes, and reducing potassium intake to prevent weakness and heart abnormalities. Major symptoms for kidney and urinary diseases and disorders include abdominal and lower back pain, incontinence and constipation. Exercise can help relieve many symptoms and help control urinary problems.

INCONTINENCE

The partial or total inability to hold urine in the bladder or fecal matter in the rectum. It is usually a symptom or condition of an underlying disorder.

There are different types, including urge incontinence, stress and overflow incontinence, dysfunction of bladder neck, weakening of pelvic floor muscles and urethra associated with pregnancy and vaginal delivery menopause, prostectomy, and obesity; all can be causes of incontinence. Urge incontinence or leakage with a full bladder is associated with reduced muscular control and bladder spasms.

Overflow incontinence or frequent and irregular urination is associated with enlarged prostate in men and prolapsed pelvic organs in women. In either case, the bladder fails to completely contract or empty because of nerve damage.

Symptoms:
Involuntary escape of urine or feces during physical activity or when coughing or sneezing. Urge to urinate frequently. Also such psychological symptoms as depression and anxiety about sexual activity, leakage, odor, and leaving the house.

ExRx:
Similar to constipation, incontinence involves the weakening of internal muscles from injury during childbirth, inactivity, or age-related atrophy. Also, enlarged prostates in men cause frequent voiding of bladder; removal of prostate causes loss of urinary control for three to twelve months after surgery. Exercise pelvic floor muscles with pelvic tilt and Kegel exercises. Practice low-impact activities and exercise such as cycling and water exercise. Avoid high-impact exercise such as tennis, running, horseback riding, dancing, and high-impact aerobics. Do not hold your breath during strength training and other stationary exercises. (See Kegel exercises, pp. 380–382.)

ːIDNEY STONES

ˌ stone, usually composed of calcium and/or hosphate, forms in the kidney or urinary ʼact.

ymptoms:
udden, severe pain in the flank that moves ›ward the groin area; may be intermittent ıd may cause vomiting and nausea.

xRx:
void such bladder irritants as alcohol, caf-ine, and carbonated beverages. Walking ɛlps the stones pass. Drink ten to fourteen asses of water a day to flush out bacteria ranberry juice works even better).

ƦOSTATE CANCER

ffects the prostate, a chestnut-sized gland rrounding neck of bladder and urethra in ales. Affects men over fifty, and represents % of all cancers; incidence increases with e. Most common in blacks; least common Asians.

mptoms:
ʼinary pain, frequent urination, and incon-ence.

Rx:
esurgery exercise—peroneal exercises; enty-four to forty-eight hours before—but-ːks squeeze, Kegel exercises (pp. 380–382). pending on degree of surgery, rehabilita-n takes between three and twelve months.

OSTATECTOMY

moval of all or part of the prostate gland h surgery that can involve cutting such surrounding tissue as the sphincter neck of the bladder.

Symptoms:
Loss of bladder control, leakage, dysfunctional bladder neck, and weakened pelvic muscles and urethra.

ExRx:
After surgery, use pelvic and perineal exercises to help restore muscle function and rejuvenate muscle cells. Men must often rely on the external sphincter muscle rather than the internal sphincter for bladder control as the latter one has been cut away, so it is important to exercise all the muscles in the area to strengthen and control the external sphincter.

PROSTATE, ENLARGED

Affects most men over age fifty; caused by age-related hormonal changes. Enlarged gland presses into bladder to distort and obstruct the flow urination. The retained urine may then form stones and cysts.

Symptoms:
Frequent urination, inability to expel all the urine in the bladder, difficulty in starting to urinate, weak stream of urine, incontinence, and in severe cases, severe abdominal pain, which requires immediate attention from a physician.

ExRx:
Antibiotics and surgery; presurgery rehab includes Kegel exercises, sitz baths; regular ejaculation. Postsurgery rehab with Kegel exercises, urinary control, and pelvic exercises for abdominal and lower back strengthen-

ing and stretching. Both the involuntary bladder neck sphincter and the voluntary external sphincter valves that provide urinary control in men are weakened during prostate enlargement and are sometimes destroyed during prostate surgery.

RENAL FAILURE

Reduction or inability of the kidneys to filter out waste products from the blood, to regulate blood pressure, and to control the body's salt and water balance. This is the final stage of kidney disease during which the patient is on dialysis, resulting in severe metabolic abnormalities including anemia, autonomic function, diabetes (30% of cases), elevated triglycerides, reduced high-density lipoprotein cholesterol (HDL), hypertension, left ventricle hypertrophy, metabolic acidosis, muscle weakness, peripheral neuropathy, and secondary hyperparathyroidism.

Symptoms:
Reduced volume of urine, upper abdominal pain, flank pain and tenderness, nausea, vomiting, breathlessness, drowsiness, and rashless itching.

ExRx:
Increasing the functional capacity of the kidneys should be the major objective for people with renal failure. Exercise training may be the only hope of increasing the functional renal capacity of dialysis patients. It can improve blood pressure control, lipid profiles, and psychological profiles in some patients. Exercise during dialysis treatment is also recommended. Gradual progression in intensity and number of repetitions is essential. For strength training, avoid heavy weights and concentrate on light weights and higher numbers of repetition. Warm-ups and stretching improve gait, balance, and coordination. Because this is a complex medical condition, your exercise program should be supervised and maintained by your kidney specialist.

META RX: LIST OF ADDITIONAL KIDNEY AND URINARY DISORDERS THAT ARE BENEFITED BY META EXERCISES

- bladder cancer
- kidney cancer
- peritonitis
- rectal polyps
- renal infarction
- testicular cancer
- urinary reflux

LIVER AND GALLBLADDER DISEASES AND DISORDERS RX

Liver problems are associated principally with alcoholism. Gallbladder disease is aggravated but not entirely caused by fatty foods. Exercise provides a substitute for the overconsumption of both these substances by offering physical stimulation and a diversion during periods when overeating or imbibing is a temptation.

Exercise is also a great rehab tool for recovering from liver and gallbladder surgery. For example, after laparoscopy (a surgical abdominal cavity exam) you will be encouraged to walk and practice hourly deep breathing and leg exercises soon after a hospital stay of twenty-four to forty-eight hours. Walking and leg exercises also help normalize your bowel movements and prevent clot formation. Although the time spent bedridden is relatively short, the residual pain from surgery requires the slow work of rehabilitation.

Cirrhosis of the Liver

Cirrhosis causes widespread destruction of normal liver cells, which are replaced by fibrous cells. Fibrous cells interfere with blood and lymph flow. Death generally comes five years from start of first signs. Men are twice as apt to contract this disease as women. Alcoholism and malnourishment are the major causes; can also be caused by hepatitis and other diseases.

Symptoms:
Stomach troubles, dull ache in abdomen, fluid retention, bloated feeling, and itchy skin.

ExRx:
Healthy eating habits, small frequent meals (six small meals instead of three large meals) help reduce bloated feeling. Recovery can occur in three weeks with proper eating, rest, and total avoidance of alcohol; four months to normal function. Exercise helps you to control your urge for alcohol and also burns off excess fat accumulations.

Fatty Liver

Triglycerides and other fats accumulate in liver cells causing liver weight to increase from three pounds up to eleven pounds. Can be caused by alcoholism, malnutrition, especially protein deficiency; also associated with obesity, diabetes, pregnancy, and bypass surgery.

Symptoms:
Massive swollen stomach; arms and chest wither.

ExRx:
Reverse with a strict diet therapy program supervised by a physician. Exercise helps reduce and control the alcohol consumption and obesity. Do strengthening exercises of the major muscle groups for arms, chest, upper back, and legs to improve blood flow to organs. When coupled with diabetes, also do cardio exercise at a moderate pace.

Gallstones

Grainy deposits of solid matter found in the gallbladder and bile duct. Gallstones form when the gallbladder is sluggish because of high cholesterol, cirrhosis of the liver, obesity, diabetes, pregnancy, fasting, or pancreatitis. Six times more common in women than men until age fifty, then occurs in equal proportions. Fatty foods do not actually cause gallbladder disease, but cause gallbladder attack by triggering the hormone that causes gallbladder contractions and bile flow blockage by stones.

Symptoms:
Severe abdominal pain, nausea, and possible vomiting.

ExRx:
As soon as you can after surgery (and hospital stay of twenty-four to forty-eight hours), walk and practice breathing techniques and gentle leg-lifting exercises every hour. Move your whole body to prevent blood clots with moderate paced, continuous motion exercises (e.g. walking and cycling). Do trunk-bending and stretching exercises to promote bowel movement and to relieve stomach pain. To avoid stomach strain, do not do leg-lifting exercises.

LIVER CANCER

A malignant tumor of the liver, which usually strikes men over sixty. There is no cure, and has a very low survival rate. Predisposed risks: cirrhosis of the liver.

Symptoms:
Weight and appetite loss, swelling of feet and legs, lethargy, and jaundice.

ExRx:
Surgery to remove the tumor and a liver transplant is sometimes performed; most commonly treated with radiation; no alcohol can be consumed. Do raised leg exercises to reduce swelling of feet.

HORMONE AND GLANDS DISEASES AND DISORDERS RX

DIABETES MELLITUS

Chronic disease suffered by fourteen million Americans in which the body produces little or no insulin or can't effectively use the insulin it does produce. Raises risk of heart and kidney disease, also gangrene. There are

SCHARLENE HERBERT

DIAGNOSIS: DIABETES

For Scharlene Herbert, fifty-two, diabetes came on relatively late in life, at the age of forty. On a trip to the southern United States, she began to notice she had frequent urination. She thought she had a bladder infection and started taking medication, but it did not help. Scharlene was also becoming dizzy but attributed that symptom to the heat.

Sometime soon after that, she was in her car driving to the bank when she went into a diabetic coma. Scharlene was able to pull into a gas station, leaving the engine running. The attendant came over to her car and knocked on her window, telling her to roll down the window and turn off the engine. In her state, Scharlene was unable to understand him.

The attendant knew her husband, as the Herberts were frequent customers of that gas station. He called her husband and told him that Scharlene was there. "She's just sitting here," her husband was told. A nurse happened to be standing near the payphone and overheard this conversation. The nurse approached the car and began speaking to Scharlene, offering her assistance. "Everything was in slow motion," says Scharlene.

The nurse was able to recognize Scharlene's problem, and she asked the attendant for some orange juice and gave it to Scharlene. "I snapped out of it," she says. The nurse told her she was diabetic.

Scharlene first went on pills for her diabetes, but she would not take her medication until her blood sugar skyrocketed, giving her blurry vision and an upset stomach. Only then would she take her pill.

Scharlene's doctor then put her on insulin. She did not want to take the insulin, and especially did not want to administer it herself, as she is sensitive to needles. She had to go two types: Type I (5%), insulin-dependent, onset occurs before thirty, body type is thin, needs insulin injections, diet, and exercise; Type II (95%), noninsulin-dependent, onset occurs after age forty, treated with drugs, exercise, and diet.

Symptoms:
At first, fatigue caused by energy deficiency; glucose-starved cells leave muscles low on energy; high blood sugar, frequent thirst and urination; unused glucose build-up (hyperglycemia) is toxic. Later on, symptoms include nerve damage, tingling, numbness, and burning of skin to loss of feeling; also, cardiovascular disease, kidney disease, and ulcerations of the skin.

ExRx:
Almost everyone with diabetes can receive some benefit from regular exercise. People with Type I diabetes should normalize their blood sugar levels, avoid or manage related problems, that is, weight, eyes, teeth and gums, skin breaks, and feet. They should avoid contact sports and sudden jarring moves that could detach a retina. Those with Type II often need weight reduction, they

---

in to the clinic twice a day, every day, to receive her injections. Finally, after six months, when she was about to leave on a vacation, she learned how to give herself the shot by practicing on an orange. Scharlene also learned how to take her own blood sugar reading, by pricking her finger.

Since the incident in the gas station in 1984, Scharlene's weight had gone from 125 pounds to 175 pounds. "You're constantly eating with insulin," she explains. It was her 1996 New Year's resolution to lose weight.

In January, she started cutting her food intake in half, literally. Whatever was on her plate, she would remove half of it. Scharlene also went on a fat-free diet and began drinking water instead of soda. Her husband had also been diagnosed with diabetes in the fall of 1995. The two of them started walking together. Every morning, the couple began taking a two and a half mile walk, lasting between forty and sixty minutes.

After three months of daily walking, Scharlene lost thirty pounds. Furthermore, with the help of moderate-paced walking, she stopped her twelve-year-long insulin usage. Now she takes Metformin and Galaborite instead. Of these drugs she says, "They don't bloat you up, and you don't have to eat all the time." With her walking program, Scharlene has also been building muscles. "I'm stronger. I don't get out of breath," she says.

After her diagnosis, Scharlene felt disabled, with little appetite for life. She went through a five-year-long depression, but things are different now. "My daughter is twenty-seven, and I can keep up with her," she explains.

Her advice to others is to watch your diet and exercise five times a week, not just the commonly recommended three. Looking back on the past, she says, "I'm more adjusted now. I'm not gonna let the diabetes control me."

must monitor blood sugar levels before exercise, and inspect their feet for infections. Also, avoid activities that cause foot stress such as basketball, hiking, jogging, and tennis. Monitor your heart rate (p. 217) and use other methods to monitor your exertion rate such as on table 15.3, Borg Perceived Exertion Scale (below). Regular continuous motion exercise at a moderate pace can cut the risk of diabetes in half (moderate exercise is 50 to 65% of your maximum heart-training rate). Glucose levels can drop even after forty-eight hours after exercising, so eat or take insulin about one to three hours before exercising. Studies show that regular exercise seems to diminish the arteriosclerosis in non-insulin-dependent diabetes (Type II) by diminishing or reducing hyperinsulinemia (insulin resistance) and also by preventing increases in the intra-abdominal adipose tissue (the fat that directly surrounds the front of the waist and stomach area. The impact of this effect is greatest if exercise is begun early in life, before the onset of irreversible vascular damage.

Be on the alert for hypoglycemic reactions during or after exercise. Exercise needs to be consistent in frequency, duration, and intensity to avoid blood sugar swings. Eat a complex carbohydrate snack thirty minutes prior to exercise to avoid hypoglycemic reaction. Carry a fast-acting sugar snack (i.e.

TABLE 15.3
BORG PERCEIVED EXERTION SCALE

6-20 Scale		*0-10 Scale*	
6		0	nothing at all
7	very, very light	.5	very, very weak
8		1	very weak
9	very light	2	weak
10		3	moderate
11	fairly light	4	somewhat strong
12		5	strong
13	somewhat hard	6	
14		7	very strong
15	hard	8	
16		9	
17	very hard	10	very, very strong
18			
19	very, very hard		

candy) in case of hypoglycemic reaction.

Diabetes is a metabolic disorder. Whereas obesity is the central problem for Meta prevention, diabetes is the central one for Meta therapy. Diabetes is a good example of a disease that can be prevented, controlled, or managed with exercise. Diabetes has many symptoms that can be helped with exercise.

Overweight patients should work toward a balance of the ratio of fat to lean tissue in their bodies. Diabetics must use exercise to balance the level of insulin against blood sugar. If your blood sugar swings too low, you must consume more carbohydrates or sugar. Your blood sugar must be normalized before you exercise because exercise burns blood sugar. The exercise itself must also be administered in a balanced dose. When symptoms are too severe, exercise must be easy to moderate. Therefore, eat food and take medication before you exercise. For less severe cases, exercise more vigorously. The severity of diabetes is associated with the number of complications including high blood pressure and eye disorders (i.e. retinopathy and peripheral vascular disease). If these eye disorders are present, vigorous exercise can send blood pressure higher and rupture blood vessels in the eyes.

To avoid increasing pressure on the eyes, refrain from such high-risk impact activities as parachute jumping, scuba diving, or sudden and strenuous exercise such as heavy weight-lifting. Also, avoid high-impact and weight-bearing exercises to avoid aggravating any neuropathy of the feet.

Exercise can help control both Types I and II by helping to manage blood sugar levels and reduce life-threatening complications (e.g. high blood pressure, heart disease, kidney disease, nerve damage, impotence, blindness, and amputations).

If you do not already have higher than normal blood pressure, you can practice vigorous exercise (65 to 85% of heart-training rate). If you have high blood pressure, exercise in the heart-training zone of 50 to 65%. Diabetes medications do not generally affect blood pressure, heart rate, or exercise tolerance but such heart medications as beta blockers or bronchodilators can have an effect.

After diabetes is in an advanced stage, moderate exercise can still strengthen the fragile body without undermining its defenses.

Hypothyroidism in Adults

A condition characterized by low levels of thyroid hormone, which is more common in women than men. Onset usually occurs between ages forty and fifty. Mostly caused by the body developing an autoimmune disorder against its own thyroid gland. This causes the thyroid to reduce the thyroid hormone production. Can also be caused by iodine deficiency.

Symptoms:
Fatigue, forgetfulness, cold sensitivity, weight gain, constipation, and sometimes goiter.

ExRx:
Take thyroid hormone replacements, and exercise regularly including leg lifts and trunk bends to prevent constipation and promote weight loss.

Hypothyroidism in Children

When treated before age three, children usually develop normally. If untreated after age two, can lead to irreversible skeletal abnormalities, a delay in sexual maturity, and can inhibit normal brain development.

Symptoms:
Respiratory difficulties, inactivity, excessive sleepiness, growth retardation, short stature, and obesity.

ExRx:
The child will need lifelong medical treatment. Focus on the child's strengths with such stimulating activities as playing ball, crawling, and somersaults.

META RX: LIST OF ADDITIONAL HORMONE AND GLAND DISORDERS THAT ARE BENEFITED BY META EXERCISES

- Addison's disease
- Graves' disease
- Hodgkin's disease
- malignant lymphomas
- pheochromocytoma
- pituitary tumors

Female Reproductive Diseases and Disorders Rx

Major symptoms include nausea, lower back pain, hot flashes, flushing, shortness of breath, and depression.

Breast Cancer

This is the most common woman's cancer after lung cancer, usually occurring after age fifty. Early detection increases survival rate. More often found in left breast and in upper part close to arm.

Symptoms:
Lump is found in breast or underarm; sometimes accompanied by itchiness. Pain occurs with an advanced tumor. Weak arm and upper torso muscles.

ExRx:
Surgical procedures include: lumpectomy, partial mastectomy, total mastectomy, and modified mastectomy. After surgery, do MuSkel Rehab stretching and strengthening exercises for chest, arm, shoulder, and back (see Chapter Fourteen).

Infertility

Inability to conceive a child after at least one year of regular sexual intercourse. The cause may be functional, anatomic, or psychological. This is not just a female problem.

Symptoms:
Anxiety and emotional distress.

ExRx:
Aerobic exercise has been shown to cause weight loss, which leads to significant improvement in pregnancy and ovulation among anovulatory obese women. For men, the impact of exercise is not yet known.

Inflammation of the Vulva and Vagina

Can occur at any age. Common causes are vaginal infection (i.e. protozoan, fungal, bacterial, and viral), vulvar infection, parasites, trauma, poor hygiene, and allergic or chemical irritations. The vagina and vulva are in close proximity and an inflammation of one can cause an inflammation of the other.

Symptoms:
Discharge, itching, and urinary or intercourse pain.

ExRx:
Take medications and/or cold compresses or sitz baths for itching from acute vulvar inflammation; severe cases may require warm compresses. Avoid tub baths with oils or soap bubbles and wear cotton underwear. Change out of wet clothes and bathing suits immediately after activity. Choose an exercise position—standing, seated, or prone—that puts the least pressure on the inflamed area.

MENOPAUSE

Changes in multiple body systems caused by aging, declining ovarian function, and reduced estrogen levels. Onset is usually between forty-five and fifty-five, or because of illness or surgery. There are three types: (1) physiologic (normal), (2) pathologic (premature), and (3) artificial. During and after menopause, women may experience the onset of many other ailments and disorders including arteriosclerosis and osteoporosis. Osteoporosis (bone loss) begins at about age thirty-five and women at that age lose approximately .5% bone mass per year. During menopause, bone loss accelerates to .6% per year. Without proper care and exercise, a postmenopausal woman can lose almost 10% of her bone mass in fifteen years.

Symptoms:
Cessation of menstruation, depression, dry, itchy skin, irritability, hot flashes and/or night sweats (60% of cases), vertigo, fainting, rapid pulse, shortness of breath, flat libido, vaginal dryness, frequent urination, poor memory and concentration, and anxiety.

ExRx:
Estrogen therapy helps prevent osteoporosis by reducing bone reabsorption and decreasing bone loss. These are also the benefits of such regular weight-bearing exercise programs as walking and stepping machines. Also, smoking cigarettes increases the risk of heart disease of women taking estrogen. Exercise allows smokers on estrogen to either quit or cut back, thereby reducing the risk of heart disease or other blood-clotting diseases.

Exercise may mimic the effects of estrogen therapy by controlling the physical and emotional symptoms and thereby reducing the side effects associated with estrogen, including vaginal bleeding, nausea, breast tenderness, and uterine cramps. Also, it may reduce the risk of endometrial cancer.

Exercise may alleviate some symptoms of menopause and also allow you to take a lower dosage of estrogen or allow its use over only a short-term period. The lowest possible dosage also reduces cancer risk. A short-term, low-dosage estrogen prescription reduces the cancer risk by nearly 85% of the normal risk of a five-year, high-dosage prescription.

Lifelong weight-bearing exercises will have helped to stockpile bone mass in your earlier years and may fortify you against and slow down the process of bone loss and maybe even increase bone mass and density. The best weight-bearing exercises are walking, stair climbing, aerobic dancing, and skiing. The least effective are swimming and floor or lying-down exercises.

Regular exercise also improves many menstrual symptoms—pre- and postmenopausal—including cramping, water retention, mood swings, headaches, and backaches.

Natural pain relief is provided by the secretion of beta-endorphins with levels increasing after twenty minutes of continuous exercise. Menstrual cramping can also be relieved by stretching the lower abdominal area. (Also see premenstrual syndrome, p. 374.)

Ovarian Cancer

A malignant tumor of the ovaries, which spreads rapidly and gives few early warnings. Only 40% of women survive for five years. Predisposed risks include family history of ovarian, breast, or uterine cancer.

Symptoms:
Early menopause, hot flashes, headaches, palpitations, insomnia, depression, and excessive perspiration.

ExRx:
Surgery to remove the ovaries and any other surrounding affected tissue, sometimes including the uterus is necessary with ovarian cancer; also chemotherapy and radiation. A regular exercise program will provide a feeling of well-being and reduce pain and side effects of the chemo and radiation treatments. Begin exercising as soon as possible after the surgery, doing stretching, deep breathing, and relaxation techniques first and progressing to weight-bearing exercises as your body recovers.

Ovarian Cysts

Noncancerous sacs of fluids and semisolids on ovaries. Depending on the severity, these may have to be removed surgically.

Symptoms:
Range from none to mild; sometimes pelvic and lower back pain, painful intercourse, and vaginal shrinkage.

ExRx:
Presurgery: Do stretching exercises for abdomen, groin, and lower back; also, the pelvic tilt. After surgery: increase exercise and activity level gradually over four to six weeks.

Painful Menstruation and Menstrual Cramps

Hormonal imbalance causes increased uterine contractions and other symptoms during menstruation. Affects 10% of high school girls, and is a leading cause of school absenteeism; it causes 140 million work hours to be lost every year by adults.

Symptoms:
Severe menstrual cramps, nausea, headache, and sometimes diarrhea.

ExRx:
Bending and leg-lifting exercises; stretching, strengthening, and circulatory exercises for the abdomen, trunk, lower back (including the pelvic tilt); stretch and relax uterine muscles surrounding muscle tissues in the back and lower back areas.

Premenstrual Syndrome (PMS)

Various symptoms that sometimes occur seven to fourteen days before menstruation.

Symptoms:
Cardiovascular: irregular heartbeat and palpitations; nervous system: clumsiness, dizziness, headache, seizures, slurred speech, and numbness or tingling in the hands; digestive: abdominal bloating, hemorrhoids, nausea, and water retention; muscles and joints: backache, joint pain and swelling, muscle aches, and a stiff neck.

ExRx:
Relieve symptoms with exercise including cycling, swimming, and relaxation techniques. Practice child pose and the sponge posture (p. 376), trunk-bending and stretching exercises

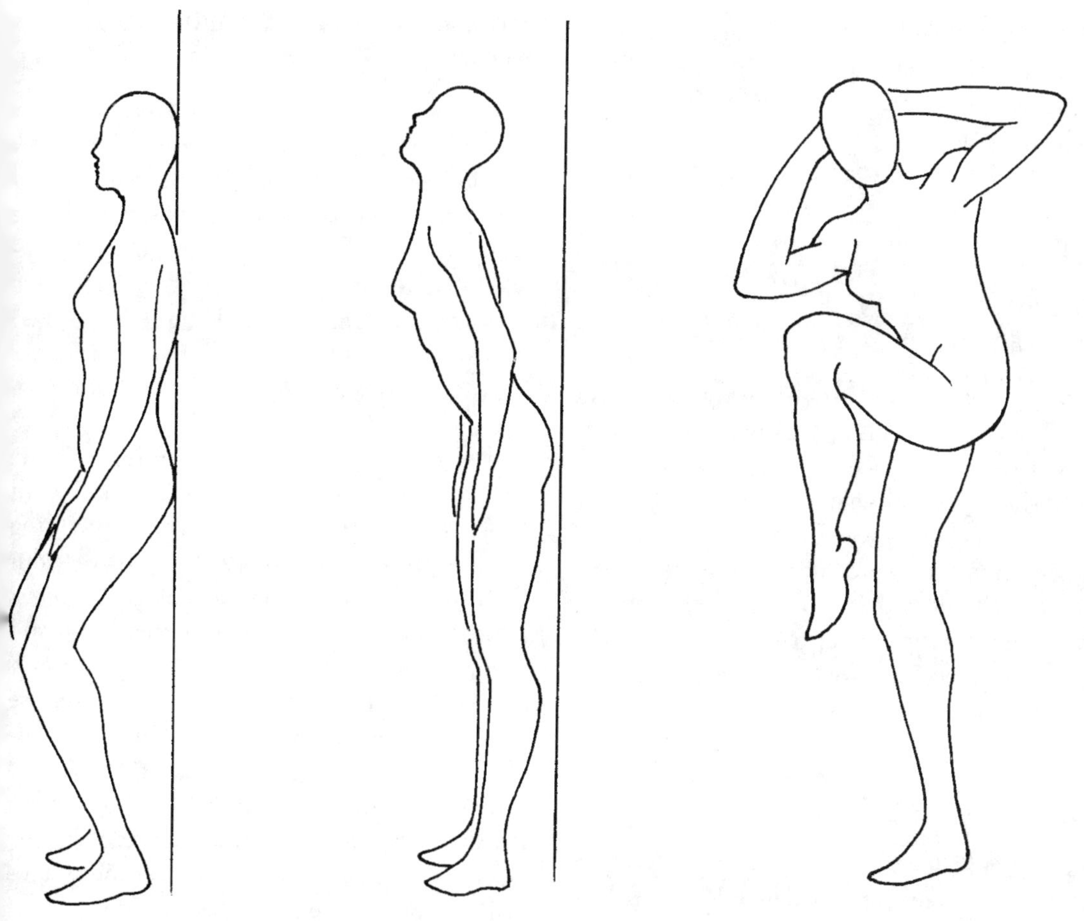

Trunk Bending and Stretching Exercises

(above). Avoid caffeine and alcohol to avoid insomnia and nervousness. Aerobic exercise has been shown to improve concentration and reduce depression during PMS.

PMS includes a wide variety of physical symptoms, and is most prominent during the child-bearing years from twenty-five to forty-five. Perhaps no other medical condition benefits more from therapeutic exercises, which can relieve a great variety of the associated symptoms. The overall therapeutic prescription is regular vigorous aerobic exercise—twenty minutes or more daily during the seven to fourteen days before your period to increase the beta-endorphin levels.

If you're out of shape or overweight, it may be difficult to exercise vigorously. In this case, low-intensity, moderate-paced exercise for up to sixty minutes will produce similar effects. Exercise in this manner until you are better conditioned for more vigorous, concentrated exercise.

You can also do cramp-specific exercises such as the bent-over stretches (pp. 378–380) to provide immediate relief. These exercises work on the abdominal muscles surrounding the uterus as well as the reproductive organs themselves. Yoga postures and such "soft exercise" as tai chi can also help relieve pain and symptoms.

The following yoga postures—the "child pose" and the "sponge posture"—are positions that will help you relax at rest.

The Child Pose:

Do a deep knee bend and bring your buttocks as close to your heels as possible; if necessary, widen your foot placement for stability. Your arms should remain relaxed by your sides with your fingers lightly touching the floor for stability. Bend forward until your forehead touches the floor. Feel your spine stretching. Hold this posture for up to six minutes. Do not do this posture if you have knee pain or injury.

The Sponge Posture:

Lie on your back with your arms and legs bent at the knees and spread-eagled. Relax as you slowly breathe in and out with your eyes closed. Hold the position for as long as you are comfortable.

META RX: LIST OF ADDITIONAL GYNECOLOGICAL DISORDERS THAT ARE BENEFITED BY META EXERCISES

- cervical cancer
- uterine cancer
- vulvar cancer

MODERATE-PACED EXERCISE FOR META REHAB AND THERAPY

The pace of your continuous exercise deter mines how fast your body burns calories pe minute. A moderate pace means moving you legs at the rate of sixty to ninety steps (or rev olutions when cycling) per minute. System wide, Meta therapy and rehab is done at slow (fifteen spms) to moderate (sixty spms pace. For many chronic problems, this pace continued throughout a cardio exercise pro gram, too.

Pace determines exercise intensity, th rate at which you burn calories, and you heart-training rate. Therefore, monitorin your exercise pace helps to control you body's reaction to overexercising (i.e. too fa a heart rate, heavy or labored breathing, an profuse sweating). But exercise pace is no necessarily the sole determinant of exercis intensity. You can maintain a slow to mode ate exercise pace and increase the exercis intensity by increasing the work load or wo effort by pacing your workout in the slight higher intensity range of forty to ninety ste or leg or arm movements per minute.

A vigorous exercise pace of ninety to on hundred twenty spms/rpms produces a high calorie burn rate, but it can also use more your glycogen or sugar stores. For diabetic this means increased insulin secretion. Lo to moderate-intensity exercise lessens th reaction and also allows you to eat and drin while you are exercising without causing stomach upset. As a result, a vigorous pa may be more suitable for nondiabetics. If yo are overweight, but nondiabetic, however, yo should still be concerned about such vigorou paced exercises as jogging and jumping rop which can put too much stress on the musc oskeletal system and can also jar some of your internal organs. In this case, the alternative to vigorous-paced, high-impact exercise is weight-loaded or resistance exercises.

Weight-loaded or resistance exercises can also raise your calorie burn rate without putting you at a greater risk of musculoskeletal injury. Weight-loaded exercise also increases the work load on bones helping to stimulate them to absorb more calcium and other nutrients. See General Rehabilitation Guidelines and Procedures and Weight-loading Schedule below for more specific instructions.

General Rehabilitation Guidelines and Procedures

Phase I: For Acute Injuries

1. After surgery, the physical therapist will use either active- or passive-assisted exercise. Passive will consist of four to six major range of moving the injured body area in the four ranges of motion: flexion, extension, supination, and pronation.
2. After you are able to move the injured area unassisted, the physical therapist will supervise unassisted ROMs and then isometric exercises on the muscles that are connected to the injured body area.

Phase II: For Moderate to Severe Injuries

1. When you are able to move the injured body area and you can do isometric exercises with your own strength and without undue pain, begin Phase II exercises.
2. Phase II exercises (bend/extend, flexion) are those that let you bend and strengthen the body area through the full range of its motion.

Phase III: For Mild Injuries

These involve dynamic exercises to strengthen muscles as well as stretch them through a full range of motion. They also involve regaining balance and motor-sensory pronation. After this phase is completed, you may begin the three levels of preventive and conditioning exercises in Part Two.

WEIGHT-LOADING EXERCISES

The amount of weight that you add depends on your own body weight and on your muscle strength and size. Here are the general guidelines. In general, do not use any weights until your doctor or physical therapist says that it is okay. Weight-loading exercises can then be added in Phase II and III of the rehab schedule.

WEIGHT LOAD/REPETITION SCHEDULE

	LOAD	REPETITIONS
Phase I	No weight	determined by MD or PT
Phase II	See schedule	1–5
Phase III	See schedule	6–12

WEIGHT-LOADING SCHEDULE

USE FOR PHASES II AND III

TYPE OF WEIGHT	AMOUNT OF WEIGHT SMALL FRAME	MEDIUM FRAME	LARGE FRAME
Hand-held	0–¼ lbs.	¼–½ lbs.	½–1 lbs.
Ankle	0–½ lbs.	½–1 lbs.	1–5 lbs.

Abdominal, Lower Back, and Pelvic Control Exercises

Use the following exercises to help with digestive and reproductive problems such as stomach and menstrual cramps and lower back pain. Bending and stretching helps circulate blood and oxygen to the affected area(s) thereby providing some pain relief.

Bent-Over Stretches

This following series of stretches and relaxation exercises help to relax and strengthen the muscles in the abdominal and midriff areas. They alleviate symptoms from premenstrual tension, digestive disorders, constipation, as well as kidney and bladder disorders, by relieving muscle contractions and increasing muscle strength and control.

Abdominal Curl

- Lie on your back with both knees bent
- Slowly curl up as you slowly inhale
- Reach forward with your arms and shoulders; try to raise your head and shoulders about three to twelve inches off the floor or bed

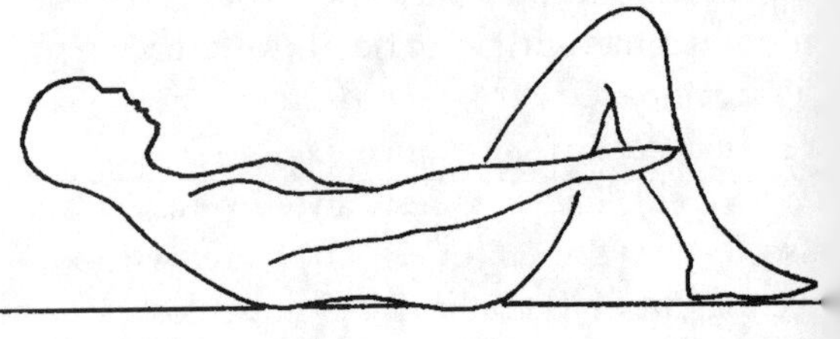

Abdominal Curl

- Hold for three to five seconds
- Slowly curl back down as you exhale

Lying Leg Slides

- Lie on your back with your knees bent and feet hip-width apart and flat on the floor
- Flatten your back by tightening and pulling your stomach muscles in.
- Hold the position while you slowly slide one heel down along the floor until your knee is only slightly bent
- Feel the contraction in your lower abdominal muscles
- Pull your heel back toward you until your knee is slightly bent
- Repeat on the other leg
- Repeat on each leg three to twelve times

Lying-down Pelvic Tilt

- Lying down in the flat-back position, pull your abdominal muscles in and slowly raise your tailbone off the floor
- Continue lifting your lower back off the floor one vertebrae at a time until you have reached your mid-back

- Slowly roll your back down one vertebrae at a time until it is flat against the floor again
- Repeat three to twelve times

Seated Lower Back Stretch

- Sit halfway back in a sturdy chair; stretch your legs out, keeping your knees slightly bent
- With your arms relaxed and resting on your thighs, lean back and touch the back of your chair
- Rest for three to five seconds
- Now, inhale as you raise your arms out in front of you; use your stomach muscles to pull yourself up so you're sitting up straight
- Repeat up to twelve times

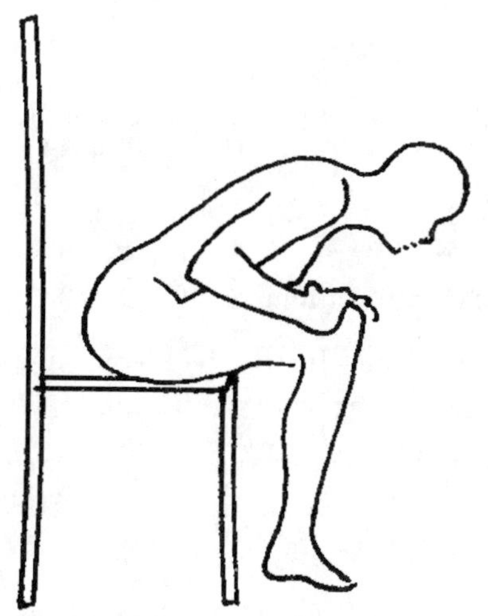

Seated Lower Back Stretch

Seated Stretching

- Sit halfway back in a sturdy chair with your feet apart and parallel to the chair legs
- Lean forward as you gently grab your thighs above the knees with your hands, fingers pointing inward
- Lean forward and raise your shoulder to your ears keeping your back straight
- Take a deep breath
- Exhale forcefully through pursed lips as you pull in your stomach muscles and let your back round; hold for three to five seconds and release
- Repeat one to three times

Front Abdominal Standing Stretch

- Stand with your feet parallel and hip- to shoulder-width apart; with elbows out, clasp your hands behind your head
- Lift your left knee toward your right elbow; hold for a second or two
- Keep your knees slightly bent and lower your leg
- Now, lift your right knee to your left elbow, hold, and lower again
- Repeat one to three times

Back and Hip Standing Stretch

- With your hands on hips, stand with your feet shoulder-width apart; keep your knees slightly bent
- Bend forward as far as you can; return to the start position

- Next, bend to the right as far as you can; return to the start position
- Now, bend backward as far as you can; return to the start position
- Bend to the left as far as you can; return to the start position
- Repeat one to three times

Standing Stretch

- Stand with your back and heels against a wall
- Inhale as you bend your knees and flatten your back against the wall
- Now, squeeze your buttocks and pull in your stomach muscles
- Hold this position for three to five seconds and exhale
- Inhale as you straighten your knees and arch your back; hold for one to three seconds
- Repeat one to three times

Please note: Do not do this stretch if you have back pain.

Kegel Exercise

Invented by a gynecologist, Dr. Arnold Kegel, these exercises strengthen the pelvic floor muscles—a sling-shaped set of muscles that run from the pubic bone to the tailbone. These also include the anus, the urethra (bladder opening), and the vagina or penis. You use your pelvic floor muscles to move your bowels, hold back urination or ejaculation, and in women, to tighten the vagina.

By developing muscle tone and strength in this area, you can use these muscles to hold back urine in the case of incontinence. First, you have to learn to identify and isolate the pelvic floor muscles from the others nearby, such as abdominals and buttocks. To begin, practice this exercise while you are urinating: When you are half finished, try to slow down or stop the flow without tensing the stomach, buttocks, or leg muscles. Keep trying each time you urinate, until you successfully stop the flow. Hold for a moment and then release the flow. This exercise will help you to identify the pelvic floor muscles so that you can perform the following Kegel exercises more effectively. Over a six-week time period, practice the slow and fast Kegel exercises, building up from three to nine repetitions to 100 repetitions.

Slow Kegel

- Women: Squeeze your vaginal muscles by pulling them up and in; men: Squeeze your anus muscles by pulling them up and in
- Hold this squeeze contraction for four seconds; breathe in and out through your nose while holding the contraction
- Relax the contraction, exhaling out
- Repetitions: beginners, one to three times; intermediate, four to eight times; advanced, nine to twelve times
- With your hands, feel your muscles to check that you are keeping abdomen, buttocks, and thighs relaxed

Fast Kegel

- Repeat the slow Kegel exercise using contractions of only one to three seconds in length

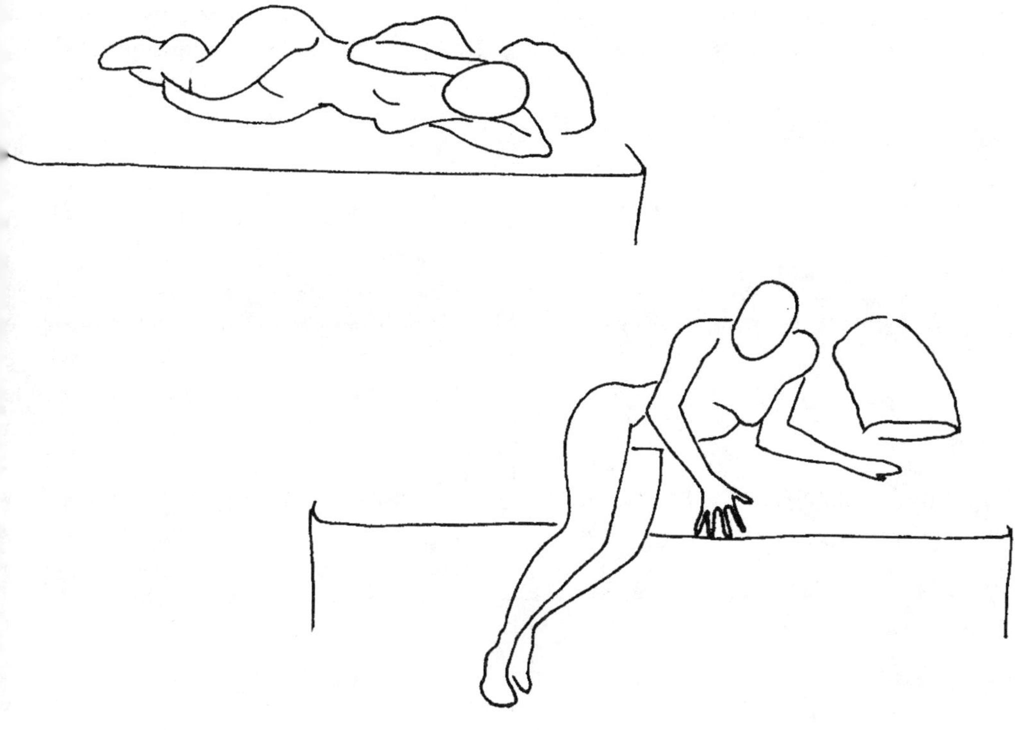

Kegel Exercise

- Relax for one to three seconds
- Repeat, using the same numbers of reps as for the slow Kegel

Kegel for Coughing, Sneezing, or Laughing

- Before you cough, sneeze, or laugh, contract your pelvic floor muscles: squeeze, pull up, and hold in your anus or vaginal muscles
- Hold the contraction as you sneeze, cough, or laugh (cough or laugh for one to three seconds)
- Stop coughing or laughing and relax your muscles
- Repeat one to three times

Please note: Because sneezing is spontaneous and unpredictable, practice this exercise by coughing and laughing. As you become more adept at those, you will also be better able to tighten your pelvic floor muscles on the spur of the moment for a sneeze.

Kegel for Lifting Objects and Changing Body Position

Please note: This Kegel technique for urinary leakage can be added to bracing technique for lower back protection when lifting heavy objects.

For Lifting:

- Stand close to the heavy object and place your feet hip-width to shoulder-width apart

- Bend your knees as you lean forward to reach for the object, keeping your back straight at all times
- Contract your pelvic floor muscles (if you have lower back problems, also contract your stomach muscles as you grab the object)
- Keep muscles contracted until you have lifted and placed the object down

For Changing Body Positions:

- Brace your pelvic floor and lower back muscles before rolling to one side
- Push yourself up with your arms to raise yourself from either a seated or lying-down position
- Lower your legs off the bed and place both feet flat on the floor
- Hold the contraction until you have raised up fully, and then relax

EXERCISE FOR CONSTIPATION AND HEMORRHOIDS

Both exercise and diet can promote better bowel movements and can also help reduce hemorrhoids, which are aggravated by frequent constipation. Eating a high-fiber diet (accompanied by plenty of fluids) is itself an exercise for the digestive system, stimulating the colon walls to produce muscular contractions so that stools can move out of your system. Otherwise, stools just sit there, drying out and hardening, and becoming more difficult to pass. A bulky, softer stool will trigger colonic contractions for easier elimination.

Exercise, particularly moderate to vigorous exercise, speeds up the transit time of bowels partially by boosting the hormonal secretions that make the bowels work. It also keeps blood from pooling in veins such as those that develop into hemorrhoids. Leg lifts, sit-ups, torso bends and twists, and abdominal-strengthening exercises also create intra-abdominal pressure which can help to relieve constipation. Any exercise that causes abdominal activity, for example sports with knee lifts or trunk turns, will also strengthen stomach muscles and aid in better bowel movements. Stretching and strengthening exercises that twist or bend the trunk area can also help energize a lazy colon. Forward bends compress the abdomen; torso twists rotate the abdominal wall, which pushes the stomach contents along the intestinal tract. Additionally, deep breathing exercises lift the diaphragm, massage the intestine, and help you to relax tense muscles.

Knee Lifts

- Raise your knees to your chest, either alternating one leg at a time in the standing position or with both knees at the same time in the seated or lying-down positions
- Inhale as you raise the knee(s)
- Exhale as you press them further toward your chest
- Inhale as you lower back to the starting position
- Repeat one to three times

Forward Bends

- Lying on your back or seated on the edge of your chair, exhale and slowly bend over or curl up, bringing your head toward your knees

- Inhale as you return to the stretched-out position
- Repeat one to three times

Please note: If frequent movement is painful, you can also remain bent over, taking deep breaths as you hold the position.

Torso Twists

- Exhale as you turn your torso to one side
- Inhale as you return to the center position
- Now, turn your torso to the opposite side
- Repeat one to three times

Please note: You may also hold each twist for a few counts of deep breathing.

PREGNANCY RX

Pregnancy is included with the Metabolic health system because it involves a woman's body gaining more weight than is normal. Similar to running a marathon, the act of delivering a child involves a tremendous amount of physical strength and stamina. But for most women, running is not a viable exercise solution because the act of running can jolt and jar the uterus and may cause complications in the pregnancy. Walking is a much better option for physical activity during pregnancy.

For inactive women, pregnancy is a condition requiring a therapeutic or rehab level of exercise, and only in few cases can women follow a preventive level program.

Studies show that women who exercise regularly before and during pregnancy have quicker deliveries and shorter hospital stays. Because they cope better with the pain and hard exertion of childbirth they require less medication. Also, regular exercisers gain less excess weight during pregnancy and get back in shape much more quickly.

Studies show that women who regularly exercise (e.g. brisk walkers) experience less discomfort during pregnancy (e.g. swelling of legs, leg cramps, fatigue, shortness of breath, mechanical strain from postural change) than pregnant women who don't exercise. Low-intensity exercise does not cause fetal weight loss, change in fetal heart rate, or fetal behavioral patterns. Moderate to high-intensity exercises, however, can produce lower birth weights.

Pregnancy is not the time to start a new exercise program, especially a rigorous one. Doctors recommend that if you have been inactive before your pregnancy, the best exercise you can do is a slow to moderate walking program, including some stretching and posture training. Posture exercises, especially pelvic tilts, will help to eliminate or control constipation, hemorrhoids, and heartburn. Good posture will also strengthen the abdomen and lower back, which is important because your center of gravity shifts forward as your baby grows bigger, stretching your abdominal muscles and tightening or shortening your back muscles.

Performing pelvic tilts helps prevent back pain and improves posture by strengthening abdominal muscles and stretching out lower back muscles. Low-impact aerobic exercise will help you strengthen your heart to better handle the extra blood circulating in your system. Avoid high-impact exercises because the hormones associated with pregnancy have loosened your joints and softened your ligaments to create the space and flexibility needed for a growing baby. Thus, your joints are more prone to injury because they are

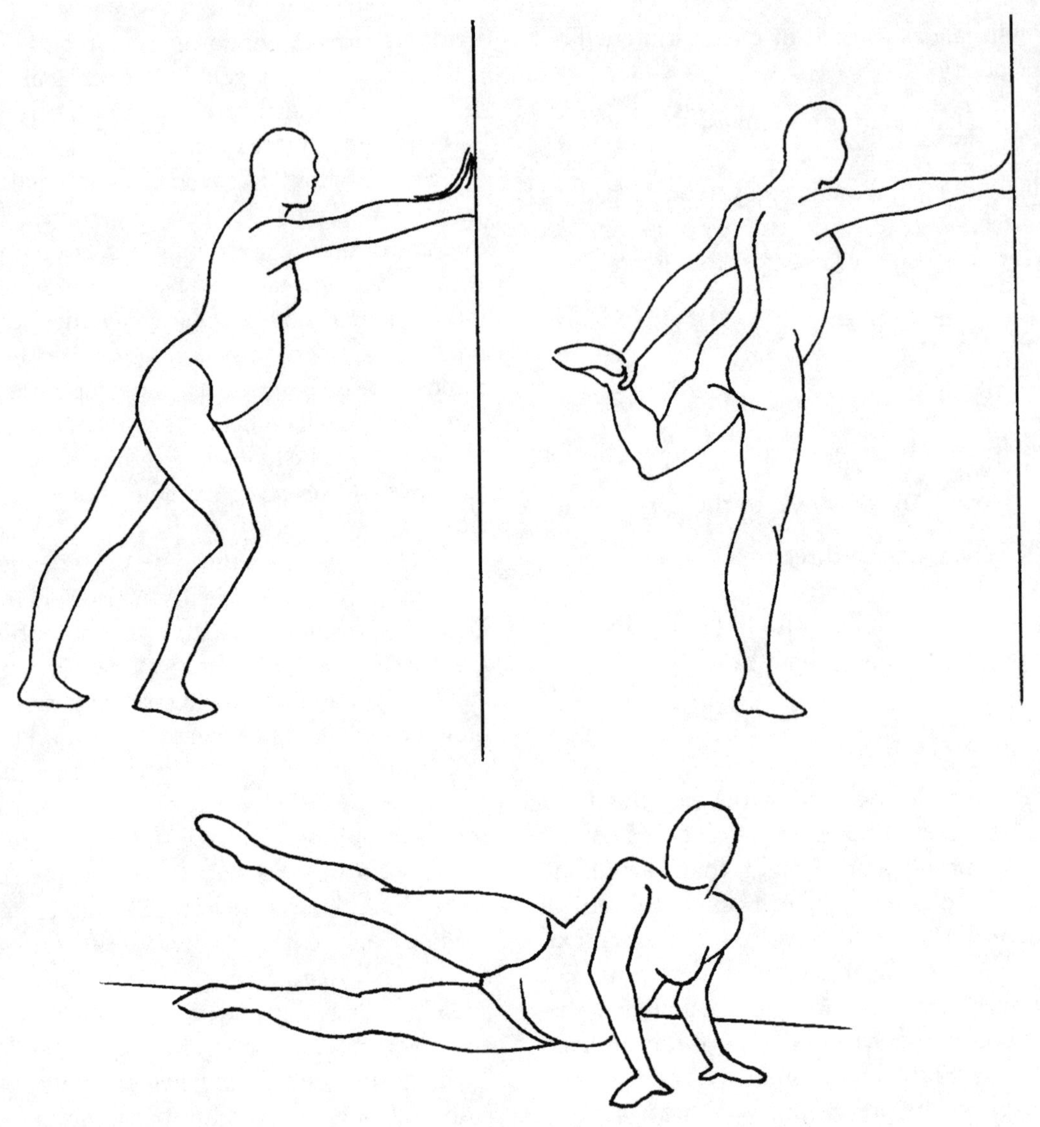

Pregnancy Stretches

loose and carrying a greater weight load.

Consulting with your doctors (both your obstetrician and your g.p.) will allow you to choose from a variety of exercise programs presented in this book. She or he should consider your health status and physical condition. If you are overweight or are going to have more than one baby, mild stretching and ROM exercises might be all you will be able to do. Consider doing a monitored prenatal exercise program sponsored by your local hospital or health club. Also, postpartum mothers can follow a similar rehab exercise prescription as for cardio patients.

On the following "DON'Ts" list are any xercises or activities that involve high-npact, bouncing, or jerking moves along ‹ith other exercise "don'ts" tips. The exercise DOs" are listed first, and contain tips for xercising while you are pregnant, which will ıelp you move your body in safe, healthy ‹ays without injuring yourself or your baby.

)Os:

- Do rest frequently between exercises or whenever you feel you need it
- Do keep your heart rate in the range of 50 to 65% of maximum, or approximately ninety to 140 beats per minute
- Do gentle, extended warm-ups and stretching exercises before and after any aerobic exercise
- Drink plenty of water and other liquids
- Stop exercising and consult with your doctors if you have any unusual symptoms, including back pain, pubic pain or bleeding, dizziness, fainting, irregular heartbeat, palpitations, or difficulty in breathing

DON'Ts:

- Don't exercise in hot and humid places
- Don't exercise while lying on your back (i.e. prone) or your stomach (i.e. supine)
- Don't exercise on hard or slippery surfaces
- Don't do any ballistic (i.e. jerky or sudden) motions
- Don't do any jumping or hopping movements
- Don't allow yourself to become out of breath

Pelvic Tilt

Please note: The pelvic tilt exercise is an important abdominal and back stretching and strengthening exercise. It is very important for anyone whose stomach muscles have been weakened or stretched by inactivity, obesity, or pregnancy. As a postural correction exercise, you should use the pelvic tilt anytime you catch yourself arching your back too much, or as a stretching exercise to reduce muscle tension in your lower back. But don't use it for severe lower back pain; wait until rest and medication have healed your back so you can perform the exercise relatively pain-free. The pelvic tilt can be performed in any of three positions: lying down, sitting, or standing.

- Tip your pelvis upward by holding (bracing) your stomach muscles in as you tuck your buttocks under your body (this flattens out the hollow or arch in your back)
- Hold the position for three to five seconds and release
- Repeat the exercise eight to twelve times, relaxing a few seconds between repetitions

POSTNATAL REHAB EXERCISE

This exercise program is similar to any other rehab program, in that you gradually increase the amount and level of exercises over a six-week rehab period. Aerobic or continuous motion exercises will assist you in shedding any extra pounds gained during your pregnancy. Practice the pelvic tilt in the prone position as a type of rehab sit-up. As your

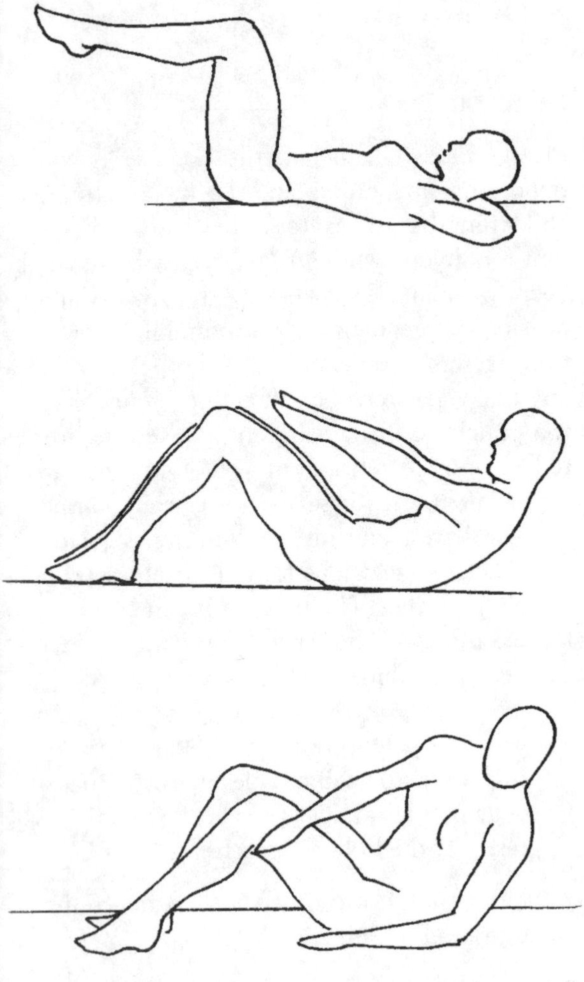

Postnatal Exercises

abdominal muscles become stronger, do the stomach and side curl exercises from the prone position.

STRETCHING AND POSTURE TRAINING

Week One

Continue practicing the pelvic tilt to strengthen and stretch your stomach and lower back muscles. You are also ready to sta strength training for your postural muscles.

Weeks Two through Six

Gradually introduce each of the remainin posture training exercise positions: lying seated, and standing. (See pp. 40–47).

WARM-UPS

Week One

Practice the full set of ROM exercises on page 171–179 at a slow to moderate pace in th lying-down, seated, or standing position, goin slowly when a full range of motion seems diffi cult. Repeat exercises one to three times.

Weeks Two through Six

Increase the number of repetitions (up to twelve) of your program according to you own personalized rehab schedule.

Stretching and Strengthening

Practice Kegel exercises (pp. 380–382) to pre vent incontinence problems and help keep the vagina elastic. Squeeze off the urine flow hold, and release in a series of three to twelve repetitions. Also, do lying down rehab abdominal and back exercises (pp. 202–203 209–211, 378–379).

The following specific exercises can begin at week one and can continue as long as they are effective.

Leg Lifts

- Lie on your back with your legs stretched out and your knees slightly bent
- Pull your legs toward your stomach until your knees are bent at a 90-degree angle

- Tilt your pelvis forward as you flatten out your back
- Repeat one to three times
- Practice by extending your legs out a little farther each time, making sure your back stays flat and does not arch
- Later, to add more resistance, do raised leg lifts

aised Leg Lifts

- Lie on your back with your knees bent at a 90-degree angle and lower back pressed flat against the floor
- Raise your legs with your knees pointing straight up to the ceiling
- Now, lower your legs back down to the start position
- As your stomach muscles become stronger, pull your knees in closer to your chest for extra resistance
- Repeat one to three times

lease note: Avoid doing this exercise with raightened legs, as it puts too much stress on our back.

tomach Curls

- Lie on your back with knees bent at a 90-degree angle
- Tilt your pelvis forward to flatten your back
- Stretch your arms out toward your knees and inhale
- Tuck your chin to your neck and exhale as you roll your head, shoulders, and upper back up off the ground; hold for a few moments
- Slowly, lower yourself back down as you inhale
- Repeat one to three times

Side Curls

- Lie on your side with your knees bent at a 90-degree angle
- To work your oblique muscles, alternate reaching your arms across your chest to the opposite knee as you sit up
- To add more resistance, cross your arms over your chest. Vary this by holding your arms out by the side of your chest
- Repeat one to three times

Abdominal, Hip, Pelvis, and Groin Injuries Rx

Not confined to sports injuries, arthritis, disk disease, kidney stone and hernia pain, prostate and bladder surgery, and a variety of infections of the abdominal and genital organs may also radiate into the hip, pelvis, and groin area. Functional abnormalities of the feet and legs can also affect this area. Exercise therapy can help alleviate pain and help rehab injured areas after either surgery or treatment.

Acute Abdominal, Hip, Pelvis, and Groin Injuries

Avulsion Fracture in the Pelvic Area

A violent muscle contraction causes a stretch or tear of the various tendons that are attached to the bones in the pelvis, hip, or

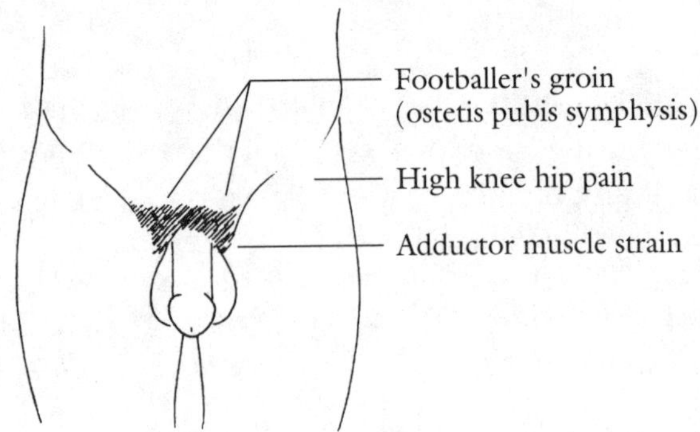

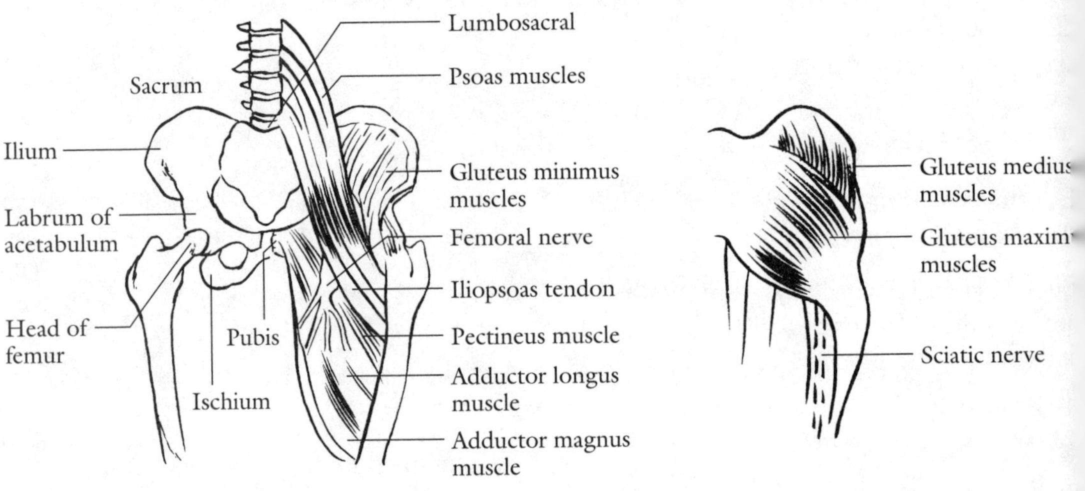

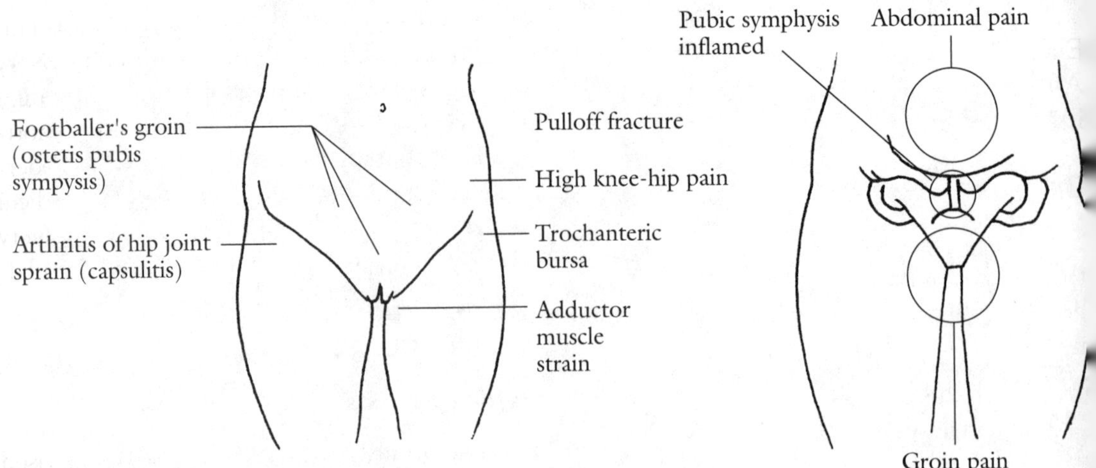

Groin Injuries

groin area. In growing children, it can also involve the tearing off of a portion of the bone. This injury often occurs during football, soccer, jumping, and sprinting.

Symptoms:
Severe pain and disability.

ExRx:
Rest and ice. Begin Phase II Rehab exercises when pain subsides, or ten days after injury. Continue rehab exercise for at least four to six weeks, and then begin the preventive exercises for another three months before returning to sports and vigorous exercise.

Blunt and Penetrating Abdominal Injuries

Life-threatening hemorrhage and shock from automobile accidents, contact sports, falls, stabbings, or gunshots; possible damage to organs.

Symptoms:
Severe pain radiates beyond the abdomen all the way to shoulder.

ExRx:
After your condition has stabilized, start with Phase I MuSkel and Cardio Rehab.

Groin Strain

Stretching or tearing of the adductor muscle that runs from the inner thigh up to the pubic bone. Caused by forcefully drawing your leg inward, as in a inside kick (soccer) or a goalie's save (hockey).

Symptoms:
Stabbing pain and inability to move the leg inward.

ExRx:
Prevent by strengthening the adductors with leg exercises, p. 338–339. Rehab with rest, ice, and immobilization. For a first-degree injury (mild), start with Phase III Therapeutic exercises; recovery takes about two weeks. For a second-degree injury (moderate), start with Phase II Rehab; recovery takes about four to six weeks. For a third-degree injury (severe), start with Phase I Rehab; recovery takes about six to eight weeks.

Hip Flexor Strain

A pulling or tearing of the iliopsoas muscle, located where the tendon attaches to the inner side of the top thigh bone. Caused when muscle tries to contract while the leg is pulled, extended, or trapped (e.g. your leg is hit when trying to kick a soccer ball).

Symptoms:
Stabbing pain when you try to lift your leg or loss of strength if it is a complete tear.

ExRx:
For mild strains, rest and ice, and begin therapeutic exercises when pain subsides. Recovery is in two to seven days. Exercise with swimming (no straight-legged kicks), stair climbing, short-stepped walking, and light cycling. For moderate to severe strains, rest, ice, and seek medical attention. Practice Phase II Rehab for recovery in one to two weeks. Rehab Phases I and II bring about recovery in four to six weeks.

Hip Fracture

A cracking or breaking of the hip joint caused by a severe blow or by thinning of the bone (see osteoporosis, p. 307). Most common in elderly people and auto accident victims; less common as a sports injury, except in racquet sports when players slam sideways into walls (squash) or fall sideways to the floor.

Symptoms:
Pain in the hip, difficult or impossible to stand or walk.

ExRx:
Regular exercise reduces the chances of bone fracture in case of injury by thickening and thereby strengthening the skeleton, and also by improving coordination to help prevent accidents in the first place. Avoid sudden moves that twist your body in the opposite direction of your foot movement. A fracture is a medical emergency—it can cause the death of the ball of the hip joint if not given proper medical attention. After joint-replacement surgery or immobilization, Phase I Rehab. Focus on strengthening the muscles that surround the hip joint, so that they will provide extra support and protection for the joint, after injury has healed. Continue on to Phases II and III when these do not cause pain and after your doctor or physical therapist has given you an okay.

Hip Pointer

A contusion to the iliac crest, the bony protrusion of the hip, caused by hitting it sideways. Occurs mostly as a football, hockey, and other sports injury.

Symptoms:
Pain, spasms, possible paralysis, inability to turn trunk or flex the hip.

ExRx:
Prevent by wearing protective pads. Treat with ice, compression, and massage. When pain subsides, do therapeutic exercises or Phase II Rehab, whichever can be done within your pain thresholds. Recovery takes about one to two weeks.

Overuse Injuries

Groin Tendinitis (Adductor Muscle)

An inflammation of the tendon insert of the largest groin muscle (the adductor) attached to the pubic bone. The adductor muscles are basically the groin muscles, which stretch from the pelvis down to the lower part of the thigh bone. They allow you to draw your leg outward from your hip. This injury is caused by repeated driving of the hip inward as in running, soccer, and hockey.

Symptoms:
Pain in groin radiates to inside thigh.

ExRx:
Strengthen the hip adductor muscles. Cease pain-causing acvitities and reduce repetitive adductor activities by substituting with other exercise such as cycling. For mild cases, begin therapeutic exercises immediately. For moderate to severe injuries, begin Phase I Rehab within a week. Sometimes, surgery is required to trim inflamed tendons. In mild to moderate cases, there is a two- to four-week recovery; a severe case may take several months.

Hip Flexor Tendinitis

An inflammation of the tendon insert of the illiopsoas muscle and sometimes the bursa sac beneath it. Caused by weight lifting from squatting position or by high jumping, hurdling, and kicking.

Symptoms:
Groin pain, especially when you raise the knee against resistance.

ExRx:
Cease the aggravating activity that caused the condition and substitute with walking, bicycling, or stair climbing. Depending on the severity of the injury, start with Phase I or II Rehab.

OSTEITIS PUBIS

Inflammation of the disk that connects the sides of the pubic bone. Caused by repetitive contraction of the inner thigh muscles. Occurs in distance running, weight lifting, soccer, football, and after prostate and bladder surgery.

Symptoms:
Pain in pubic bone that can radiate into the thighs and abdomen, which can be felt when raising your legs against resistance.

ExRx:
Phase II Rehab exercises can begin within three to five days after the pain subsides or after surgery.

SNAPPING HIP SYNDROME

A variety of symptoms resulting from the illiotibial band snapping over the outside hip bone. Causes trochanteric bursitis. It can be caused by hurdling, gymnastics, or dance.

Symptoms:
May feel and see the hip pop or snap; pain in hip area.

ExRx:
Prevent by stretching tight muscles. Cease aggravating activity and seek medical attention. Start Phase II Rehab as soon as pain subsides, with a recovery in about six weeks.

STRESS FRACTURE AT TOP OF THIGH BONE

Just below the ball of the hip joint, caused by repetitive pounding or impact to the lower part of the leg. Caused by long-distance running on hard surfaces. If untreated, it can lead to a complete fracture in adults and death of the hip joint in children from the termination of blood supply.

Symptoms:
Gradual increase in groin and outer thigh pain, which can radiate to the knee. Also, the pain may increase when hip bone is pushed against. Accompanied by limping and limited hip motion.

ExRx:
Prevent by reducing running distances and by running on softer surfaces. Treat by ceasing to run and avoiding weight-bearing activities. Start Phase II Rehab when pain subsides. Recovery can take from two to three months.

TROCHANTERIC BURSITIS

The inflammation of the bursa sac located over the hip joint. Caused by friction from repetitive contraction of hip muscles, primarily in running.

Symptoms:
Pain at top of outer thigh especially when moving leg sideways (abduction).

ExRx:
Cease running or other activities that caused the injury; ice, massage, and seek medical treatment. Doctor may drain bursa, prescribe anti-inflammatories, or physical therapy for hip muscle tightness. Strengthen the gluteal muscle while stretching illiotibial band. Begin Phase II Rehab exercises as soon as possible.

Abdominal, Hip, Pelvis, and Groin Rehab Exercises

Phase I Abdominal, Hip, Pelvis, and Groin Rehab Exercises are used after surgery and are done with a physical therapist. Phase II Rehab Exercises are used for moderate or severe injuries. If you have been exercising at Phase I, start Phase II when you are able to move the injured area on your own. Phase III Rehab Exercises are used for mild to moderate injuries. Start Phase III when you can do Phase II without pain.

Phase I Abdominal, Hip, Pelvis, and Groin Rehab (with a Physical Therapist)

Start five days to three weeks after surgery or after immobilization period determined by your doctor or surgeon. A physical therapist assists with ROM and isometric exercises. You will first try to use your own strength to move the injured area (active-assisted exercise). If pain is too severe, the physical therapist will use passive-assisted exercise.

Phase II Rehab (at Home)

Use the following exercises as a starting point for rehabilitating moderate to severe injuries. Do these exercises two to three times a day building up to between ten and thirty repetitions. Also use lower back and thigh exercises to rehab and condition the hip, pelvis, and groin area.

Seated Hanging Leg Turns

- Sit on a table or on a telephone book placed on a chair with thighs supported and lower legs dangling, hip-width apart
- First, slowly rotate your legs inward until you touch your toes; pause
- Next, slowly rotate your legs outward until you touch your heels
- Repeat each turn five times building up to thirty reps; do one set a day building up to three

Prone Knee to Chest Pull

- Lie on your back
- Pull your bent knee toward your chest, alternating your injured and healthy legs
- Use your hands to pull your knee closer to your chest for a greater stretch
- Repeat five times building up to thirty reps; do one set a day, building up to three

Standing Knee to Chest Pull

- Stand with your feet shoulder-width apart
- Raise your knee toward your chest, alternating your injured and healthy legs

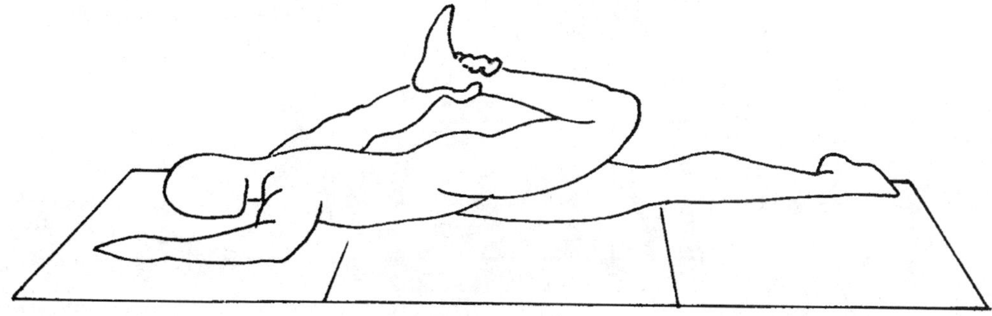

Lying Heel to Buttocks

- Repeat five times building up to thirty reps; do one set a day building up to three

Lying Heel to Buttocks

- Lie face down on a floor or mat
- Alternately bend back each of your legs, pulling the heel toward your buttocks with the opposite hand
- Repeat five times building up to thirty reps; do one set a day building up to three

Lying Lateral Leg-Lifts (Beginner or Advanced)

- Lie on your back, hands resting away from the sides of your body
- Beginner: slide the injured leg outward, then inward
- Advanced: lift the injured leg two to three inches off the ground, and then move the leg outward, then inward
- Next, slide (beginner) or lift (advanced) the healthy leg two to three inches off the ground and move it outward, then inward
- Repeat five times building up to thirty reps; do one set a day, building up to three

Leg Swings

- Stand next to a wall and brace your hand against it
- Swing your outside leg across your inside leg toward the wall; pause
- Next, swing your leg across and out, away from the wall
- Repeat five times building up to thirty reps; do one set a day, building up to three

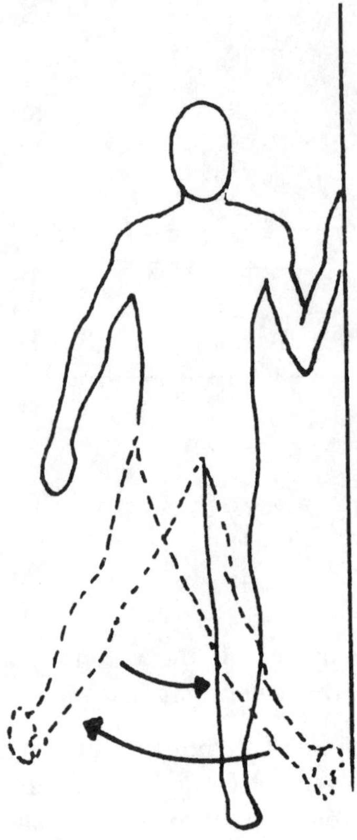

Leg Swings

Seated Resisted Leg Crosses

- Attach an ankle weight or wrap a belt or tubing around your ankles for resistance
- Sit on a table or other raised surface with your thighs supported and your lower legs dangling
- Spread your legs forcing your ankles outward; hold for five to ten seconds
- Repeat the exercise three times building up to ten reps; do one set a day building up to three

Seated Weighted Lateral Ankle Raises

- Attach an ankle weight to your injured leg
- Sit on a raised surface with your thighs supported and your lower legs dangling
- Raise your injured leg inward and upward; hold for five to ten seconds
- Repeat five to ten times on each leg; do one set a day, building up to three

Phase III Rehab

Lying Raised-Leg Lifts

- Lie face down with your upper body resting on a bench or table and your legs hanging off the sides
- Alternately raise and lower the injured leg and the healthy leg
- Repeat five times building up to thirty reps; do one set a day building up to three

Standing Weighted Leg Raises

- Stand with your feet shoulder-width apart and parallel to one another, ankle weights attached
- Raise the knee of the injured leg waist-high; hold five to ten seconds
- Lower your leg; rest
- Repeat five to ten leg raises; change legs and repeat; do one set a day building up to three

Lying Weighted Leg Raises

- Attach ankle weights to both legs
- Lie on a table or bench with your upper body supported and legs dangling
- Raise your injured leg with knee slightly bent; hold for five to ten seconds; lower it back down
- Repeat five to ten times; change legs and repeat; do one set a day, building up to three

CHAPTER 16

Cardio Rx

Exercise Solutions for Cardiovascular and Respiratory Systems

HEART, VESSELS, AND LUNGS

Cardio Rx offers a systemwide exercise prescription for disorders of the heart, blood vessels, and lungs. This comes in the form of walking, cycling, and water exercise routines including breathing, chest, and diaphragm relaxation exercises. You can use cardio therapy for any breathing difficulties affected by nose and throat injuries or any condition in which you have been bedridden for more than thirty days.

First, find a specific exercise prescription under the cardio disorder for which you have been diagnosed, then practice one of the three phases of Cardio Rehab. Your doctor will prescribe the appropriate phase based on testing the overall condition of your heart and lungs. Generally, you can practice Phase II or III exercises for mild to moderate arterial or vein blockages or such impediments as angina, asthma, intermittent claudication, or sinusitis. But, for such severe conditions as heart attack or lung surgery and other disorders involving severe respiratory distress or damage, Phase I will be your probable starting point.

Common cardiovascular treatable symptoms include chest tightness or pain; extreme fatigue; muscle pains in the chest, calves, arms, and neck; dizziness in response to exertion; shortness of breath, numbness and tingling in hands and feet; and swelling in the legs and arms. The primary treatable symptom of cardio-related problems is fatigue.

ANCER CARE AND CARDIO RX

any cancer patients report that fatigue and :haustion—not pain—is the most common mptom that they experience during and ter their cancer treatment. Fatigue has a ımber of causes, among them the depression ıd anxiety that result from a cancer diagno- ;. Another is from the cancer treatments. ırgery, chemotherapy, and/or radiation ther- ›y alone or together can leave you exhaust- l for weeks and months, sometimes even ears. The cancer itself, especially if it is lvanced, can reduce the numbers of oxygen- ırrying red blood cells and the infection- ghting white blood cells, further fatiguing ›ur body.

Exercise therapy and rehabilitation for ıncer patients involves a number of health 'stems. If the surgery involves damage to ıch muscles as those in the neck and chest ea, MuSkel rehab exercises are also pre- ribed. Initially, Psyche Rx exercises will also elp to cope with the trauma of the disease iagnosis. Next, moderate Cardio Rx exercis- ; will help to maintain stamina during and fter treatment. **Abandoning exercise may nly complicate your cancer.** You need that xtra energy that exercise (within limits) can rovide! Contact the Nursing Society at 388) 4-ANEMIA for additional help on oping with cancer-related fatigue. For physi- al rehab after surgery, see Chapter Fourteen, IuSkel Rx. For depression and anxiety, see Chapter Seventeen, Psyche-Immune Rx.

The major portion of this chapter is bro- en down into three areas, which are: (1) eart and blood vessel diseases and disorders 2) lungs and breathing diseases and disorders, nd (3) nose and throat diseases and disorders. ach of these three areas is followed by an lphabetic listing of the diseases or disorders found under that category. Symptoms are then described for each disease or disorder, which is followed by an ExRx for that specific ailment. You will note that some of the more common, more rehabilitative disorders and injuries have many exercises associated with them, while other diseases (e.g. prostate cancer, kidney stones) will have only a few exercises associated with them. If you feel you want more exercise than what is given with any ExRx, consult Parts I and II of this book and practice those preventive exercises that are associated with the body system or area that you are rehabilitating. Remember: Always start at a lower level and work your way up to your own personal optimum level. Do not turn your rehabilitative exercise therapy into a competition with anyone—including yourself. That is the surest, fastest way to injury, pain, and setbacks on the road to recovery.

WARNING: Although many over-the-counter and prescription pain relievers are prescribed for reduction of pain caused by injuries, do not take any pain relievers before exercising as they tend to mask pain, which can cause further injury resulting from overexercising or overusing an injured body area or part. Take the medication as directed, after exercise and when you are more stationary. Awareness of an injury is key to healing it!

HEART AND BLOOD VESSEL DISEASES AND DISORDERS RX

ANEURYSM

A severe blockage and enlargement of an arterial wall or a weakening of the main arteries in the abdomen, chest, and brain. If aneurysms are not surgically repaired, they can rupture and cause death.

Symptoms:
Enlargement is often without symptoms. In some cases, however, there is radiating pain and shortness of breath.

ExRx:
After consulting with your doctor, you may need surgery as well as medication and, afterward, Cardio Rehab exercises. In general, you should slow down your activities and monitor your blood pressure to keep it at a safe and steady level by exercising moderately, eating sensibly, and reducing stress. You can also exercise to lose excess weight, which will also help alleviate the condition.

Aerobic exercise should be done at a slow to moderate pace: do water exercise, stationary cycling, strolling or slow walking, and bowling, instead of jogging, running, or swimming. Your heart rate should not exceed 100 beats per minute. Because regular swimming, jogging, and running cannot be easily practiced at low-intensity levels, they may also cause respiratory stress. Take your own blood pressure regularly and follow your doctor's guidelines. Monitor your circulation by examining your feet and legs for changes in color (e.g. too red or too pale), temperature (e.g. too hot or too cold), or for tingling or numbness. Stop exercise when you experience such severe symptoms as headache, chest or abdominal pain, extreme restlessness or anxiety. If strength-training is possible, practice with light weights that do not not exceed three to four pounds.

ANGINA

An advanced symptom or condition of coronary artery disease (CAD), which indicates high risk of heart attack.

Symptoms:
Feeling reminiscent of severe indigestio squeezing or pressure on chest, induced physical or emotional stress. Episodes of le than five minutes may be accompanied nausea, sweating, and vomiting. Sympton can last ten to twenty seconds and occasio ally up to thirty minutes or more.

ExRx:
See Cardio Rx Exercise Guidelines, p. 42
To reduce symptoms, the need for medic tion, and to slow down the progress of angi incurred from inactivity and weight gai increase the amount of regular aerobic exe cise that you do. Although patients wi unstable angina should avoid exertion, stu ies show that in the cases of stable angin when three or more hours of exercise a done per week, and are combined with a lo fat diet, the progression of coronary arte disease can be slowed down after one year practice. It has also been shown to reduce t frequency and duration of painful and sile ischemic episodes. While there is no ev dence yet on improving the longevity of ang na patients, physical exercise, when do with comprehensive medical care (i.e. drug proper nutrition, and psychological counse ing) does improve cardio circulatory functio for various work tasks, and, in some cases, th pain threshold for patients both before an after bypass surgery. Exercise also decrease your at-rest heart rate, your systolic bloo pressure, and rate pressure, while increasin the overall heart stroke volume, physic work performance, and oxygen pulse.

As with high blood pressure, exercise als has a direct effect on angina. Angina is a sig that not enough blood flow is reaching th heart because of a temporary or parti ɔstruction of the arteries by a buildup of atty deposits or a spasm that restricts blood ow.

Stable angina is chest pain that is pre-ictable in frequency and duration and can be elieved with exercise, rest, and nitroglycerin. is not linked to physical exertion. With egular exercise, stable angina episodes ecome less severe.

Unstable angina, however, is chest pain hat is triggered by even minimal activity and ecomes worse over time. It can be brought n by mild exertion and cannot be easily elped with exercise.

Exercise relieves stable angina by dilating r opening blood vessels, increasing blood flow, nproving your oxygen-from-blood extraction bility, and increasing the heart's pumping abil-y. This last benefit is reflected in a lower heart ate, both resting and during steady exercise, hich means your heart makes less of an effort ɔ circulate blood through your body.

With angina, your chest pain or tightness vill help you regulate your exercise pace and ntensity. You don't necessarily need to stop vith chest pain, but just slow down so that our heart is getting enough blood. The esults can be remarkable. If you have chest ain when your heart rate is 120 beats per ninute, for example, when you walk a twen-y-minute mile, then regular exercise may educe your heart rate to 105 beats per ninute for the same pace—well below the eart rate at which you feel chest pain.

The best exercises for stable angina are ontinuous motion exercises that raise the eart rate into the aerobic-training zone. This should be done gradually, using exercise vith intensity rates that can be easily ncreased or decreased in response to chest ɔain, such as walking, stationary biking, rowing, and skiing on exercise machines. Doctors often recommend taking nitroglycerin before you start exercising to increase blood flow. Also, extra time (ten minutes) should be taken to warm up and cool down your body, so that your blood flow is not increased abruptly, but gradually. Over the long term, angina patients who exercise regularly reduce chest pain episodes and their need for medications.

Angina episodes are more apt to occur with vigorous physical exertion than moderate. At the beginning of your exercise program (the first six weeks), "too vigorous" may be jogging, hill walking, lawn mowing, and such physical labors as snow shoveling, chopping wood, or changing a flat tire. More compatible exercises are strolling and walking on flat ground, nonimpact or slow-motion aerobics, gardening, painting, or window cleaning. These activities can be graded with a specific heart rate or level of blood pressure.

Harsh weather (too cold, windy, hot, humid, or muggy) can also increase the intensity of your exercise routine and can bring you closer to an angina episode. Avoid cold air that may cause a reflex spasm or constriction of coronary arteries. Air that is too hot and humid can cause breathing problems when exercising and should also be avoided. Also, **never exercise after a heavy meal** as this can cause stomach cramping and can make your heart work too hard trying to digest and exercise at the same time.

You should always be prepared to reduce the intensity of any exercise that has caused chest pain and, in turn, spend more time on all nonpainful exercise routines, building up their pace and intensity at the rate of five extra minutes per routine per week.

Arterial Occlusive Disease

The aorta and its major branches are blocked or narrowed.

Symptoms:
High blood pressure; blockage of carotid (neck) artery leads to stroke; blockage of femoral (leg) artery leads to calf pain (intermittent claudication), cool legs, or foot pain. Feet pose serious problems because they are the farthest from the heart and suffer the most from poor circulation.

ExRx:
For mild: Walking exercise and stationary cycling helps slow down onset of symptoms. Stop smoking, keep your blood pressure under control, do raised foot exercises, and practice foot care. For moderate or severe cases, drug therapy, and surgery will probably be necessary.

Atherosclerosis

A disease of the arterial wall in which the inner layer thickens, narrowing the channel, and impairing blood flow. Also known as hardening of the arteries.

Symptoms:
Stems from poor circulation and starts at your extremities, the first symptoms sometimes being cold feet or numb fingers. The disease can then progress through a series of ever-worsening symptoms and disorders, including fatigue, high blood pressure, irregular heartbeat, angina, and, unchecked, eventually leads to heart attack or stroke.

ExRx:
Aerobic and circulatory exercise helps burn off excess fat and keeps it from clinging to arterial walls. It also helps develop the secondary bloc vessel system to improve overall circulation.

Blood Clot in a Vein (Thrombophlebitis)

Phlebitis is an inflammation of a vein that ca lead to the formation of a thrombus (a bloc clot within a blood vessel). The clot may the either block circulation or detach and mov to lodge elsewhere. This can lead to a fat pulmonary embolism. Predisposing risk include prolonged bed rest, trauma, surger childbirth, and use of oral contraceptives.

Symptoms:
Severe localized pain, swelling, and decrease circulation.

ExRx:
Wear nonskid footwear and support stockings; avoid prolonged sitting or standing blood thinners may be prescribed by physician.

Leg exercises, such as walking and wate exercise, can improve circulation and pro mote healing, and can prevent such complications as pain, swelling, and leg ulcers.

Leg raises also help. Elevating your leg helps gravity move excess fluid out to hel promote healing, and also reduces th amount of work your leg muscles have to d to draw down nutrients and oxygen from you respiratory and circulatory systems.

Buerger's Disease (Thromboangiitis Obliterans)

A rare, inflammatory, occlusive disorder causing lesions and blood clots in small- an medium-sized arteries, which reduces bloo flow to the legs and feet. Usually affect

DONALD WHELAN

DIAGNOSIS: ATHEROSCLEROSIS

For Donald Whelan, a seventy-one-year-old former international businessman and manufacturer, atherosclerosis is the family disease. His brother died of a massive heart attack at the young age of forty-seven, and his sister died of heart disease at fifty-one. Both his mother and father also died of atherosclerosis.

Donald began to show signs of the disease in 1990. His doctor gave him a stress test, and the readout indicated an anomaly. An angiogram was performed (a cathode was inserted into his femoral artery and dye was injected into his bloodstream), which revealed narrowing sections in the arteries. However, his doctor felt they were not serious enough to require angioplasty.

Two years later, when Donald was preparing for an archaeological trip to northwestern China, his doctor put him on beta-blockers. Donald went on the drug, went to China for the summer and had no trouble while there. When he came back, further tests were run, and they showed severe blockage. Angioplasty was then performed. Angioplasty has a 60% success rate, and Donald was one of the 60% whose arteries stayed open.

He stayed healthy through 1993 and 1994. Donald kept a daily record of his heart rate, by wearing a heart monitor. An avid hiker, he hiked down a hill on January 6, 1995 and felt a "hot discomfort" in his chest. That day, he ended up in the emergency room, where another angiogram was performed. The doctors found six arteries closed up. Donald had a sextuple bypass. "Because of my conditioning, I was home in four and a half days and released by the surgeon in one month and released by the cardiologist in four months," he explains.

Two months after the massive heart surgery, Donald enrolled in a rehab program and began his workouts. Still on beta-blockers, his workout begins with forty minutes on the treadmill, including a five-minute warm-up period. While on the treadmill, he goes from a 0% grade to between a 15 and 20% grade, advancing one degree per minute until reaching the maximum, then decreasing one degree per minute until he is back down to 0.

Next, he uses the arm-pedaling machine for five minutes, then on to the rowing machine for five minutes at 110 to 120 watts. When he stops rowing, his heart rate drops thirty-two beats in sixty seconds. It's because of his conditioning, Donald says. After the rowing, Donald moves to the wall weight machine, whose pulley weights adjust to work Donald's triceps, biceps, chest, and back muscles. He does six positions at twelve and a half pounds, with thirty reps—three sets of ten—at each position. To end his workout, Donald cycles for fifteen minutes, the last five minutes being a cool-down period. In all, it is an eighty-minute workout, and he does it every Tuesday, Thursday, and Saturday.

On Mondays, Wednesdays, and Fridays, he goes to the Catalina foothills in Arizona for a three and a half mile hike, which gives him an even workout—first going uphill, next hiking on a flat section, and then downhill. Donald averages fourteen and a quarter minutes per mile while hiking.

Jewish men, ages twenty to forty, who smoke heavily. Smoking further constricts blood vessels and slows blood flow.

Symptoms:
Cramp-like pains on instep of foot; at the beginning, the feet are cold, pale, and numb; later the feet are red, hot, and tingling.

ExRx:
Stopping smoking is essential. Avoid such triggers as emotional stress, injuries, and exposure to extreme temperatures. Exercise may aggravate; if so, relieve by rest and leg-elevation gravity exercises (such as prone leg raises) to fill and drain blood vessels. Practice heel-toe rolls for instep pain as well as foot therapy exercises. Proper foot care and well-fitting shoes are also very important.

Bypass Surgery (See Heart Surgery)

Cardiac Tamponade

Blood enters sac around heart, causing pressure on heart muscle. Tamponade may occur in pericarditis; can also be caused by blood and blood clots surrounding the heart after heart surgery.

Symptoms:
Breathlessness, low blood pressure, and distended neck veins.

ExRx:
Requires drainage by needle or surgery. If blood clots are present, an anterior thoracotomy (open-chest surgery) may be performed to remove them. Cardio rehab may be done after surgery.

Cardiomyopathy, Dilated

An enlarged heart, which is the result of extensively damaged heart muscle fibers that cause the heart to contract poorly. Can be caused by alcoholism or a vitamin or mineral deficiency.

Symptoms:
Shortness of breath, fatigue, chest pain, palpitations, edema, and dry cough.

ExRx:
Avoid alcohol and reduce your salt intake. Encourage other family members to learn CPR in case of an emergency. Bed rest, steroids, and an aerobic and circulatory exercise routine tailored to your individual tolerance. As a relaxation technique and to promote greater intake of oxygen, do breathing exercises in the lying down position.

Coronary Artery Disease (CAD)

Loss of oxygen and nutrients to the heart caused by diminished blood flow through the arteries. More common in men than women, CAD is a western hemisphere epidemic. Stress and cigarette smoking aggravate the various types of arteriosclerosis, causing fat and fibrous plaques to narrow the arteries.

Symptoms:
Angina-type chest pain, with a tightness in the chest that radiates to the arm, neck, jaw, and shoulder blades.

ExRx:
Control cholesterol levels with a diet low in cholesterol and saturated fats; if inactive, return to exercise gradually doing noncom-

petitive activities, for example swimming and walking. Slow down any exercise when you feel side stitches or fatigue. Stop exercise when experiencing chest pain, cold sweats, or dizziness. Avoid extreme hot or cold weather, wind, humidity, heavy pollution, and high altitudes. Don't exercise when feverish or when you don't feel well. Your exercise routine should be tailored to the results of your heart tolerance test.

HEART ARRHYTHMIA REACTION

A slower- or faster-than-normal heartbeat, which can occur with anti-arrhythmia drugs, antidepressants, beta-blockers, drugs that lower cholesterol, and during exercise.

Symptoms:
Fatigue, dizziness, fainting, palpitations, and chest pain.

ExRx:
Exercise under doctor's supervision at a low to moderate pace (keep your heart rate between twenty and thirty beats per minute below the heart-training zone.

HEART ATTACK (MYOCARDIAL INFARCTION)

Literally, death of the heart. One of the arteries fails to deliver enough blood to the part of the heart muscle it serves, resulting in reduced blood flow and local tissue destruction. There are more than one million heart attacks every year in the United States, with about one-third of them being fatal. Males are more likely to suffer a heart attack than females, with other predisposed risks being cigarette smoking; aging; high-fat, high-cholesterol, low-fiber diet; stress; obesity; high blood pressure; diabetes; and genetic factors.

Symptoms:
Persistent crushing chest pain that may radiate to the arms, back, or neck and be accompanied by sweating, clamminess, nausea, vomiting, and loss of consciousness.

ExRx:
Post-heart attack: A twelve-week exercise program including walking, biking, swimming, and special Cardio rehab warm-ups. Do not exercise or have sexual intercourse without your doctor's approval, or if you are tired, upset, or if you have either consumed alcohol or a big meal.

The best rehab continuous exercises that put the least strain on the heart are walking, cycling, and water exercise because they can be regulated for a gradual increase of the work load on different muscle groups. They also distribute the work load over the whole body. Allow twelve weeks to build up from a fifteen-minute to a forty-five-minute exercise period. Practice extended warm-up and cool-down periods of five to ten minutes each. Avoid strengthening exercises during the recovery period, concentrating instead on stretching before and after continuous exercises. Use ROM exercises as an unstressful way to warm up individual body areas. Use a slow walk or step-in-place as your total body warm-up. A slow walking pace is forty to sixty steps per minute (spm), moderate is sixty to ninety (spm), and brisk is ninety or more (spm).

HEART FAILURE

The heart is unable to pump a sufficient amount of blood to the lungs and the rest of the body at the necessary rate. There are two types: left-sided failure (caused by high blood pressure, hyperthyroidism, heart valve defects, and anemia) or right-sided failure (almost always caused by hypertension, but also can be the result of a heart valve defect). Can also be caused by a severe heart attack.

Symptoms:
Left-sided heart failure affects the respiratory system with shortness of breath caused by fluid buildup in the lungs, also night sweats accompanied by an attack of breathlessness. Right-sided heart failure has more symptoms throughout the body, with swelling of limbs and extremities (especially legs and ankles), enlargement of the liver, and indigestion-like symptoms.

ExRx:
Rehabilitate with medication, rest, and slow walking. Depending on amount of heart muscle damage, aerobic exercise may be tolerated by only a few heart failure patients, with most only being able to do slow-paced circulatory exercises.

HEART SURGERY

Any surgical procedure or operation performed on the heart. One of the most complicated heart surgeries is the triple (or more) bypass; one of the less complicated is a heart valve replacement. Coronary bypass surgery is also one of the most common heart surgeries and is sometimes used for the treatment of severe angina. In this operation, a long vein is taken from the leg and sewn into the aorta or diseased vessel below the blockage, thus bypassing the trouble spot. Another very complicated operation is a heart transplant in which a diseased heart is replaced with a healthy heart.

Symptoms:
After surgery, and depending on the amount of disease and the type of heart surgery, there will be varying degrees of healing-type pain, with soreness surrounding the surgical incision.

ExRx:
At the hospital, within two days after most heart surgeries (check with your doctor and surgeon), you can do simple ROM exercises in bed. During the next two days, do seated ROM exercises. For the next eight days, take short walks of up to ten minutes a day. If necessary, walk with shuffle steps. Rest after ten minutes. Another ten minutes can then be spent on the stationary cycle or walking some more.

At home, continue the ten-minute walk and/or stationary cycle regimen for at least three to four weeks. On long car trips, stop every hour to walk and stretch for one to ten minutes. For the first six weeks, you shouldn't push or pull anything heavier than five pounds to allow your breast bone incision to heal. Return to work or normal activities on a half-day basis, gradually building up to full days.

HEART VALVE DISEASE

Mechanical disruption of blood flow by valve narrowing, incomplete closure, or position slippage. Can lead to heart failure and chronic problems requiring surgery.

Symptoms:
Shortness of breath, fatigue, and heartbeat irregularities.

ExRx:
Low-impact, moderate-intensity aerobic exercise; avoid isometric exercise, especially for leaking valves. After surgery, use Cardio Rehab, p. 421.

HIGH BLOOD PRESSURE (HYPERTENSION)

Blood exerts too much pressure against artery walls. Affects 15 to 20% of North American adults. Can cause stroke, heart disease, and kidney failure.

Symptoms:
None until severe, then headache. The first stage of symptoms of the illness are not really physical symptoms that you can feel, but higher than normal blood pressure caused by the blood putting too much pressure on your artery walls. Left unchecked, these artery or tube linings become "frayed" and begin to accumulate plaque fats that can reduce or block the passage of blood through the arteries. Eventually, these blockages can cut off oxygen and nutrients to the heart muscle and the brain, resulting in one of two of the three major killers: heart attack or stroke.

ExRx:
To prevent, exercise regularly and eat a low-fat, low-sodium diet. Studies show a direct relationship between regular exercise and lower blood pressure (see Chapter Eleven). After the disease has set in, exercise has a positive suppressive effect on elevated blood pressure while you move or exercise. This effect is especially beneficial for reducing mild hypertension. It may also help to reduce the dosage needed of antihypertensive drugs. Some drugs such as beta-blockers may reduce your exercise performance and impair the conditioning response. In addition to a regular exercise program, continuous motion exercises that are effective include walking, rhythmic ROMs, stationary cycling, swimming, and extra-long warm-ups and cool-downs. Practice Cardio Rehab exercises at a level determined by the stages or severity of your hypertension.

HYPERTROPHIC CARDIOMYOPATHY

A thickening of the heart walls (muscle).

Symptoms:
Reduced blood circulation, fatigue, fainting, and dizziness.

ExRx:
A slowed down exercise program (see Slow-Motion Exercise, p. 423), especially when mixing with drug therapy.

INFLAMMATION OF THE HEART MUSCLE

Can be acute or chronic and can occur at any age. It is caused by viral, bacterial, or parasitic infections as well as immune reactions.

Symptoms:
Fatigue, shortness of breath, and heart palpitations.

ExRx:
Manage symptoms with massage, stretching, anti-inflammatory agents (e.g. aspirin). The limits on your activity are not permanent; engage in recreational activities that are not physically demanding until you regain strength and capacity for more intense exercise.

INFLAMMATORY HEART DISEASE (PERICARDITIS)

Inflammation of the sac around the heart. May be caused by infection, cancers of the chest area, high dose radiation to chest, autoimmune chest diseases, or arthritis.

Symptoms:
Malaise, fatigue, joint pain, sharp sternum (chest bone) pain that radiates to neck, shoulder, back, and arms.

MONELLE LUMSDEN

DIAGNOSIS: HOLE IN THE HEART; OPEN HEART SURGERY

Monelle Lumsden, a performer and exercise instructor who teaches five aerobic dance classes per day and helps her clients weight train, was born with a hole in her heart. Monelle says she had been an exercise enthusiast all her life and had been teaching exercise classes for ten years before this serious problem was even noticed by doctors. She was forty-one when it first became noticable.

December of 1993 was a particularly stressful time for Monelle. Not only was she carrying her full load of classes, she was also doing fashion shows. It was during that hectic month that Monelle noticed her heart skipping beats and alternating between a slow and a fast rhythm. Additionally, Monelle, who describes herself as being "energetic from morning to night" began feeling tired and dragging by five or six p.m.

As these symptoms persisted, Monelle went to see her doctor in February. Her doctor performed an echocardiography (an ultrasound technique to form images of the heart to aid in diagnosis) and found that Monelle's heart was enlarged, stressed, and had a hole in it that measured over one inch. Monelle would have to have open heart surgery to repair the hole before the end of the year.

Although the hole had always been present in Monelle's heart, prior to that December, she had exhibited few of the symptoms, such as low blood pressure, fatigue, and the most common symptom, shortness of breath, so it is no surprise that doctors had misdiagnosed her as having a minor heart murmur (occasional extra beats), which is a common problem and really nothing to worry about. Often during her childhood, however, minor colds would deteriorate into bronchitis, which, at the time of the echocardiography, was discovered to be the result of added stress on her lungs caused by a misdirected vein (caused by the hole in her heart) that was spilling blood into her lungs.

Monelle had open heart surgery to fix the hole and to redirect the misdirected vein. The vein repair ended up taking longer than expected, and, as is always possible during open heart surgery, Monelle had a stroke. She, the energetic aerobics instructor, woke up to find her whole left side paralyzed. Her doctors said that it would be at least a year before she was able to move it at all.

But Monelle would not have it that way. She was determined to not only walk again, but to return to teaching aerobics and exercise as soon as possible.

Monelle began physical therapy two days after her surgery. At first, the therapy consisted mostly of deep body massage, stretching, and shiatsu (accupressure) to stimulate blood flow. As some strength returned to her muscles, Monelle did resistance exercises with her therapist in which the therapist would slowly direct Monelle's arms or legs while Monelle resisted the motion. From this, she progressed to slowly moving her limbs on her own, then with bungee cords for tension, and finally, with weights.

In addition to the paralysis from the stroke, Monelle woke up with a frozen shoulder, which is paralysis of the shoulder resulting from nerve and bone damage caused by the splitting open of the rib cage for open heart surgery. To correct this, she constantly did the resistance exercises on her pectorals, deltoids, and trapezius muscles. Getting her elbows to touch in front of her with her arms bent was the hardest part, but she was determined to be able to move her arms without pain.

Monelle was able to walk with the aid of a walker within eight days following her surgery. She went home—not to a rehabilitation center—after eighteen days without having taken any medication aside from what she was given immediately following the surgery. Her physical therapist visited her at home twice a week.

Toward the latter part of September, however, the swelling of her left leg, which the doctors at the hospital had attributed to postsurgery water retention, had not gone down despite the diuretics she had been prescribed. She went to her own doctor, and an x-ray revealed that she had another common complication of open heart surgery—pericarditis, or, the filling of the pericardium (the sac that surrounds the heart) with fluid. The two and a half additional weeks that Monelle had to spend in the hospital not only slowed down her recovery, she was also unable to continue her rehabilitation exercises because any strain on the heart would put her in jeopardy of further surgery.

Fortunately, the fluid was removed without further complications, and Monelle returned home in mid-October and resumed her physical therapy. By November, she was able to walk with a cane, but her goal was to be able to walk without any aid in time for the holidays. She did her Christmas shopping with the cane, but would walk around the house without it.

By mid-December Monelle had achieved her goal of walking without the aid of a cane and decided it was time to start doing step aerobics again. Her doctor recommended that she do ten minutes of step, rest for five minutes, and then ten more minutes of step. At that pace, which she maintained for two weeks, Monelle's heart rate was about 120 beats per minute when she exercised.

At the end of two weeks, Monelle added five minutes to the second half of the exercise routine, so that she was stepping for ten minutes, resting for five, then stepping for fifteen more. While stepping, her heart rate hovered around 130 beats per minute. Finally, after two weeks at that pace, Monelle was able to step for twenty minutes straight and maintain her heart rate above 140 beats per minute—within the aerobic range.

By then it was mid-January, five months after Monelle's initial surgery. On January 15, her birthday, Monelle met with a client and worked out, though not aerobically. One month later, on February 15, Monelle led two step aerobics classes. By April, she was up to full steam—four classes per day.

When jokingly asked if she thought that the hole in her heart would possibly have been diagnosed sooner had she not been in such good shape all along, Monelle readily answers in the affirmative, but also adds that in such a situation, the recovery would not have been so easy and complete . . . if she would have even made it to surgery.

Along with exercise, however, Monelle's will, her determination to work her way back to full physical health (which was undoubtedly strengthened by her exercise regimen), played a major role in her recovery. "You've got to get your head in gear, then get your body in gear," Monelle advises anybody recovering from a physical calamity. "The earlier you start, the harder you work, the better."

ExRx:
First, treat the underlying disease. Manage the symptoms with massage, stretching, and anti-inflammatory agents (e.g. aspirin). After antibiotic treatment, use slow to moderate walking or stationary cycling exercise to regain strength.

Intermittent Claudication

Claudication is a cramp-like pain in one or both legs, which develops while walking and is caused by a blockage (arteriosclerosis) of the arteries that are supplying blood and oxygen to the legs. Affects 3% of the population. A symptom of peripheral vascular disease.

Symptoms:
Calf pain during walking and other leg activities.

ExRx:
First, if you smoke cigarettes, you must stop. Then practice a regular exercise routine. Exercise therapy is superior to drug therapy because it has fewer side effects. In the early stages, regular walking is the best exercise. Later, other circulatory exercises (e.g. dancing, jogging) can be practiced when the walking regimen is well established. Use a therapeutic or intermittent walking program (i.e. walk until calf pain sets in, rest, and then start walking again when the pain subsides). This will gradually increase the walking distance before the calf pain occurs and you have to rest.

Myocardial Infarction (See Heart Attack)

Peripheral Vascular Disease (PVD)

Although not as severe a health threat as coronary artery disease (CAD), 50% of PVD patients also have CAD. Cigarette smoking is a big factor in contracting PVD. The nicotine in cigarettes acts as a potent vasoconstrictor. One cigarette can reduce blood circulation to your feet, toes, and fingers by as much as 40%.

Symptoms:
Leg pain and cramping; cold extremities and bluish color.

ExRx:
Walking to the point of pain or nonweight-bearing exercise. Consult with your doctor before beginning a regular exercise program.

CARDIO RX: LIST OF ADDITIONAL HEART AND BLOOD VESSEL DISORDERS BENEFITED BY CONTROLLED BREATHING EXERCISES

- aortic aneurysms of the abdomen
- ischemia
- leukemia, acute
- leukemia, chronic lymphocytic

Postural Hypotension

This low blood pressure problem is sometimes the result of either antidepressants or antihypertensive medicines causing the blood to pool in the lower extremities. Can also be caused by diabetes, or a sudden, severe injury, which results in shock.

Symptoms:
Dizziness, faintness, and risk of falling when rising from a lying or sitting position.

ExRx:
Avoid staying in a prone position too long, it can aggravate dizziness. Keep your head and feet elevated when lying down. Before rising, stimulate blood flow to your heart by practicing heel-toe rolls, flexing your ankles and feet to shins five to twelve times. Practice isometric exercises for lower arms and legs to stimulate blood flow back to your heart, for example, tense and relax your arm muscles by making a fist, then tense and relax your abdomen and buttocks muscles. (See isometric exercises, pp. 299 and 348.)

RAYNAUD'S DISEASE

About half a million people, mostly women between the ages of fifteen and forty-five, experience Raynaud's, a form of vein constriction wherein the hands, fingers (especially), toes, and feet, when exposed to cold air or even touching something frozen, have an exaggerated cold response. Leads to skin damage. When the symptoms happen with no underlying cause, it is called Raynaud's disease; if there is an underlying disorder or cause, it is referred to as Raynaud's phenomenon.

Symptoms:
Numbness and tingling in fingers and toes, which first turn white from loss of blood circulation, then blue as oxygenated blood returns, and finally red as vessels dilate and blood surges back into the fingers and toes. This response to cold can also cause pain and numbness as blood vessels essentially go into spasm and constrict excessively to restore circulation.

ExRx:
Practice heel-toe rolls (p. 177), hand exercises (pp. 233–236), warm water exercises, and circulatory exercises. Avoid activities that put pressure or cold on the fingers (e.g. typing, weeding, snow skiing, water sports, and swimming in cold water). Wear warm clothes and gloves, don't smoke cigarettes, and get plenty of rest. Circulatory exercise increases the blood flow to your extremities thus relieving the pain and numbness while conditioning your veins to accept a greater flow of blood even while you are at rest.

VARICOSE VEINS

Overfilled, distended, and twisted blood vessels. Mostly found in the legs and calves; affects more women than men.

Symptoms:
Bulging veins in the leg; sometimes no pain or discomfort; in others, severe aches in the affected areas, swelling of the feet and ankles, and itching. In women, symptoms can be worse just before menstruation.

ExRx:
Leg-based exercises (especially if the varicosity is in calf muscle), such as walking. Stronger leg muscles help to push blood back up to the heart and a stronger heart muscle increases speed of blood flow. Exercise therapy slows down progress of this condition. In severe cases, surgery may be needed; after surgery, exercise helps prevent the condition from recurring. Practice heel-toe rolls, p. 177; wear support stockings.

LUNGS AND BREATHING DISEASES AND DISORDERS RX

Smoking is the leading cause of lung cancer and, ultimately, severe lung damage. It also causes bronchitis and emphysema, aggravates asthma and allergies and complicates menopause and arterial disease. In the early stages of smoking, aerobic exercise can offer a substitute for the nicotine stimulation provided by smoking. In many cases, smokers who take up exercise find it easier to quit smoking later on. The longer you smoke, the more addictive the habit becomes, and requires psychological therapy, as well as cardio exercise therapy.

Quitting smoking has both physiological and psychological implications. Exercise provides a healthy substitute for the stimulating effects of smoking by bringing more oxygen to the brain, making you more alert and focused, while providing a diversion or break from concentrated activity.

Smoking produces vascular spasms which impede blood circulation. A single cigarette can reduce circulation up to 40% in the fingers, feet, and toes. Quitting smoking reduces the need for surgery in 90% of the circulatory diseases.

Adult Respiratory Distress Syndrome (ARDS)

Fluid builds up in lungs; can result from a massive sympathetic discharge caused by a brain injury, hypoxia, or from an increase in capillary permeability. Can be fatal, but patients can make a full recovery with treatment.

Symptoms:
Lungs stiffen, shallow breathing, and shortness of breath.

ExRx:
At first, medical attention and use of a mechanical ventilator. With a doctor's okay, practice breathing exercises and begin Cardio Rx Rehab to gain physical conditioning, page 421.

Allergies (Airborne)

Airborne allergies are reactions to irritants (e.g. pollen, mites, dust, mold, cigarette smoke, animal fur) that produce nasal congestion and eye inflammation. Some are seasonal, for example, hay fever; others are year-round, for example, dust, mites, and animal fur. Approximately twenty million sufferers in the United States.

Symptoms:
Sneezing, runny nose, nasal congestion, itchy red eyes, sore throat, headache, and hives. Also "allergic shiners" (dark circles under the eyes).

ExRx:
Long-term drug therapy. Allergy sufferers should conserve their energy, and do relaxation techniques, and slow to moderate activities. Don't exercise heavily during an allergic reaction. Physical activity can clear sinuses during allergy attack, but the effects are temporary.

Avoid or eliminate sources of the allergens through air filters, air conditioning, and frequent vacuuming. Exercise indoors in a clean environment (e.g. health club) during the allergy season. Aerobic exercise and indoor exercise clears nasal congestion, coughing, and other symptoms temporarily. Exercise also can clear passages for better breathing during exercise, so don't avoid exercise because of symptoms. For some, exercise may induce asthma symptoms, which requires pre-exercise prophylactic use of a bronchiodilating inhaler.

Vigorous exercise can be an effective way to control nasal congestion because the increase in blood flow to the nasal area gets water circulating through the nasal mucus. You will probably feel relief five minutes into the exercise period, and that relief will last for a half hour or more after exercising. The following is a list of tips for exercising with allergies:

- Bring your handkerchief or tissues, because you'll want to blow your nose so that breathing will be more comfortable
- Avoid exercising in air that contains such irritants as smog, pollen (counts are lowest between two and five p.m.), and humidity
- Breathe through your mouth until your nasal passages are clear
- Use your antihistamine before you begin exercising to clear your air passages
- Exercise in a dehumidified air environment, unless you are allergic to air-conditioned or overheated air
- When exercising outdoors, wear a scarf or mask on your face to filter the air or warm up cold air before it enters your lungs
- If either cold or hot air gives you an allergic reaction, then breathe through your nose (it's a built-in dehumidifier)
- If exercising gives you an allergic reaction (i.e. exercise-induced anaphylaxis), you may need to exercise with a friend and also inject yourself with adrenaline from a carry-along kit; in this case, do slow to moderate exercise
- Don't eat for at least four hours before exercising to avoid food triggering the attack

If you are in rehab, you may have to gradually build up your breathing capacity. If you continue to experience nasal blockage, you may have to work around the mucus buildup.

Asbestosis

Chronic lung disease caused by inhaling asbestos fibers, which then fill and inflame the lungs. This is probably the most pervasive work-related disease.

Symptoms:
Shortness of breath with exertion or rest, rapid breathing, dry cough, and finally respiratory failure.

ExRx:
Cannot be cured, but you can relieve respiratory symptoms with breathing exercises, conservation of energy, and relaxation techniques (see Cardio Rx Exercise Guidelines, p. 421.)

Asthma

Asthma is an immune disorder which strikes the lungs. Breathing passages become inflamed, narrowed, or blocked, and then overreact to various stimulants from within or outside the body. This causes wheezing, coughing, chest tightness, and even life-threatening respiratory failure. Half of all sufferers are under age ten; affects twice as many boys as girls. Asthma is actually a severe type of allergy, and untreated allergies can progress to asthma.

Symptoms:
Shortness of breath, wheezing, coughing attacks, and chest tightness. A severe attack may not respond to drugs, and in this case the patient should seek medical attention immediately.

MARY PIERCE

DIAGNOSIS: LUNG TRANSPLANT; ALPHA-1 DEFICIENCY

Mary Pierce had an onset of asthma at thirty, when she began having trouble breathing. Breathing became so difficult that she had to quit skiing and playing tennis. Mary also quit smoking cigarettes, thinking that would cure her troubles. When smoking cessation had no effect, Mary went to the doctor. At that point, she had only 17% of her lung capacity left and had dropped fifty pounds, down to a malnourished ninety-nine pounds.

On her fortieth birthday, she was diagnosed with an inherited, chronic, and usually fatal disease—Alpha-1 deficiency (A-1). Mary's doctor told her that her only option was a lung transplant, but she didn't want to take such a drastic step before exploring other options. Her dropping weight was her immediate concern. She began to do research and found that 50% of lung patients lose weight from protein malnutrition—their bodies use up all their nutrients just trying to breathe. Eating, especially protein, is hard on their bodies because they have a difficult time metabolizing what is eaten.

Mary read books on vitamins and began to eat "tons" of them. She also ate several small, high-fat meals a day. The Omega-3 and Omega-6 oils in fat reduced her lung inflammation, as did the Alpha-1 enzyme, which she lacked. Mary took nightly IVs of a high-fat diet while still eating as much as usual during the day. Even when she finally hit 120 pounds, she was burning 2,400 calories just by sitting quietly—that's over 1,000 times more than a normal person would.

Finally, her regimen worked and Mary achieved a close to normal weight. "I had stopped the disintegration," she explains. She was achieving her goal of staying alive as long as she could until she had to have the transplant operation—and until they found a donor for her.

Happy with her progress, Mary bought a bicycle and began biking twenty minutes a day, but her lungs impeded her workout somewhat. As soon as her heart rate hit about 110 bpm, she had to stop.

One night in 1993, Mary had a dream about her long-dead mother. Mary had almost forgotten what her mother's face looked like, it had been so long. In the dream, her mother hugged her, then pushed her away "as if I had something to do." The next day Mary received

ExRx:
Practice relaxation techniques, pursed lip breathing, and coughing exercise techniques to clear passageways of mucus. Because similar exercise prescriptions apply to both asthma and allergies, also see allergies, p. 410.

Asthma sufferers live with the recurring fear of having attacks of severe breathlessness. This may make them shy away from exercise out of fear of having chest tightness and a wheezing attack right in the middle of exercising. But a regular aerobic exercise program a call from the University of Michigan. They told her that they had a pair of lungs for her. She had the operation on April 3, 1993.

The day after the transplant, she took her first deep breath in fifteen years and started to cry. She thought, "My life is fulfilled." Mary began biking and walking every day, because she no longer had restraints on her lung capacity. "I couldn't even sit down. I wanted to be in motion," she says. Mary wanted to try everything she couldn't do before. She went to a gym and took water aerobics and step aerobics classes. She also began lifting weights.

Mary says she wishes she had been lifting weights all along. Those with A-1 have a hard time with aerobics because the lungs give out. But many lung patients are given Prednisone, the main side effect of which is osteoporosis. Resistance training not only preserves bones, but actually increases the bone mass and density.

A year after her transplant, Mary heard about the US Transplant Games, sponsored by the National Kidney Foundation. The games are done in Olympic style, and when Mary heard about them, she thought to herself, "I can ride a bike."

Mary began training, riding thirty to forty miles per day, and won two bronze medals at the games in Atlanta. Her next goal was to go to the World Games. She started training but had a hard time raising the money to go. The Alpha-1 Foundation told her to keep training and not to worry about the money: They would raise it. And they did. Because the Foundation had believed in her and funded her, Mary had extra reason to bring home a medal, and she did—this time it was gold. She also took sixth in the race-walk event.

Mary became increasingly interested in promoting Alpha-1 deficiency awareness. A-1 is as common as cystic fibrosis, but is usually misdiagnosed as asthma, bronchitis, or emphysema until it is too late to do anything about it. Now Mary works with Team Alpha-1, which travels the country organizing Alpha-1 and transplant patients to go out for bike rides. The Alpha-1 patients often ride with oxygen on their backs. The events raise money for the Alpha-1 Foundation and also raise public awareness of the often fatal disease, which usually affects the lungs, kidneys, or both. Team Alpha-1's regular program starts in June all over the country.

Mary has added racquetball to her sports competition list and has climbed Mt. Rainier. She is presently organizing a climb of Alaska's Mt. McKinley.

actually helps control the symptoms of asthma by strengthening the lungs and giving the asthmatic person control over breathing. Along with medication and monitoring, exercise actually opens the chest and eases breathing.

Choose one or more of the following three aerobic or respiratory-conditioning exercises. Each has special advantages:

1. Indoor swimming offers an environment of warm, humid air, which is not as great a trigger as many other environments.

2. Mall-walking offers graded walkways for easy warm-ups and cool, pollen-free air.
3. Intermittent activity. Start-and-stop exercises and sports may induce fewer symptoms than such high-intensity continuous exercises as jogging and rowing.

The following is a list of exercise tips for asthma sufferers:

- Premedicate before exercise, for example, to reduce airway sensitivity, take two puffs of an inhaled bronchodilator with cromolyn sodium
- Carry your dilator with you to ward off attacks
- Practice slow belly-breathing exercises; shallow, rapid breathing acts as a stimulant for an attack; deep breathing strengthens your diaphragm muscles
- If or when vigorous exercise is not possible, start with relaxation exercises, for example breathing during stretching, which enables you to breathe easier by first releasing muscle tension

Black Lung (Miner's Asthma)

Progressive lung disease caused by prolonged inhalation of coal dust particles, which causes fibrous tissue to form that damages lungs and impedes breathing. There are two types: simple black lung and complicated black lung.

Symptoms:
In simple black lung there are no symptoms, especially in nonsmokers. With complicated black lung there is shortness of breath, cough, and phlegm, in addition to complications, which include pulmonary hypertension, enlarged heart, and emphysema.

ExRx:
Prevent further physical deterioration by staying moderately active, pacing yourself, and practicing relaxation techniques. Serious cases require chest physical therapy including coughing techniques and increased fluid intake. See Cardio Rx Exercise Guidelines (p. 421) and relaxation techniques (pp. 244–248).

Chronic Bronchitis and Emphysema

Chronically blocked breathing passages, which affects 1.7 million Americans. Predisposed risks include smoking cigarettes, air pollution, allergies, and respiratory infections.

Symptoms:
Coughing, difficulty breathing with minimal exertion.

ExRx:
Quit smoking cigarettes; smoking cessation may reverse this condition. Treat with controlled coughing exercise or exercise in cool, purified air. Avoid overexerting yourself by scheduling rest periods and distributing active periods throughout the day.

Similar to asthma, chronic bronchitis and emphysema can cause severe breathing disabilities and destruction of lung tissues. These diseases cause increased mucus production that blocks air passages and impedes the function of cells that digest disease-causing organisms. This causes inflammation, destroys air sacs in the lungs, and leads to abnormal fibrous tissue growth in the bronchial tree.

Early intervention can stop and even reverse this process.

Chronic Obstructive Pulmonary Disease

Collectively, asthma, emphysema, and chronic bronchitis are three chronic lung diseases that affect over seventeen million Americans. They are more common in men than women, probably because until recently men were heavier smokers and also took more jobs in those industries (i.e. mining, steel production, and so forth) that exposed them to air pollution and lung carcinogens.

Symptoms:
See asthma; also chronic bronchitis and emphysema.

ExRx:
These severe forms of breathing disorders require you to more frequently practice coughing and breathing exercises to conserve your energy and clear your breathing passages. Keeping your lungs free of mucus will prevent infection or further deterioration of your condition, allowing you to physically condition your body, and improving your breathing capacity for greater amounts of physical exertion.

Common Cold

Acute viral infection. Children usually get more colds than adults. Predominant during colder months, and the rainy season in the tropics.

Symptoms:
Nasal congestion, headaches, and achy joints.

ExRx:
Rest, relaxation, and increase your fluid intake. Any form of moderate-intensity exercise will stimulate blood to travel to the nasal and sinus area. (However, because this is an infection of the respiratory system, it is probably best to avoid swimming and other water exercise or sports until the infection has passed.) This fresh flow washes away stagnant mucus and bacteria and helps clear nasal passages to reduce swelling, pressure, and pain. This works for a number of disorders involving nasal congestion, such as allergies and asthma, as well as sinusitis, colds, and the flu. Exercise also stimulates air flow through the nose, throat, and lungs, which causes these muscles to contract and expand. This muscle action also moves mucus and other waste products out.

Cor Pulmonale

A chronic heart condition involving the enlargement of the right side of the heart as a result of chronic lung disease. Lung disease and damage causes resistance to blood flow through the branches of the pulmonary artery, which, in turn, causes increased pressure in the pulmonary artery (pulmonary hypertension). The strain placed on the heart may eventually cause right-sided heart failure. Of patients who have cor pulmonale, 85% also have chronic pulmonary disease; 25% of these eventually die. Affects more middle-aged men than women.

Symptoms:
Chronic cough, shortness of breath on exertion, wheezing, fatigue, weakness, drowsiness, and alterations of consciousness.

ExRx:
Rest often, and practice breathing exercises as prescribed by a doctor.

Cystic Fibrosis (CF)

An inherited, genetic, chronic lung disease; the glands that line the bronchial tubes produce an excessive amount of thick mucus causing recurrent lung infections. There is also failure to produce certain enzymes that break down fats and help to absorb their nutrients into the body. Because of this, CF is also associated with malnutrition. Usually diagnosed during early childhood; it affects both sexes equally, and incidence is high in persons of northern European ancestry. Causes sterility in males, but not in females.

Symptoms:
Wheezy respirations, stunted growth, salty sweat, dry cough, shortness of breath, chronic lung infections, abnormally fast breathing, and inability to gain weight. Eventually these problems can lead to a collapsed lung and emphysema, a condition in which lungs overinflate and lose their elasticity.

ExRx:
The goal of treatment is to help the child lead a normal life as long as possible. Physical therapy includes chest, aerosol therapy with postural drainage (special positioning of the body), and breathing exercises several times a day to help remove mucus and lung excretions. Studies have shown exercise reduces the abnormally high nasal mucus in resting CF patients and helps improve lung function in males.

Emphysema (see Chronic Bronchitis and Emphysema)

Flu (Influenza)

Acute viral infection of the respiratory tract, which is very dangerous to the elderly.

Symptoms:
Symptoms usually last for twenty-four to forty-eight hours and usually include a nonproductive cough, fever, and fatigue; there is usually a three- to five-day recovery period.

ExRx:
Bed rest, walk around room, and practice rehab reconditioning exercises. Light to moderate regular exercise seems to make the body more resistant to bacterial and viral infections. Strenuous exercise is not likely to have this effect because heavy breathing, especially in confined spaces, can increase your infection risk. If you already have a cold or flu, you should not exercise, but instead recover first, and begin your exercise routine when you start to feel better. Exercise at a low-intensity level at first, taking time to rest and clear your nasal passages.

Legionnaires' Disease

A bacterial infection, which is an acute form of pneumonia. Affects more men than women, from middle-aged to elderly. Smokers are three to four times more likely to contract this disease.

Symptoms:
Bloody cough, shortness of breath, accompanied by widespread muscle pain and weakness.

ExRx:
Treatment includes coughing and deep breathing exercises. Long bed rest also requires Cardio Rx Rehab (also see pneumonia, p. 417).

Lung Cancer

One of the most prevalent forms of cancer in the United States. Mainly caused by cigarette smoking. Some survive five years, but prognosis is generally poor. It is the most common cause of cancer death in men and the second most common cause (after breast cancer) in women. Largely preventable, 80% are smokers over age forty. Cigarette smoking risks include: the number of cigarettes smoked per day, how early in life the patient started smoking, the nicotine content in the cigarettes that were smoked, and the depth of inhalation. Other risks include family history of lung cancer and working with asbestos or other carcinogens.

Symptoms:
None at beginning, but later a smoker's cough, accompanied by shoulder pain.

ExRx:
Quit smoking cigarettes to prevent or when diagnosed. After surgery, chemotherapy, or radiation, practice ROMs to prevent stiffness. Begin Lung Rx Rehab and Cardio Rx Rehab, see Cardio Rx Exercise Guidelines, p. 421.

Pleural Effusion

An accumulation of fluid between the pleural layers, which lie between the lung tissues and membranous sac (pleura) that protects it.

Symptoms:
Shortness of breath and chest pain.

ExRx:
Fluid removal with needle or a tube promotes deep breathing. Practice controlled breathing exercises, relaxation techniques, and gentle stretching.

Pneumonia

Acute lung infection, which is the sixth leading cause of death in the United States. Persons with normal lungs and an adequate immune system can fully recover. Death from pneumonia is common because it is often a complication of many other serious diseases or injuries.

Symptoms:
Coughing, chest pain, fever, shaking, chills, and respiratory failure.

ExRx:
Often requires extensive bed rest; stretching and strengthening can begin in bed in either the prone or seated position. Post-bed rehab, Cardio Rx (p. 421).

Pneumothorax (Collapsed Lung)

An accumulation of air in the pleura—membranes that enclose the lungs. Occurs in otherwise healthy adults (mostly men) in the twenty- to forty-year-old range.

Symptoms:
Sudden sharp chest pain and shortness of breath.

ExRx:
A small pneumothorax in an adult does not usually require treatment; a larger pneumothorax can call for the removal of air with a needle or suction tube. After surgery or treatment—bed rest with careful monitoring of vital signs, blood pressure, pulse rate, respiration. Begin Cardio Rehab (p. 421) after the condition is stabilized and with a doctor's approval.

Pulmonary Edema

Abnormal accumulation of fluid in veins and capillaries in lungs; can be local (following an injury) or general (in heart failure).

Symptoms:
Shortness or exertion of breath, coughing, attacks of respiratory distress; breathing is easier when upright.

ExRx:
Do relaxation techniques (see pp. 244–248). Practice breathing and coughing exercises while sitting up.

PULMONARY EMBOLISM AND INFARCTION

An embolism is a blockage of an artery by a blood clot, air bubble, a piece of tissue, and so forth, which is in the bloodstream. Infarction is the death of an area of tissue caused by lack of blood supply. There are six million cases of pulmonary embolism per year, causing 100,000 deaths. Predisposing risks include a long-term bed rest, emphysema or chronic bronchitis, congestive heart failure, vein inflammation, varicose veins, pregnancy, obesity, cancer, and taking oral contraceptives.

Symptoms:
Labored breathing, accompanied by chest pain.

ExRx:
Ten to fourteen days of treatment, surgery, and use of antiembolism stockings. Rehab with Cardio Rx, p. 421.

RESPIRATORY ACIDOSIS

Sudden failure in ventilation reduces carbon dioxide removal from the lungs, which causes increased blood acidity. Predisposing risks include bronchitis, asthma, prescription or illicit drug desensitization of respiratory center, central nervous system trauma, neuromuscular disease, or airway obstruction.

Symptoms:
Headache, weak muscles, and sometimes coma.

ExRx:
First, treat the cause because the prognosis depends on severity of the underlying condition. Severe cases may require both Nervous System Rehab (see Chapter Seventeen) and Cardio Rehab (p. 421).

SARCOIDOSIS

A rare, multisystem, granulomatous disorder that produces swelling of lymph nodes, lung problems, and skeletal, liver, eye, and skin lesions. Onset usually occurs between ages twenty and forty, strikes women twice as much as men. Blacks also have a genetic predisposition. There are two types: acute and chronic.

Symptoms:
For acute type: painful joints and muscles, lymph node enlargement, muscle weakness, breathlessness, cough, skin eruptions, and fatigue. For chronic type: fever, painful joints and muscles, numbness, painful bloodshot eyes, and a facial rash.

ExRx:
Acute type resolves within two years; chronic is a lifelong illness. Exercise is used along with medication and diet to help treat symptoms. Also avoid direct sunlight. May require Cardio Rehab (p. 421); also see Chapter Fourteen, MuSkel Rx, and Chapter 13, Age Rx.

SILICOSIS

Most common fibrotic lung disease (i.e. lung disease caused by the inhalation of air containing silica dust), has a high incidence of emphysema and tuberculosis as a result. Affects many sandblasters, tunnel workers, and ceramic workers. Prognosis is good, unless disease progresses into fibrotic form, including pulmonary hypertension or tuberculosis. Acute form develops after one to three years of exposure to silica, which accelerates after ten years.

Symptoms:
None or shortness of breath with dry cough, which progressively worsens.

ExRx:
Relieve respiratory symptoms through steam inhalation and chest therapy. Increase your exercise stamina with regular activity such as walking.

TUBERCULOSIS (TB)

A bacterial infection, which causes granulated tissue in the lungs with a consistency similar to crumbly cheese. Predisposed risks include crowded living, silicosis, alcoholism, compromised immune systems, diabetes, aging, and close contact with someone who has TB. Correct drug treatment provides excellent prognosis.

Symptoms:
None in some cases; in others, chest pain, mucus cough (sometimes with blood), weight loss, and fatigue.

ExRx:
Drug therapy, then Lung Rx Rehab, p. 423.

CARDIO RX: LIST OF ADDITIONAL LUNG INJURIES AND BREATHING DISORDERS THAT ARE BENEFITED OR REHABILITATED BY EXERCISE

- blunt chest injury
- bronchietasis
- nasal congestion
- near drowning
- pleurisy

NOSE AND THROAT DISEASES AND DISORDERS

The nose and throat are the breathing passageways that allow air to flow into the lungs. When they are blocked, breathing difficulties and symptoms, such as shortness of breath, occur. Nose and throat conditions may also include sore throat and difficulty swallowing. Breathing exercises (see p. 166) can help improve breathing both before and after diseases and disorders.

ADENOID ENLARGEMENT

A fairly common childhood condition, which involves an excessive growth of tissue in the upper part of the pharynx that connects the nasal passages.

Symptoms:
Obstructed breathing including frequent snoring, prolonged nasal congestion, and nasal speech.

ExRx:
Surgical adenoid removal. After surgery, nose and mouth breathing exercises (p. 166).

LARYNGITIS

Acute or chronic inflammation of the voice box (larynx); can be an isolated condition or part of general respiratory infection. Causes include viral infections, too much talking or shouting, inhaling smoke and pollutants, allergies, and alcoholism.

Symptoms:
First, hoarseness; later, loss of voice, pain when swallowing, and an overall ill feeling.

ExRx:
Avoid overuse of voice; treat bacterial infection, gargle with warm salt water to soothe throat, use cough and sore throat medication, and avoid cigarette smoke and talking. The larynx can be conditioned similar to other muscles with proper posture techniques and exercises. These include learning to speak, cheer, and shout, using proper breathing and speaking techniques. Practice upper body posture exercises (p. 158), chin tuck (p. 160), and diaphragm breathing exercises (p. 167).

SINUSITIS

Swollen or blocked nasal cavities.

Symptoms:
A build-up of sinus pain and pressure; can lead to excessive headache pain.

ExRx:
Exercise stimulates mucus flow, which flushes out bacteria and clears air passages. It also shrinks swollen blood vessels, and this relieves the sinus pain and pressure.

When the headache pain is excessive, try extended warm-ups and stretching exercises to relieve the headache before proceeding to the aerobic and/or circulation exercises. If this does not work, medication or rest may be required before you continue.

SORE THROAT

Inflammation of pharynx, which is the passage between the mouth and esophagus. Widespread with adults who use tobacco or alcohol, or who have chronic sinus infections, allergies, and coughs.

Symptoms:
Difficulty swallowing, pain, rawness, and dryness in the throat.

ExRx:
Quit smoking cigarettes, rest and avoid cold air. Because aerobic or strenuous exercise may aggravate a sore throat or related condition, practice such low-intensity continuous exercise as walking or cycling. Until condition has passed, also avoid swimming and water exercise as these may also aggravate a sore throat.

VOCAL CORD NODULES AND POLYPS

A small lump of tissue (nodule) or stalk-like growth (polyp) that forms on the vocal cords. Caused by abuse of the voice box (improper speaking or shouting techniques), especially in the presence of an infection. Voice box abuse leads to scarring and permanent hoarseness. Predisposing risks include smoking cigarettes, allergies, and dry climates.

Symptoms:
Coarse, difficult breathing; husky and hoarse voice, but painless.

ExRx:
Use of a humidifier combined with speech therapy (voice rest, training to reduce intensity and duration of voice production) eliminates continuing and recurring nodules and polyps.

CARDIO RX: LIST OF ADDITIONAL NOSE AND THROAT DISORDERS AND INJURIES THAT ARE BENEFITED BY EXERCISE

- nasal fracture
- nasal papillomas
- nasal polyps
- nosebleed
- septal perforation and deviation
- throat abscess
- tonsillitis
- vocal cord paralysis

CARDIO RX EXERCISE GUIDELINES

The best preventive Cardio exercise prescription is to maintain a strong heart muscle, good breathing capacity, and good circulation. Such exercises as walking, cycling, and low-impact aerobics, which promote blood flow by using repeated and continuous movements of major muscle groups (legs, arms, and shoulders working together) can offer these benefits. Local exercises, such as stretching and strengthening, do not provide enough continuous blood flow to improve cardiovascular health. The best cardio exercise is either circulatory or aerobic.

Aerobic exercise is vigorous arm-leg exercise done at a heart-training rate of 60 to 85% of the maximum heart-training rate. Aerobic exercise provides the benefit of strengthening the heart muscle itself.

Circulatory exercise is slow to moderate in intensity, and combines arm-back-leg exercise done at a heart-training rate of just above the resting heart rate of 40% up to 60% of the maximum heart-training rate (see Monitoring Your Heart Rate, p. 217). Even though circulatory exercises need not raise your heart rate into the so-called aerobic training zone, they are still beneficial because they increase the blood flow through your arteries and veins, and contribute to better blood vessel health. They should definitely involve your calf muscle, which acts as a second heart by pumping up the blood that tends to pool in your lower extremities.

The basic cardio exercise prescription consists of continuous major muscle exercise movements in a regular exercise program. These are done for circulatory system health at a slow and moderate pace, and for heart muscle and lung health at a brisk pace. If you are predisposed to cardio health problems, the Cardio Ex program (in Part Two) can help you slow down, reverse, or stop the progress of your heart disease.

The Cardio Ex Prevention Program is designed to strengthen your heart and lung muscles while improving your circulation. Basically, you are increasing your body's capacity to process oxygenated blood—this is called endurance, which helps to slow down or prevent the onset of circulatory and breathing disorders. Preventing such diseases as high blood pressure or emphysema can, in turn, protect you against heart attack, stroke, and heart failure.

The Cardio Rx Therapy Program is designed to provide therapy for mild to moderate circulatory and breathing disorders, for example intermittent claudication, sinusitis, varicose veins, angina, and asthma. For those with family histories of high blood pressure, its onset can be delayed by being a regular cardio exerciser. The best therapeutic exercise is to restart your circulatory system and consistently send your blood to and from all your muscles and organs. With this exercise foundation, you can return to cardio health and then practice the preventive exercises. You should also use Cardio Rx Therapy if your cardio system rates III or IV on the severity scale. Use this program for mild to moderate disorders or for symptoms that require exercise therapy (e.g. after a prolonged bed rest).

Cardio Rx Therapy employs continuous exercising of your arms and legs and has a direct effect on blood pressure and blood flow. During circulatory exercise, blood pressure goes up slightly, but over days and weeks of exercise practice, it drops.

Cardio Rx therapeutic exercise is done at a slow to moderate pace with frequent rest periods whenever you feel pain or discomfort. It relieves the pain from arterial blockage in the chest, neck, and lower leg areas.

The Cardio Rx Rehab Program is the exercise program for post-heart attack patients, for those who have advanced symptoms of coronary heart disease, or people who are recovering from surgery for aneurysms. Postrehabilitation, you can either continue with the therapeutic program if there are still some problem areas, or go to the preventive program. You can also use Cardio Rx Rehab if your cardio system rates IV or V on the severity scale. Use this program for severe disorders and symptoms including aneurysms, blood clots, hypothermia, heart attack, or heart surgery (e.g. valve replacement, bypass, angioplasty). Use this program, too, for postoperative rehab or if you have had extended bed rest (two weeks or more). Of course, for both therapy and rehab, you should consult your physician before beginning any exercise.

The Cardio Rx Therapy and Prevention Program takes care of cardio disorders that have been diagnosed and already have shown some of their disabling symptoms. The exercise prescriptions help alleviate them and, in some cases, reverse the effects of the disease. The difference in the three approaches (i.e. prevention, therapy, and rehab) is related to the amount of exercise you can do and the speed and intensity at which you can build up your blood flow without suffering and muscular pain.

Bed Rest, Extended

Cardio Rx Therapy is not only for heart patients, but anyone who has lost their cardiovascular endurance because of extended hospitalization or bed rest (two weeks or longer), immobilization (e.g. body cast), or from such illnesses or treatments as chemotherapy, surgery, and so forth. It is also for those who are out of shape because of being inactive for one year or more. Cardio Rx Rehab provides long-term exercise prescriptions for rebuilding the cardio system after heart attack and heart surgery.

Even though all forms of exercise can serve as long-term relaxation therapy, stretching and muscle tightening exercises can relax the muscles and contribute to relaxing the mind. These exercises, for example the slow-motion circulatory exercises, can be practiced by those who cannot overexert themselves or are still in need of rest.

Relaxing, Prone or Seated

Lie down in bed or sit upright in a chair and close your eyes. Breathe slowly and evenly. The greater the physical stress or impact of training, the deeper your breathing must be initially. As you calm down, breathing will become normal. Now, consciously tighten and relax the muscles all over your body, one muscle group at a time. Start with the face muscles, then go on to the hands, legs, and feet.

SLOWING THE EXERCISE SPEED

How fast you exercise affects both your ability to exercise and the rate of your recovery. When doing a therapeutic or rehab program, slow-paced exercise can be more effective than moderate- or fast-paced exercise because it causes less pain and fatigue. In other words, taking it slower helps you take it longer. To complete your program, it may be necessary to slow down or rest in between exercise segments.

SLOW-MOTION EXERCISE

Vigorous exercise can become too difficult or even hazardous with certain health conditions that cause fatigue, shortness of breath, irregular heartbeat, or joint movement pain. In such cases, patients should practice doing their exercises at a substantially slower rate. The benefits of improved circulation, calorie burn, and muscle stretching and strengthening can still be obtained, they just take longer.

Slow exercise is practiced at one to five seconds per repeated move. It looks like you have been filmed with a slow-motion camera. Posture training, ROMs, warm-ups, and continuous motion exercises all lend themselves to the slow-motion approach. You should slow down when you have conditions that cause fatigue, dizziness, or joint pain. In most cases, it's better for your health to move more slowly than not at all.

STOP-AND-GO EXERCISE

As a rehab or therapy cardio patient, you should monitor your discomfort symptoms whenever you exercise. The following is a short list of monitoring tips:

- Don't exercise if you have a fever or don't feel well
- Don't exercise in extreme cold, hot, or windy weather; high humidity; heavy pollution; or at a high altitude
- Slow down exercising if you have muscle cramps, a side stitch, or if you are excessively out of breath or feel fatigued
- Stop exercising immediately if you feel chest pain, dizziness, a cold sweat, nausea, heart palpitations, heart fluttering, or an abnormal heart rhythm. Seek medical attention immediately.

LUNG AND BREATHING RX EXERCISE GUIDELINES

BREATHING DIFFICULTIES

Exercise prescriptions should match the severity of the symptoms. Lung and breathing disorders range from shortness of breath to severe chest pain and hyperventilation.

Lung Rx Therapy covers breathing disorders of a temporary or mild to moderate variety. Sinusitis, nasal congestion, mild allergies and asthma are among the conditions that can be treated with Lung Rx. These conditions usually require some breathing and coughing therapies, but also can be handled by doing moderate forms of aerobic and circulatory exercise.

Lung disorders of a severe nature, for example recovery from lung surgery, adult res-

TABLE 16.1
WALKING SCHEDULE

	Phase One	*Phase Two*	*Phase Three*
Intensity	*Very Slow*	*Slow*	*Slow to Moderate*
VO_2 Max (%)	40–50	50–60	60–70
METs	1–2 (very light)	2–3 (light)	3–5 (fairly light)
Speed (steps per minute)	5–20	20–30	30–45
Duration (min per day)	1–3	3–5	5–15
Distance	⅛ mile	¼ mile	½ mile
Frequency	daily	daily	daily
Mode	without arm swing	straight-arm swing	bent-arm swing

piratory distress syndrome, chronic bronchitis, emphysema, and pneumonia, require special breathing exercises before, in between, and after slow circulatory exercise.

Most exercise prescriptions involve taking control of your breathing action and are usually done in conjunction with other medical treatments. If your condition is severe, you may have to avoid deep breathing exercises.

Moderate Breathlessness Techniques

Exercise can help you control respiratory symptoms and problems such as moderate breathlessness and coughing. Monitor the severity of your symptoms. If possible, postpone exercise, and rest or reduce your exercise intensity. Follow the following specific exercise guidelines for breathlessness or coughing:

- Don't exercise when you are emotionally upset or during an asthma or coughing attack
- Exercise in warm, dehumidified air and avoid breathing cold, overly dry, or polluted air; wear a face mask in cold air, if necessary
- Take sips of water to keep air passages moist during exercise

- Use pursed-lip breathing to control breathlessness
- Monitor your breathing intensity using the talk test (i.e., if you can't talk continuously without having to gulp for air in between words, you are working too hard. Slow down your pace) and by rating your perceived exertion level
- Practice longer, more gradual warm-ups
- Emphasize exercise duration (length of time) instead of exercise intensity
- Reduce breathlessness though muscle relaxation exercises
- Improve breathing capacity with deep breathing, chest expansion, and trunk strengthening exercises
- Breathe in through your nose and out through your mouth with each exercise repetition
- Don't hold your breath
- Avoid overhead arm-strengthening exercises to avoid overtaxing your respiratory system
- Start with slow repetitions of one to three reps per exercise and build up to twelve to fifteen reps before adding any additional weight or resistance
- Expand your heart and lung capacity with aerobic exercises at moderate to vigorous pace accompanied by rhythmic breathing
- Breathe rhythmically, taking as much time to exhale air as you do to inhale it
- Practice intermittent exercise of short physical duration followed by short rests
- Be sure to relax your neck and shoulder muscles to allow for maximum air flow especially when the level of exertion increases, for example, as with stair climbing or brisk walking.

SEVERE BREATHLESSNESS TECHNIQUES

Sit up, hyperextend the neck, lean forward with mouth open and tongue out, and breathe with nostrils flaring. For severe breathing problems, see illustration page 167.

BREATHING COLD AIR

Cold air makes it much more stressful to exercise if you have heart or lung disease. Inhaling cold air causes the lungs and arteries to constrict and perhaps go into "reflex spasm." Cold also causes the body to conserve body heat. Blood vessels constrict ("vasoconstriction") so blood can remain in your vital organs to keep them at normal temperature. This also causes your blood pressure to rise and makes your heart muscle work harder. If you are not heart healthy, you may experience ischemia (obstruction of arterial blood flow to the heart), angina, or both. Vasoconstriction also causes your extremities to begin to cool off.

CONTINUOUS BREATHING EXERCISE THERAPY

Your lungs respond well to exercises that require you to breathe rhythmically and continuously. Vigorous arm-leg exercises increase your rate of breathing and work your lungs, diaphragm, and abdominal muscles.

With lung and breathing disorders, you can combine breathing (see pp. 166–168), coughing (see p. 168) and postural drainage techniques to clear passages, so you can continue exercising. If your breathing disorders are severe, you will have to start with the Cardio Rx Rehab program, p. 421.

SHORT-TERM BREATHING TECHNIQUES

You can use pursed-lipped breath (p. 167), nose or mouth only breath (p. 166), as well as coughing exercises, for diseases that have shortness of breath, coughing, and other nose, throat, and breathing difficulties.

CHAPTER 17

Psyche-Immune Rx

Exercise Solutions for Mental, Emotional, Sexual, and Immune Systems

THE PSYCHE-IMMUNE SYSTEM

This chapter covers prescriptions for emotional, mental, immune, and sexual disorders. The body area covered is the "mind," that is, the brain and less materially, the inner self and the immune and sympathetic nervous system. Unlike the physical nervous system, the sympathetic nervous system affects body functions through thoughts and emotions. Primary symptoms of the sympathetic nervous system include muscular tension, breathing and heartbeat irregularities, stressful physical reactions (especially pain), and body temperature changes.

The Psyche-Immune exercise prescriptions are focused on managing stressful reactions related to traumatic events. Body area exercises include relaxation exercises (see Body Area Muscular Tension Exercise, pp. 246–247) for specific muscle groups. Anxiety, depression, fatigue, fear, insomnia, irritability, low self-esteem, irrational repetitive behaviors, and psychosomatic pain are among the symptoms that can be successfully treated with exercise. It can even help with mental illness and mental retardation.

Refer to the specific psychological or immune disorder for which you have received a medical diagnosis. Then, follow the specific Rx exercises—including those that cover your other body systems.

The major portion of this chapter is broken down into five areas, which are: (1) mental and emotional diseases and disorders, (2) medication side effects, (3) immune diseases and disorders, (4) sexual disorders, and (5) wrist, hand, and finger injuries. Each of these three areas is followed by an alphabetic listing of the diseases, disorders, or injuries found under that category. Symptoms are then described for each disease, disorder, or injury, which is followed by an ExRx for that specific ailment. You will note that some of the more common, more rehabilitative disorders and injuries have many exercises associated with them, while others (e.g. atopic dermatitis, premature ejaculation) will have only a few exercises associated with them. If you feel you want more exercise than what is given with any ExRx, consult Parts I and II of this book and practice those preventive exercises that are associated with the body system or area that you are rehabilitating. Remember: Always start at a lower level and work your way up to your own personal optimum level. Do not turn your rehabilitative exercise therapy into a competition with anyone—including yourself. That is the surest, fastest way to injury, pain, and setbacks on the road to recovery.

WARNING: Although many over-the-counter and prescription pain relievers are prescribed for reduction of pain caused by injuries, do not take any pain relievers before exercising as they tend to mask pain, which can cause further injury resulting from overexercising or overusing an injured body area or part. Take the medication as directed, after exercise and when you are more stationary. Awareness of an injury is key to healing it!

MENTAL AND EMOTIONAL DISORDERS RX

What happens in your brain, your body, as well as your external environment can influence your state of mind and emotions. The body reacts in both a physical and psychological way to these stimuli. Thus, physical and psychological therapy can work hand in hand.

The old theory of psychological change was that *insight* preceded *change*. Increasingly psychologists now view mental illness as a "vicious circle" that can be broken by taking small, manageable, but positive steps toward a goal. A resolution to start an exercise program is one of them. Fellow exercisers can also lend support. A friend who already exercises can help you get started so that you don't have to be on your own at the beginning. Another solution is to just start walking. Walking is a common activity that serves as an excellent entry platform to all other exercises. For a depressed person, an exercise program might start with simple stretching exercises combined with slow walking, for example, and gradually progress toward more strenuous exercise. In severe cases of depression, however, exercise alone may not be enough and medication may be required to balance the patient's brain chemistry.

STRESS AND EXERCISE

Emotional or mental stress produces many physical symptoms, such as hyperactivity, muscle tension, and fatigue. These symptoms can, in turn, complicate an underlying illness or disorder. A regular exercise program can provide both an anchor and a structured model for coping with the stresses of everyday living, work, and marriage. Exercise also provides tools for mental and emotional control. Control of one's physical well-being, which comes with strength, endurance, and flexibility, can translate into mental well-being.

For reducing a moderate amount of stress, exercise can be the primary—sometimes the only—solution. For higher levels of stress and tension, exercise can be used in tandem with counseling and drug therapies.

MENTAL ILLNESS AND EXERCISE

Mental illness is a form of imprisonment in varying degrees. To maintain even a minimum physical balance, exercise is crucial. Even the severely mentally ill should be kept physically active while being treated. Most in-patient psychiatric units and institutions have recreational therapy programs; sometimes, it is be essential to their accreditation.

Similar to other organs we have discussed, the brain needs sufficient blood flow for physical nourishment (i.e. oxygen and nutrients), and also physical stimulation for sharper mental activity. Improved brain function (e.g. clearer thinking) can affect emotional disorders by improving a person's perception of reality in much the same way that healthier food makes the mind more alert and able to think faster and more accurately.

ADDICTION (SEE DEPENDENCY)

ALCOHOLISM

Addiction to alcohol; the chronic inability to stop consuming alcoholic beverages or drinks.

Symptoms:
Amnesia, mood swings, depression, violent behavior, hostility, denial of problem, upset stomach, poor hygiene, and frequent infections and injuries (e.g. bruises, burns, and fractures).

ExRx:
You can begin a rehabilitative exercise program to rebuild your health at the same time that you start seeking therapy for your addiction. You can start with low to moderate levels of exercise, including walking and ROMs, and build up from that base. As you grow stronger, your resolve to quit drinking alcohol will also grow stronger. Exercise strengthens the body and mind, aids in behavior modification, and rehabilitates the body during and after abstinence and detoxification.

ANOREXIA NERVOSA

This is a sometimes fatal eating disorder. Self-starvation is induced by the irrational fear of gaining weight; affects mostly young women, but increasingly more men and older women also show signs of this disorder. May occur with or without a bulimia eating disorder. Causes are psychological as well as cultural. Studies show that sports and exercise can be a significant part of this disorder for some women.

Symptoms:
Irrational fear of gaining weight or getting fat, compulsive exercising, depression, severe weight loss, and anemia.

ExRx:
Anorexia should be treated as a psychological eating and exercise disorder because patients with this disorder have unrealistic ideas about eating, nutrition, and exercise. They consequently undereat and overexercise, and often need to have specific prescribed limitations on each of these activities. The illness has a high mortality rate—6% of patients die. Traditionally, the last stages of weight loss are treated in a hospital or institutional setting where regimented eating behavior modification with rewards is employed. Some patients can benefit from this type of regimented eating and exercise discipline, but an exercise regimen for those patients who are severely

debilitated by the disorder cannot be done because any excess calorie burn would be counterproductive and dangerous. Strength-training therapy can help by maintaining and redistributing body weight into aesthetically appealing muscle. Nutritional counseling should be balanced with a limited exercise regimen of two to three hours a week at the maximum.

ANXIETY

A nervous reaction to stressful threats to your well-being, including those that accompany disease and injuries. It is a natural reflex to things we fear, but chronic, baseless anxiety is a disorder.

Symptoms:
Sweating, heart palpitations, muscle tension, fatigue, and high blood pressure.

ExRx:
Regular aerobic exercise, circulatory exercise, and deep-breathing exercises release muscle tension all over the body. Studies show that aerobic exercise is better than nonaerobic exercise in treating anxiety and that a negative mood swing in the first five minutes of exercise shifts to positive after ten to fifteen minutes. (Also see general anxiety disorder, panic attacks, and stress.)

APNEA (SEE INSOMNIA AND APNEA)

ATTENTION-DEFICIT DISORDER (ADD; HYPERACTIVITY)

The inability to focus attention on key tasks or to engage in such passive activities as learning, reading, and listening. Present at birth, but usually disappears after four years of age. Can be a physiological brain disorder.

Symptoms:
Disruptive behavior, organizational difficulties, moodiness, inattentiveness, impulsiveness, in addition to being easily distracted.

ExRx:
No cure, but drug therapy and behavior modification can lessen and control symptoms. Exercise, sports, and physical games can also channel excess energy into a focused activity and leave the child more relaxed. Aerobic exercise, hiking, and running all are big energy expenders. Organized, focused activity is much more important for the ADD child than quantity of activity.

BIPOLAR DISORDER

Characterized by mood swings that shift to either euphoria or depression. There are two types; Type I is a continuous depression with occasional euphoric episodes, which mostly affects women between the ages of twenty and thirty-five. Type II is defined by depressive episodes and mild, low-grade mania, that is, hypomaniac episodes. These disorders are generally divided into unipolar and bipolar types. The most common type are unipolar, which are depressions that occur periodically; with unipolar disorders the patient returns to a normal level of stability. The bipolar patient, however, swings between episodes of hyperactive behavior combined with ongoing, nonstop thought processes (manic phase) and incidents of fairly severe depression. Some patients will have a series of manic episodes early in life, followed by a long depressive era later on. This disorder is highly individual; exercise prescriptions should be tailored to each patient.

Symptoms:
Manic episodes of hyperactivity combined

with sleeplessness, inability to eat normally, and distractibility; followed by depressive episodes, sluggishness, withdrawal, and negative thinking.

ExRx:
Lithium or drug therapy may be necessary. Start exercising with short periods of less strenuous exercise, such as stretching only, and progress gradually to a more strenuous routine, for example strengthening and cardio exercise. This approach is better than doing just aerobic exercise during sluggish periods. Relaxation exercises during hyperactive periods also help even out mood swings.

BULIMIA

An eating disorder characterized by binge eating followed by purging (vomiting) or fasting. Affects mostly women, but is increasingly found in men, too.

Symptoms:
Hyperactivity, excessive exercise, weight fluctuations (sometimes dramatic), and depression.

ExRx:
Combine exercise with responsible eating. Use deep breathing exercises (p. 245) and relaxation exercises (pp. 244–248) during anxious or negative thinking episodes. Noncompetitive sports or exercise with a friend will help quell competitive and compulsive exercise urges.

CREATIVE BLOCK

A temporary inability to think through a problem to a final satisfactory solution.

Symptoms:
Nervousness, depression, and irritability.

ExRx:
Aerobic and circulatory exercises increase blood and oxygen flow to the brain elevating moods and awareness. Exercise offers diversion, distraction, or distance—allowing the mind to work subconsciously on the problem. Many poets, writers, and thinkers have been inspired during their jogs or walks.

CONVERSION DISORDER

The temporary loss of a body function (e.g. loss of vision, inability to move or swallow) for a short duration, which has no physical cause, but rather is the result of an unresolved psychological conflict. This disorder usually lasts a short time and is not life-threatening.

Symptoms:
Sudden disability or loss of function; can be related to a stressful event or to apathy.

ExRx:
In addition to psychotherapy, relaxation training can ease the transition back to normalcy. Because a conversion disorder is short-term, exercise can help to snap a person out of it. For example, passive-assisted exercises by a physical therapist can help a conversion-paralysis patient regain function. Some doctors recommend activity and exercise following relaxation training.

DELUSIONAL DISORDERS

Fixations on false beliefs (e.g. feelings of persecution) that interfere with social relationships, but usually do not interfere with a person's job or thinking ability. Affects men and women, mostly between ages forty to fifty-five.

Symptoms:
Anxiety, relentless criticism, jumbled responses, social isolation, and depression.

ExRx:
Psychotherapy and antipsychotic, antidepressant drugs. Practice deep-breathing and relaxation exercises; exercise in groups or with a partner; develop an exercise support system. Increased circulation is undoubtedly helpful to productive brain function.

DEPENDENCY

An addiction to substances or chemicals; most often a misguided form of pain or emotional stress relief. Alcohol, drugs, and other such chemicals as the nicotine in cigarettes reduce the brain's levels of norepinephrine, a neurotransmitter essential for emotional stability.

Symptoms:
Frequent use of a substance (e.g. cocaine, alcohol, prescription narcotics) can lead to low self-esteem, fatigue, nervousness, and loss of appetite. Muscles and the heart can weaken and atrophy. Also, high blood pressure, frequent colds, and infections occur because the addiction weakens the immune system; can also cause elevated cholesterol levels. There are usually withdrawal effects upon abrupt cessation of the substance.

ExRx:
A progressive exercise program rehabilitates the whole body and provides an alternative means of combating the symptoms and effects of dependencies. The length of time you have been addicted must be considered (especially if longer than one year), but generally start with gradual exercise. Relaxation, deep-breathing, and circulatory exercises reduce the physical reaction to withdrawal symptoms and stress, and can divert you from negative thinking. At the same time, damaged body systems, neurotransmitters, and your weakened heart and muscles start growing stronger, which will make your body feel better and will help clear your mind.

DEPERSONALIZATION DISORDERS

Persistent episodes of mind/body detachment with feelings of loss of self-awareness or of a body part.

Symptoms:
Anxiety accompanied by a feeling that life is not real; also depression, speechlessness, dizziness, obsessive contemplation, and fear of going insane.

ExRx:
Combined with ongoing, cognitive therapy, exercise can help you anchor yourself in physical reality, which brings you back from your extreme, detached-from-life viewpoint. Exercising the body area and limbs that feel detached can bring back the feeling of connection to your body. Relaxation and deep breathing are also important and can be used as a type of mild hypnotherapy. In a rested and safe, trancelike state, past events can be recalled, helping to quiet anxious responses.

DEPRESSION

A recurring syndrome of negative thinking and recalling of unpleasant events and thoughts, which can have psychological or physiological causes. It can also be a reaction to the diagnosis or incidence of other such diseases as cancer and heart attack. Depressive disorders afflict 5% of Americans; 2% have major depression. Major depression is characterized by feelings of persistent sadness and hopelessness that interfere with work and relationships and in some cases can lead to suicide if left untreated. May be a result of major life change or family loss. Can also be caused by a deficiency of neurotransmitters in the brain.

Symptoms:
Mental tension, feelings of hopelessness, and perpetual sleepiness and fatigue. Major depression symptoms can include lethargy, sadness, anger, anxiety, inability to concentrate or think clearly, sleeplessness or sleeping too much, loss of appetite, and suicidal thoughts.

ExRx:
Short-term exercise therapy can help the mind to relax because the body is relaxed. Circulatory exercises (e.g. such slow-motion activities as strolling and tai chi) divert a person's mind from negative thinking while relaxing the body. Aerobic exercise can elevate the mood to eliminate mood swings by raising the metabolism and increasing blood and oxygen flow to the brain. It may also release pain-killing compounds, called endorphins. Finally, an exercise program itself provides a sense of accomplishment and increases your feelings of self-worth.

It is difficult to feel depressed in the middle of a vigorous exercise routine. Warming up your body, breaking a sweat, and breathing heavily changes your physical state, and the effects last for at least twenty minutes after you stop exercising. Over the long run, depression may be easier to head off in its early stages, and is difficult to treat if allowed to persist. Unfortunately, major depression occurs even in athletes. Exercise may help, but it is not a perfect protection. In advanced or severe cases, progress slowly by gradually increasing the duration and intensity of your exercise sessions and by seeing a doctor and a psychiatrist.

Disassociative Fugue

A change of consciousness that may last for hours or days causing the sufferer to wander away from familiar surroundings.

Symptoms:
Sudden personality change, travel, or violent episodes.

ExRx:
Reorganize your routine to avoid any triggering events, and develop coping techniques. Regular exercise (e.g. relaxation and deep-breathing exercises) can calm and relax the body so the mind can recall events and learn to understand its distressed state.

Exercise Addiction

Practicing too much exercise or sports to avoid personal responsibilities and social contact. Compulsive exercise can also be related to unrealistic ideas and a distorted body image.

Symptoms:
Emaciation, many overuse injuries (e.g. pulled muscles, pinched nerves), and isolation (difficult to do any activities or exercise with friends). Those with this addiction spend five to six (or more) hours a day exercising, seven days a week.

ExRx:
Seek to redefine and rebalance your life goals toward family, friends, career, and cultural development. Substitute solitary exercising with such social activities as walking or bike

ILAN BERCI

DIAGNOSIS: DEPRESSION

Ilan Berci was completing his engineering degree in 1992 when he started feeling the onset of depression. It began in earnest at his first job as a computer system administrator. "It really affected me at night," he remembers. "I couldn't sleep and would think of very scary thoughts."

Many members of his family on his mother's side also have chemical imbalances and are required to take antidepressants. After close to three years of worsening depression, Ilan was considering the same solution.

However, Ilan noticed a pattern: if he abstained from eating sweeteners, both natural and artificial, he tended to stay within the same mindset throughout the day. He started experimenting with his diet, cutting out the sugars, then milk, meat, and alcohol, until he became completely vegan (no animal or dairy products).

His doctor recommended that he also exercise to lower his high blood pressure, which was 140/90. He began weight lifting, and discovered that with his diet and exercise he could easily control his depression. He reports now that he has not so much as caught a cold since he began his program. "My family has noticed that I'm much more uplifted than I used to be and have stopped hinting for me to go on Prozac. My mother's side of the family, almost all of whom are on medication or once were, are the most impressed," he says.

Ilan works out for about an hour before breakfast in the morning. He does this three times a week: on both Saturday and Sunday and one day before work during the week. Although the amount of hours is moderate, he calls his workouts, "intense and focused." He also takes two half-hour walks a day at a moderate pace, and is an avid juggler and unicyclist.

His blood pressure is now down to 105/70. The weight lifting has taken him from 175 pounds to a muscular 210 pounds. According to Ilan, he is in the best physical shape of his life, and mentally, he is "very alert from sun up to sun down." He feels more confident and balanced because, in his own words, he is "more disciplined in diet and exercise."

riding with a friend, which will help you slowly regain some connection and perspective on how you spend your time. Also, eat a balanced diet.

Studies show that an exercise addiction can be just as serious an eating disorder as bulimia or anorexia. In place of food craving, there is an obsessive/compulsive desire to exercise. This addiction can include maintaining a schedule of intense exercise; detailed record-keeping of exercise; resisting the temptation to not exercise; feelings of guilt and anxiety when there is a lapse in the exercise schedule followed by compensatory increases in exercise to make up for these lapses; and pushing oneself to exercise even when tired or ill.

FATIGUE

A feeling of always being tired, which is both a physical and psychological symptom. If continuous, it qualifies as a disorder. (See chronic fatigue syndrome, p. 449)

Symptoms:
Poor posture, constant muscle tension, shrugged shoulders, tiredness, listlessness, lack of endurance, back pain, and sleeplessness.

ExRx:
Stimulate low energy first with posture and breathing exercises and then follow with circulatory exercises. Over the long term, build up physical endurance with a regular exercise program and normalize your body's sleep activity and rest periods to eliminate bouts of prolonged tiredness.

FEAR

Fear is a reaction to an external threat that causes a fight, flight, or coping response.

Symptoms:
Muscle tension, sweating, and rapid heartbeat.

ExRx:
Exercise can make you stress-hardy and create a demeanor of self-confidence so that you will be less apt to feel threatened.

GENERAL ANXIETY DISORDER (GAD)

Overwhelming, uncontrollable worry without a specific cause that interferes with normal living. Dissimilar to fear, GAD is an apprehensive reaction to such internal threats as repressed thoughts or unacceptable impulses.

Symptoms:
Fatigue, tendency to become angry and fearful, restlessness, rigid movements, trembling, muscle spasms, and inability to concentrate.

ExRx:
Deep-breathing exercises and slow-motion circulatory exercises are recommended. Plan and schedule exercise periods to avoid such triggering stimuli as unpleasant environments and events. (Also see anxiety, panic attacks, and stress.)

HEADACHES

Sharp, debilitating pain and pressure that can hit hard and last for days. They may be linked to your emotional state, hormone imbalance, or a head, neck, or spinal cord injury. They can also be triggered by such outside or internal stresses as anxiety and depression. There are various types with different degrees of severity including cluster, migraine, exertion, and tension headaches.

Symptoms:
Tension headaches (usually mild) are related to muscle tension in face, jaw, neck, shoulders, and back. Exertion (moderate) headaches are characterized by nausea, sensitivity to light, and a "throbbing" pain. Cluster headaches (moderate to severe) are accompanied by a need to fidget or move to provide relief. Migraines (severe) typically affect only one side of the head, but can affect both. Migraines are characterized by severe pain, nausea,

extreme sensitivity to light and sound, and sometimes visual distortions.

ExRx:
Exercise can either help or hurt a headache. Recurring headaches should be diagnosed by a doctor or headache specialist. Regular, moderate exercise of almost any kind, between headaches, can reduce the occurrence of headaches by releasing the body's own pain-killing hormones—endorphins and enkephalins. Specific body area exercises, stretching, and ROM exercises can relax the muscles in the neck, shoulders, and jaw, and cut off the source of a developing or ongoing tension headache. Practice five to eight reps of the head tilt exercise (p. 171) two to three times a day. This is also effective: Stand with your back to the wall. Place your hands behind the base of your head with your elbows touching the wall. Bring your elbows together in front of your face while tilting your head forward. Hold briefly, and return your elbows to the wall. Do five to eight repetitions two to three times a day. Next, do a series of shoulder shrugs with your arms hanging by your sides. Cluster headaches are caused by a histamine imbalance and can be helped by vigorous exercise, which increases blood flow to the brain. During an acute migraine attack, rest and quiet is the only appropriate response. Regular exercise can increase blood flow and improve blood pressure in the brain; slow walking at the first sign of a migraine may also reduce the symptons.

Hypochondriasis

Unrealistic fear of having a serious disease or exaggerating the severity and significance of aches and pains. Fear persists despite doctor's reassurances.

Symptoms:
Sleeplessness and anxiety related to the fear of being seriously ill, complaining about and misinterpreting physical sensations as serious symptoms, combined with a preoccupation with body functions, and an extensive knowledge of illnesses and treatments.

ExRx:
A doctor's evaluation and diagnosis of imagined symptoms is important to put the mind at rest, but exercise produces its own set of positive physical sensations—such as muscular contractions, movement, heavy breathing, sweaty workouts, and so forth, which supersede those of the hypochondria, and, over the long term, seem to erase them. The muscle fatigue from exercise supplants a perceived pain in a nearby area or over another area of the body. Exercise can mask or even erase symptoms by temporarily distracting the patient and providing general benefits, but strongly held preoccupations are difficult to eradicate entirely. Because the hypochondriacal patient believes that he or she has a serious illness, the ability to exercise can be used in cognitive therapy. The simple equation, "If you are well, you cannot function as a sick person," plays an important role in the psychological counseling for this disorder.

Insomnia and Apnea

A form of nighttime anxiety in which you are unable to fall asleep or stay asleep, and your muscles remain in contraction without release. These discomforts and anxieties keep you from falling asleep and getting a good night's rest. Frequent restless nights wear down the body and aggravate this sleepless condition. Insomnia can be caused by an illness; such chemical stimulants as drugs, alcohol, or caffeine; anxiety; or by a schedule change. Apnea is a type of insomnia that causes a sleep breathing disorder in which there is too much relaxed tissue in the throat. This causes breathing interruptions, snoring, and compensating chokes or loud snorts. Because it occurs hundreds of times during sleep, it results in frequent awakenings and a restless kind of sleep.

Symptoms:
Insomnia is the inability to fall asleep, tossing and turning, nightmares, early morning awakenings, fatigue, restlessness, moodiness, and lack of energy. Apnea causes restless sleep, choking or snorting during sleep, and snoring.

ExRx:
Exercise fatigues the body with muscle work accompanied by energy burn from improved circulation. Muscular tension also burns energy, but its continuation without proper blood flow causes pain and continued tension. Exercise improves the most restful phase of sleep—slow-brainwave sleep—when the body temperature drops and breathing regularizes.

By increasing the duration of exercise from one to two hours, you can make yourself more tired in order to fall asleep easier and faster. Long-term solutions include reducing your body fat, which can crowd your air passages and can cause apnea or other such sleep breathing problems as snoring. Studies show that moderate and balanced aerobic fitness has significant positive results on sleep in older men, including shorter sleep onset latencies, reduced amounts of wake-time after sleep begins, fewer discrete sleep episodes, fewer sleep stage shifts during the initial part of the night, and higher sleep efficiency. Aerobic exercise also helps adapt your circadian rhythms (your internal clock) when coping with a change in work schedules.

Low Self-Esteem

A condition characterized by having negative feelings about yourself. These negative thoughts can include your appearance, your personality, intelligence, your ability to perform, and many others. Can lead to such psychological disorders as depression or anxiety.

Symptoms:
Anxiety, fatigue, listlessness, lack of motivation, difficulty concentrating, appetite and weight change, and feelings of self-worthlessness, guilt, or shame.

ExRx:
Regular exercise elevates your mood by stimulating hormone flow (e.g. adrenaline). Exercise also directly affects the secretion of naturally occurring neuroregulating hormones, morphine-like substances called endorphins and enkephalins, which can further elevate your mood. Getting in shape is another esteem-builder; as you work out you feel and look better physically, which can boost your morale and feelings of self-worth.

Memory Loss

The lack of ability to recall information. Affects everyone to certain degrees, but occurs more frequently after age fifty.

Symptoms:
Forgetfulness; difficulties with recall and concentration.

ExRx:
Circulatory and aerobic exercises have a marked impact on strengthening recall and mental acuity. A regular exercise routine may slow down memory loss. Starting an exercise

program gives immediate benefits to short-term recall and sharpness of visual observation. Exercise energizes and revitalizes the brain as it does with any muscle or organ in the body, providing blood flow and oxygen; this assists the movement of neurotransmitters in the brain.

Obsessive-Compulsive Disorder

Repeated thoughts and defensive behavior rituals arising from efforts to control anxiety, guilt, and "unacceptable" impulses.

Symptoms:
Repetitive and persistent worry, involuntary thoughts, and negative images.

ExRx:
Treatment is usually a combination of medications, counseling, and aversion therapy consisting of exercise, sports, or other diverting recreational activity. Aversion therapy is a thought-switching or thought-stopping activity, which relieves stress by redirecting emotional energy toward recreation, exercise, or sport. When anxiety and frustration occur, they can be relieved by activities, physical movement, by in-place exercises, by moving away from the stress source, or by deep-breathing techniques.

Pain Disorder

Continuing and chronic complaints about pain without a physical cause. Mimics pain symptoms of various diseases, such as angina chest pain but without the disease. Affects more women than men, ages thirty to forty, and interferes with work and personal relationships. As in hypochondria, symptoms of pain predominate over the nonexistence of a disease. However, chronic pain syndromes are usually associated with other illnesses (e.g. depression).

Symptoms:
Range from persistent complaints to frequent hospital visits.

ExRx:
Treatment includes antidepressants, electrical stimulation, massage. Use relaxation exercise as a distraction technique, and specialized physical therapy.

Panic Attacks

This disorder is anxiety in its most severe form, including intense apprehension, terror, and fear of impending doom. Can also be associated with agoraphobia (fear of public places) or other phobias. Because of the intensity of the reaction, there is a high risk of alcohol and drug abuse.

Symptoms:
Panic episodes continually repeat and leave the sufferer shaken and exhausted. During an attack, there is rapid breathing, hyperventilation, profuse sweating and trembling, and confusion.

ExRx:
Various medications can be prescribed, including antidepressants, anti-anxiety drugs, and beta-blockers. Deep-breathing exercises relieve panic attacks while they are happening. A regular exercise program that concentrates on relaxation therapy can prevent or help reduce the number of panic attacks. Daily running or brisk walking has also helped some patients with this disorder.

PHOBIAS

A variety of personal fears that are out of proportion to the actual danger, including agoraphobia, social phobia (embarrassment in public), or other specific phobias to animals, objects, activities, or situations.

Symptoms:
Severe anxiety; dizziness and falling; feelings of unreality; cardiac distress; loss of bowel and bladder control; feelings of weakness, cowardice, ineffectiveness, or low self-esteem; and mild depression. Can also cause panic attacks.

ExRx:
May never be cured, but drug therapy and behavioral therapy coupled with such self-help physical therapies as relaxation techniques and regular aerobic activities can relieve stress and redirect excess energy caused by anxiety, fear, and panic.

POST-TRAUMATIC STRESS DISORDER

Lingering distress (more than one month) following a traumatic event.

Symptoms:
Chronic anxiety, feelings of fear and helplessness, emotional numbness, flashbacks, and sleeplessness.

ExRx:
Psychotherapy may be necessary. Practice relaxation exercises to reduce anxiety and induce sleep. Progressive desensitization—exposing the person in stages to their cause of anxiety—may also help. Use exercise support groups.

PSYCHOACTIVE DRUG ABUSE

Repeated use of drugs, legal or illegal, that cause physical, emotional, mental, or social harm. Can occur at any age; caused by inadequate coping skills, low self-esteem, or peer pressure. Drugs include anti-anxiety (e.g. valium), depressants (e.g. barbiturates), hallucinogens (e.g. LSD and PCP), narcotics (e.g. cocaine and heroin), and stimulants (e.g. amphetamines). Can lead to such life-threatening complications as AIDS, heart disease, cardiac arrest, and mental illness.

Symptoms:
Can include distress in digestive, heart and respiratory, musculoskeletal, or nervous systems; body functions are weakened. Accompanied by anxiety and agitation.

ExRx:
Drug abuse requires intense medical treatment and care, including detoxification, psychological counseling, fluid replacement, and nutritional and drug therapy for stomach distress, drug-induced anxiety, and agitation. Under a doctor's care, exercise can be used for short-term therapy and long-term rehabilitation. Regular exercise may even alleviate the problems (e.g. low self-esteem) that lead to drug abuse. An exercise rehab program can be either total in scope or concentrated on body area weaknesses caused by complications of the drug abuse (e.g. Chapter Fourteen, MuSkel Rx, for severe muscle wasting; Cardio Rx Rehab, p. 421, for heart and lung disease).

SCHIZOPHRENIA

Long-term (more than six months) disturbances in behavior, perception, thought content and form, and sense of self. Occurs in

CINDY KLAJA-MCLOUGHLIN

DIAGNOSIS: CARDIAC ARREST; TRAUMA

In August 1988, Cindy Klaja-McLoughlin was training with a friend for an upcoming 5K race when she fell unconscious on the track. Comatose and in cardiac arrest, Cindy was rushed to a nearby suburban hospital by ambulance. Doctors there told her family not to expect her to make it through the night, and her last rites were performed.

Later that evening, however, Cindy was life-flighted to the University of Pittsburgh Hospital, where the doctors informed her family that she probably would survive, but that she would also probably suffer some degree of brain damage when she finally came out of the coma. When she regained consciousness a few days later, she had little short-term memory. But after about a week, she was back to normal. She attributed her survival and recovery to her excellent health prior to the incident. But she still had several unanswered questions.

Her cardiac arrest, she found, had been caused by "idiopathic ventricular fibrillation," a disorder that causes the patient to go into cardiac arrest whenever a burst of adrenaline is released. To rectify this, a device called an automatic defibrillator was surgically implanted into Cindy's abdomen and was connected to her heart by electric wiring. The defibrillator senses when Cindy's heart rate accelerates and sends out electric impulses to slow it down and bring her out of cardiac arrest.

After six weeks in the hospital, the body Cindy had been so proud of before was now marked by surgical scars and was temporarily misshapen while it made room for the implant. Her confidence began to wane. But she made up her mind to put herself in motion, little-by-little, and two months later, in December of 1988, she was back at the Y riding the stationary cycling machine and doing circuit training. With the stationary bike, she started off riding for fifteen-minute stretches and built up to forty-five minutes by the summer of 1989. She also returned to running that summer, though not competitively. Instead, she ran a two-mile course at a comfortable pace and did not keep track of the time.

early adolescence to early adulthood in 1 to 2% of the population.

Symptoms:
Delusions, disorganized behavior and speech, hallucinations, ambivalence (conflicted feelings), as well as such generalized reactions as fatigue, anxiety, agitation, low self-esteem, and depression.

ExRx:
Long-term treatment with antipsychotic drugs relieves anxiety and agitation for some patients, such group activities as sports may be enough for others. Studies show that exercise helps improve psychological functioning in the following areas: communication, animation, personal interest, motivation, and insight into body image. It also lessens motor

Over the next two years, Cindy experimented with various cross-training exercises. Every day, she either inline skated, did step aerobics, jogged, or weight trained. Then, on Memorial Day of 1991, as she broke into a sprint, her adrenal glands sent out a little boost and sent her back into cardiac arrest. A witness called an ambulance, but Cindy's defibrillator did its work before she even arrived at the hospital, and she was released right from the emergency room. Despite her condition, Cindy still refused to give up such benefits of exercise as a higher energy levels, stamina, self-confidence, and the psychological lift from the rush of endorphins.

On the sixth anniversary of her first cardiac arrest Cindy and her husband planned a little celebration. That morning, at work, however, she suffered her third cardiac arrest while holding a cup of coffee. As she hit the ground, the coffee spilled and caused third-degree burns on her leg. But her defibrillator soon kicked in and returned her heart rate to normal. The burns were the worst of it. When she went to the hospital for tests, doctors told her that the latest cardiac arrest was probably a "sympathetic episode"—a psychosomatic throwback to her first cardiac arrest. She returned to work that very same day and even went on a two-mile walk that evening—she needed it to help her calm down.

As routine as these cardiac arrests seemed to be becoming, Cindy's third cardiac arrest did prove to be "the charm." She "realized how fragile life truly is, and that it can be taken when one least expects it." She decided to take risks and to follow her dreams, to do what she wanted rather than what was expected of her. She resigned from the corporation where she worked and went on to pursuing acting, a move for which she says exercise helped give her confidence.

In December of 1994, Cindy was fitted with a new defibrillator. A month later, she bought a cross-country ski machine and has been "hooked" ever since. She "indulges" herself by using the machine for thirty to forty minutes daily, does crunches five times a week, and does "a ton of walking" in New York City as she builds up her acting credentials along with her body.

retardation and body tension. Breathing and stretching exercises lessen anxiety and panic attacks while strength training and aerobics increase self-esteem. A regular exercise program will probably not reduce the need for drugs aimed at relieving symptoms, but it can enhance psychosocial treatment programs. Biofeedback forms of body control and deep breathing are also helpful approaches to reducing many of the symptoms.

SOMATIZATION DISORDER

The presence of a group of numerous stress-related symptoms that suggest physical disorders when there is no organic illness. More often found in women than men; this disorder has both genetic and environmental factors. Differs from hypochondria in that somatization-disorder patients focus on multiple symptoms rather than conviction of illness.

Symptoms:
Exaggerated physical complaints, multiple and often simultaneous medical evaluations for blindness, dizziness, paralysis, chest pain, and heart palpitations.

ExRx:
Care giver can help you live with symptoms. Specific exercises aimed at symptoms (e.g. relaxation exercises for muscle tension; deep breathing for anxiety; balancing for dizziness; ROMs for paralysis; stretching and isometric muscle contraction and release for chest pains) help relieve or even eliminate some of these symptoms.

STRESS

Your body's reaction to a real or perceived external annoyances and aggravation (including overwork, sleeplessness, worries about family, health, or job). When aggravated, your body readies for action: the heart rate increases; muscles tense up; blood sugar rises; breathing becomes rapid and shallow; circulation to the skin and digestive system diminishes and increases to the muscles of the legs and arms.

Symptoms:
Muscle tension, tension headaches, irritability, fatigue, propensity to rush and hurry, panic from "too much work, too little time," and insomnia.

ExRx:
Obtain greater degrees of stress relief by increasing intensity and muscle involvement: from breathing, ROMs, and stretching to slow-motion circulation and low-intensity aerobic exercise. Exercise as prevention can make your body stress-hardy by reducing the time period of your stressful reactions (e.g. anxiety, fear, and muscular tension), and also by raising your stress threshold, making you less apt to have a severe stressful reaction. Exercise can even reverse stressful symptoms by slowing down and deepening your breathing, and by relaxing your muscles through tension and release. Exercise and relaxation reduce the stimulation of the adrenal gland, which produces stress hormones (e.g. adrenaline). Stress lowers norepinephrine levels in the brain; exercise boosts them up again. For obvious reasons, the best stress-reducing exercise is noncompetitive.

STUTTERING

Repeated hesitation and delay in uttering words; the inability to control your speech by not being able to pronounce certain words sometimes caused by too much tension in the mouth and vocal cords as you try to speak. Stuttering is not a dysfunction of the tongue and lips; it is a neurological disorder. The muscles of the tongue and lips merely obey the inappropriate orders of the brain.

Symptoms:
Excessive tension in the vocal cords and muscles involved in speech causes an attempt to make sounds that the locked vocal cords cannot create. Anxiety and frustration is accompanied by puckering lips and poking teeth with tongue to form words.

ExRx:
Specific relaxation techniques and retraining techniques are most useful, but overall body relaxation and breathing exercises may help over the long term. Two basic ways to exer-

cise include breathing techniques and tension-control exercises. Avoid weight lifting and other strength-training exercises that produce excessive muscle tension in the neck. Practice posture training and relaxation exercises of the muscles of the head and neck, as well as of the major muscle groups of the whole body. Relaxing the major muscles that surround the vocal cords can help the vocal cord muscles relax. Deep-breathing exercises while talking can help. Practice airflow technique—just before you talk, inhale, and blow out a short, silent stream of air. This temporarily relaxes your vocal cords before you start to talk. (Also see Head and Neck Rx, pp. 275–280, and upper body posture training in Chapter Seven.)

MEDICATION SIDE EFFECTS RX

The use of many medications has become standard practice for treating many diseases and conditions. They are often used to man-

TABLE 17.1
MEDICATIONS, SIDE EFFECTS, AND EFFECTIVE EXERCISES

Medications	*Side Effects*	*ExRx*
anticonvulsants; antidepressants; antipsychotics; hypnotics; sedatives	dizziness	balancing exercises; regular exercise
anticonvulsants; antidepressants; antipsychotics; hypnotics; sedatives; diuretics; antihypertensives	confusion/depression	relaxation exercise
antidepressants; antihistamines; antihypertensives; antipsychotics; beta-blockers; benzodiazepines	fatigue/weakness	aerobic exercises; increased physical activity
antiglaucoma agents; antiasthmatic agents; bronchodialators	increases in heart rate	relaxation exercise; intermittent exercise
antipsychotics; advenergics; adrenergics, levopopa; antidepressants	involuntary muscle movements	stretching; relaxation exercises
antipsychotics; antihypertensives; diuretics; narcotic analgesics/nitrates; levodopa; antidepressants; vasodialators	postural hypotension	balancing exercises; seated exercises
antichlorogenics; barbiturates; benzodiazepines; chlormazines; diuretics; phenothiazines	urinary incontinence	pelvic floor exercises

age symptoms such as pain, breathlessness, and depression. Exercise can help reduce the dosage of many medications and therefore the side effects associated with overconsumption of the medications.

ENERGY DRAIN

Many drugs can cause fatigue for purely physical reasons. Chemotherapy drugs, for example, cause anemia (which also causes fatigue) for a few days or weeks, as do alpha- and beta-blockers by suppressing the heart rate during exertion. Drugs must be metabolized (digested) by the body, or else they may attack body tissues (e.g. chemotherapy) and cause the need for repair. However, subjective symptoms of fatigue, lethargy, and so forth should not be equated with the energy required for metabolism. When the body works on itself for repair, digestion, and healing, it can also drain its own energy reserves.

Symptoms:
Fatigue and muscle weakness.

ExRx:
Regular exercise builds up energy reserves, similar to charging you car's battery, giving you a greater reserve with which to combat the side effects of drugs and the body's repair process. Exercise also permits lower dosages of many drugs and shortens the recovery time.

MEDICATION INTERACTIONS

Reactions, both during and after exercise, caused by prescribed medications. The reactions, linked to blood flow, heart rate, breathing, and body temperature, should be discussed and planned for with your doctor. Some medications, such as those for heart conditions, orthostatic hypotension, diabetes, and high blood pressure, are actually prerequisites for starting to exercise.

Symptoms:
See Table 17.1 for symptoms involved with medications.

ExRx:
To prevent symptoms, cool down gradually and over a longer period (five minutes or more, until your rate of breathing is back to normal, approximately twelve to twenty breaths per minute). Use exercise to prevent the dizzy or nauseous feeling you get when raising and lowering your head, as with bending over and straightening up. Raise your head more slowly and regain your balance before going on to the next exercise.

OVERHEATING REACTION

Some drugs interfere with the vasodilation (the relaxation of blood vessels) that allows more blood to flow to the skin surface where it can release your body heat. These medications are called heat-blockers. Other such drugs as antidepressants, antihistamines, chemotherapy drugs, decongestants, diuretics, glaucoma drugs, reanticholinergics, and some tranquilizers increase body heat by interfering with sweating or the brain's ability to regulate body temperature. These are called heat-makers. Drug reactions can cause heat stroke in summer and frostbite in winter.

Symptoms:
Nausea, sweating, and faintness.

ExRx:
Avoid getting overheated by reducing the intensity of your workout in extreme temper-

tures; drink fluids frequently. Avoid mineral loss—especially electrolytes (e.g. calcium, sodium, potassium, and magnesium) by drinking vegetable or tomato juice, even chicken soup. With heart disease drugs, drink electrolyte-enriched sports liquids and tepid, not cold, water.

IMMUNE DISEASES AND DISORDERS RX

Immune disorders cut across almost all the body's health systems. Common symptoms are fatigue, joint pain, and itchy skin. Many can be triggered or caused by psychological and physical stress. Regular exercise and relaxation exercise techniques can provide long- and short-term solutions to helping reduce or control the symptoms.

A trend has been shown in medical and scientific studies that light to moderate exercise increases your immune responses, while heavy, intense exercise training, including overtraining, may lead to immune suppression or even malfunction. This may explain the recurrent infections that competitive athletes experience during periods of maximum training and competition stress. Over the long run and during periods when there is no intensive activity, the infection rate might be lower. But over the short to medium term, medical literature shows that athletes are particularly susceptible to upper respiratory and skin infections.

Competitive—especially contact—sports may compromise the aspect of your immune system known as "host defense," both by reducing your physical protection and by impairing your immuno-surveillance. The skin's protective faculties are also impaired. For example, skin lacerations, vigorous sweating, and maceration of the dermis (softening or breaking down of tissue) impair the defense normally provided by the skin surface. Also, negative changes in soluble and cellular components of the immune system can increase susceptibility to infection. Finally, with strenuous training during infections, illness can heighten the severity of the disease process.

Over the short term, exercise can be used to gradually nurture and boost your immune response. In the long term, regular exercise provides a cumulative effect of making your body more stress-hardy.

ACQUIRED IMMUNE DEFICIENCY SYNDROME (AIDS)

Progressive weakening of the immune system makes you vulnerable to infections and unusual cancers. Caused by a retrovirus called HIV (human immunodeficiency virus) that infects white blood cells and others. Those who practice unprotected sex (i.e. without condoms), intravenous drug users, and blood transfusion recipients are at greatest risk.

Symptoms:
Sudden development of opportunistic infections, purple skin lesions, and fatigue. Also decreased food consumption and loss of weight and lean body mass, decreased immune system function, and body tissue wasting.

ExRx:
Too much intensity or exertion might fatigue the body, so moderate exercise is a safer bet especially when AIDS has manifested itself. However, exercise offers many benefits to the AIDS patient, including improved mental function, improved neuroendocrine function (the interaction between the nervous system and the endocrine system), and improved immune function. It also reduces the adverse

MICHAEL MCDONALD

DIAGNOSIS: AIDS

"I truly feel that I am successfully battling many of the symptoms usually associated with my illness," writes Michael McDonald, who was diagnosed with the HIV virus in 1985 and AIDS in 1992. "Although I have had some opportunistic infections, I believe my ability to recover has been greatly improved through staying active both physically and mentally."

Michael was working as a medical researcher when he found out he had HIV. He had been accepted to medical school but wanted to work in the field for a while to make certain it was what he wanted to do. Although Michael had always been physically fit—a competitive swimmer in both high school and college—after the diagnosis, he was only working and socializing. "I was working in the lab during the day and in bars at night. I was drinking—not excessively, just socially—and not paying attention to signs and symptoms," he says.

He continued seeing his general practitioner rather than an infectious disease specialist, which, he thinks in retrospect, would have helped him as his T-cell count dropped. (Recently, medication helped cure Michael of disseminated histoplasmosis, which ravages the lungs and other organs.) "But in Ohio, in 1985, AIDS was not talked about at all. It was easy for me to be in denial," he explains.

Healthy people have about 1,000 T-cells, which act as the disease scouts of the immune system, racing to check out a suspected foreign agent in the body, then calling for the killer cells to come and destroy it. HIV attacks the T-cells themselves. When there are less than 200 T-cells, the patient is diagnosed with AIDS. For the last two years, Michael has been living with no T-cells at all.

"I now have myself on a fairly regular exercise regimen to keep myself healthy," he says. Three to four times a week, Michael spends thirty to forty minutes doing aerobic exercise on a stair machine, stationary cycle, and treadmill. Then he proceeds to thirty to forty minutes of strength training using weight equipment. He does one or two sets of ten to twelve reps of

stressor-induced psychological and immunological reactions for nonsymptomatic HIV-1, and may increase CD-4 cell counts, which may slow down the disease's progress. Most important, exercise promotes a positive attitude and hardiness that appears to be so closely linked to long-term survival. People who are infected with HIV or who have AIDS should exercise regularly to build and maintain strength. This will help them manage symptoms of disease and the side effects of the many medications they take, and elevate their mood to better cope with the disease, which, at the moment, remains incurable. In Stage 1 AIDS (asymptomatic HIV positive), there are generally no limits on exercise. Strengthen muscles now to build up your reserve strength. Exercise may actually help each exercise in a full body workout, including chest presses, lat pull-downs, biceps curls, triceps extenders, leg presses, leg curls, crunches, and leg stretching.

For the last two years, Michael has also been practicing chi kung, a form of movement similar to tai chi but that focuses on meditation, breathing, and posture as well as on movement. "It's a wonderful exercise. I always thought this stuff was kooky 'til I started getting involved with it. I am taking low doses of prednisone to help reduce the swelling of Reiter's syndrome, an infectious arthritis like rheumatoid arthritis. Drugs like this take a toll on your kidneys, and using the techniques of chi kung I visualize moving chi—life energy—to that area.

"There is all this energy in the world, in the sky, the clouds and the trees. According to Chinese medicine, this energy comes in through the top of your head and moves things around. The whole thing is about balance. Nobody said it's a cure but it is a healing process," he explains.

When Michael was diagnosed with HIV, he was also told he probably only had two years to live, so he decided not to start medical school. "When I didn't die, I went back to school," he says. Rather than medical school, Michael decided to concentrate on exercise physiology.

At present, Michael is the personal trainer on a Ohio State University study, which is determining the effects of exercise on immunodeficient syndromes. So far, twenty-five volunteers have joined the twelve-week exercise program. Michael believes in the benefits of exercise for patients. "There's not one that hasn't reported a better state of mind, with less depression and anxiety. They all want to do a maintenance program. . . . People with terminal diseases are constantly stressed, facing new challenges and losing control. At the very least, exercise is a way to relieve some of that stress," he writes.

Michael also teaches water aerobics parttime and travels the country as a public speaker. Because he is at risk from infection, he makes sure to wash his hands frequently and not eat uncooked food. "We used to think that once all your T-cells were gone, you were dead. Now there are many people out there living without T-cells for many years. It takes work but it can be done."

delay the onset of symptoms. However, be cautious not to exercise too intensely because exhaustion may overtax your system. In Stage 2 AIDS (early symptomatic HIV), reduce your exercise intensity, lower your heart-training rate to 50 to 70% of max. Continue to exercise, including relaxation exercises to diminish the severity and frequency of selected symptoms. In Stage 3 (full-blown AIDS), dramatically reduce the intensity and duration of exercise. Postpone exercising until after peak fatigue periods.

ANKYLOSING SPONDYLITIS

Progressive inflammatory disease, which affects the spine and related soft tissue; begins in lower back and progresses up the spine to the neck. Bone and cartilage deteriorate; spine and joints become fused (grow together).

Symptoms:
Limited range of motion in lower spine, lower back pain, chest pain, and limited chest expansion, pain and tenderness over inflamed sites, accompanying arthritis in hips, shoulders, knees; mild fatigue; hip deformity; and curvature of the spine. Symptoms progress in stages, unpredictably disappearing and then flaring up again.

ExRx:
Practice posture exercises (see Chapter Seven, Age Ex). Avoid leaning over for long periods of time to minimize back stress. Do ROMs, back stretching and strengthening exercises, and deep-breathing exercises. Water exercise or swimming provides the best back and spine support with least amount of pain. (Also see Chapter Fourteen, MuSkel Rx.)

Atopic Dermatitis

A chronic skin inflammation with intense itching, which can appear at any age but usually strikes during infancy to early childhood and early adulthood with later flare-ups in late childhood and early adolescence. It may disappear and then reappear. Cause can be metabolic, or may be biochemical-induced and genetically linked to elevated serum immunoglobulin E levels or defective T-cell function. Affects 0.7% of population, usually those that also have allergies.

Symptoms:
Scratching intensifies itching and results in red lesions, also accompanied by severe skin infections.

ExRx:
Practice meticulous skin care, drug therapy, and avoidance of allergens. Use deep-breathing and relaxation exercises to avoid, slow down, or control stressful reactions.

PSYCHE-IMMUNE RX: LIST OF ADDITIONAL SKIN DISORDERS BENEFITED BY EXERCISE

- acne
- allergic contact dermatitis
- impetigo (bacterial skin infections)
- genital herpes
- gonorrhea

Cancer and Cancer Treatment

Not a single disease, but hundreds of diseases that involve abnormal cellular proliferation to various body areas forming tumors or masses that destroy organs and tissues. The treatments can be local or systemwide; many associated side effects, with both radiation and/or chemotherapy.

Symptoms:
Weakness and pain in the affected areas; symptoms vary with the different forms of the disease. Radiation causes loss of flexibility and mobility of joints and organs from scarring, in addition to edema (i.e. swelling of joints and limbs). Chemotherapy can cause anemia, peripheral nerve damage, cardiomyopathy, and pulmonary fibrosis (lung tissue scarring). Tolerance for exercise is often limited by lower endurance, muscle atrophy and frailty, reduced range of motion in surgical areas (chest mastectomy), and edema and gout from nerve damage to feet.

FAYE RASCH

DIAGNOSIS: CHRONIC FATIGUE SYNDROME

Faye Rasch is at present a nineteen-year-old NYU student. While still in high school, she repeatedly went to her doctor with complaints of general exhaustion and fatigue. "I'd have nine hours of sleep at night and would still be tired," she writes.

During her senior year in high school, she was diagnosed with a type of CFS called Epstein-Barr. She had to have a B_{12} injection in her shoulder once a week, which caused a lot of pain, discomfort, and also negatively affected Faye's ability to practice karate, which she began during that same year. Faye's mother did some research and found certain dietary supplements that were comparable to the injections, and Faye started taking the supplements and stopped the injections.

Faye says she has been told there is no cure for Epstein-Barr, but the vitamins and her karate are helping her manage the symptoms. She does her karate workout four times a week. It is very intense, involving kicking, punching, and blocking. There is also one-on-one sparring and going through specific forms.

Faye says karate makes her feel better. "I felt more awake after I left than when I got there," she explains.

It may have some connection to the extreme liveliness of her chosen sport, because walking on a treadmill almost puts her to sleep. Karate requires a lot of concentration and energy from its participants. "The more you stimulate your brain synapses, the more you wake your mind up," she says.

As a youth, Faye danced for exercise, but she does not recall fatigue being a problem then. "I think I didn't have [Epstein-Barr] yet," she states.

Regarding her syndrome, she says, "They tested me again recently, and it has gotten better."

ExRx:

Regular exercise may help prevent or delay the onset of certain cancers. Exercise is also an appropriate therapy for rehabilitating and maintaining the physical and psychological fitness of cancer patients as well as coping with depression and the side effects of treatments. It is very important to avoid exercising to exhaustion when you are undergoing any type of cancer therapy. The goal is to return a cancer patient to a healthy, active lifestyle and restore the function of damaged limbs and body areas as well as improve strength and endurance and increase physical reserves.

CHRONIC FATIGUE SYNDROME (CFS)

Also called "yuppie flu" because it affects mostly adults under age forty-five, 75% are usually women. It has been classified both as a medical and a psychiatric condition. Possibly a reaction to viral illness, but must be studied further as to its exercise connections and benefits. Initial studies show that CFS patients have higher perceived exertion scores in relation to their heart rates than the sedentary control subjects. May also include fibromyalgia symptoms (see p. 303).

Symptoms:
Mimics mononucleosis; usually a prolonged, overwhelming fatigue (especially after exercise), muscle weakness, low-grade fever, pain in glands, insomnia, joint pain, poor concentration and memory, irritability, depression, sleep disturbance, sensitivity to light, and frequent sore throats and headaches.

ExRx:
No known cure, but some experimental drug treatments have shown progress: antiviral—acyclovir; antianxiety—Xanex; and antidepressants—Tagamet. Best possibilities are to manage symptoms by avoiding irritants, resting, and gradually introducing a progressive, slow to moderate exercise program to both maintain basic fitness and possibly build back up to normal level. Avoid high-intensity exercise. Moderate exercise training can improve overall symptoms but watch for increased fatigue after initial training session and during the first few weeks. CFS is an extreme form of the symptoms experienced by out of shape, inactive, and often overweight people who may also smoke and drink excessively. Great care should be given in prescribing an exercise program that does not further weaken the patient. Even though CFS patients show normal muscle physiology before and after exercise and normal fatigability and metabolism at intracellular and systemic levels, there are important differences: CFS patients were unable to fully activate their muscles during intense, sustained exercise, suggesting that muscle fatigue is an important central component of CFS. Thus, low-intensity muscle strengthening and stretching, posture training, and deep breathing exercises, along with slow walking, may be enough to keep CFS patients healthy and sensibly prepare them for further exertion. Exercise may also have a psychogenic component. Slowly increase the intensity and duration of exercise. It is very important as part of bringing the patient back to an active lifestyle. (For rehab see Cardio Rx, p. 421 and Chapter Fourteen, MuSkel Rx)

DERMATOMYOSITIS AND POLYMYOSITIS

Rare, often fatal, severe inflammatory disorders that produce weakness in skeletal muscles—primarily the neck, pharynx, shoulder, and pelvic muscles—rather than distal muscles (e.g. hands and feet). Dermatomyositis is characterized by muscle weakness with skin rashes and lesions; polymyositis has the same symptoms but no rashes. Seven-year average survival among adults; 80 to 90% of children regain normal function, however. Middle-aged women constitute 66% of sufferers of these diseases.

Symptoms:
Similar to muscular dystrophy, psoriasis, and systemic lupus. There is muscle weakness, tenderness, and discomfort, which impairs normal activities (e.g. climbing stairs, raising the head from a pillow, or getting up from a chair). The first symptom is usually a red rash that erupts on the face, neck, upper back, chest, and arms. Leads to muscle contracture, atrophy, and tissue death. Nausea, weight loss, and fever can also accompany other symptoms.

ExRx:
Get bed rest during the acute phase, and apply heat to relieve muscle spasms. Practice ROMs and slow-paced, circulatory exercises during remission stage to prevent muscle contracture and to help you to regain normal muscle strength. (For rehab, see Chapter Fourteen, MuSkel Rx.)

HIVES

Eruptions on skin in reaction to drug, food, insect stings, or inhaled allergens (e.g. animal danders, cosmetics). Occurs in approximately 20% of the population.

Symptoms:
Some swelling, itching, or burning.

ExRx:
Drug therapy and preventing trigger factors. Hives does not limit exercise capacity, nor is it aggravated by exercise. Symptoms can be controlled or avoided with deep-breathing and relaxation exercises. (For rehab, see Chapter Seventeen, Psyche Rx)

JUVENILE RHEUMATOID ARTHRITIS

An inflammatory disease of joints and connective tissues. Also affects skin, heart, lungs, liver, spleen, and eyes. At any given time, it affects up to a quarter-million children under age sixteen. There are three major types: systemic, polyarticular, and pauciarticular.

Symptoms:
Vary according to type. Systemic involves mild arthritis with fever and rash, irritability, listlessness, and fever spikes. With the polyarticular type, many joints become swollen, tender, stiff; listlessness; weight loss can mimic severe rheumatoid arthritis. The pauciarticular type involves inflammation of a few joints, stiffness in morning or after inactivity periods, and imbalanced joint development.

ExRx:
Anti-inflammatory drugs, physical therapy, along with a carefully planned diet and exercise program with parent-child participation. Maintain joint mobility through ROMs, stretching, and strengthening exercises.

LUPUS ERYTHEMATOSUS

Chronic inflammation of connective tissues. Affects nine times more women than men, and can worsen during pregnancy. There are two forms: discoid lupus erythematosus (DLE), which affects only the skin and is more common; and systemic lupus erythematosis (SLE), which affects all organs and is more serious and potentially fatal. The main cause is an autoimmune dysfunction in which the body works against itself by producing antibodies against its own cells. Other causes include genetic, hormonal, and environmental factors. Physical (e.g. sunlight exposure) and mental stress also play a role, along with viral infections, in the disease's development.

Symptoms:
Recurring flare-ups—especially in spring and summer—of joint stiffness, fatigue, fever, anemia, weight loss, rashes and skin lesions, and pain in joints (similar to rheumatoid arthritis). The more serious form can cause renal failure, pleurisy, and pericarditis.

ExRx:
Protect against sun exposure during outdoor activities (wear a sunscreen, hat, clothing,

and cover-up). Practice such moderate activities as golf, gardening, walking, and some swimming. Take frequent rests. Exercise only after you are rested. Because vigorous exercise can depress the immune system, avoid high-impact, high-ballistic exercises that also put too much stress on joints; instead do moderate-intensity, low-impact exercises. Practice ROMs and frequent postural alignment exercises to protect joint mobility and reduce joint stress. Apply heat packs after exercise to relieve joint pain and stiffness. Mild symptoms usually require no or little medication (e.g. aspirin, corticoid creams for acute flare-ups, and corticosteroids. For rehab see Chapter Fourteen, MuSkel Rx and Chapter Fifteen, Meta Rx.)

Organ Transplant

A major surgery that replaces a diseased, dysfunctioning organ with a healthy organ. This surgery is performed at the end stages of organ failure for kidney, heart, lung, and also for the pancreas in Type I diabetes.

Symptoms:
Side effects of immunosuppressant medication (necessary for post-organ transplant patients) include hypertension and also muscle weakness and reduced bone density. Individuals are also typically very out of condition as the result of the progress of the disease, as well as the surgery recuperation period.

ExRx:
Exercise can still significantly improve aerobic capacity, blood pressure control, and also increase muscular strength and reduce the fat-to-muscle ratio. Watch out for early leg fatigue, then switch to upper body exercises and back to legs afterward. Nonweight-bearing, seated, or lying exercises, will help in-phase joint pain caused by immunosuppressant drugs. Gradually progress to such weight-bearing activities and exercises as cooking and even jogging. Strength-training programs should also progress at a slower rate with a lower level of repetitions: one to six per exercise.

Psoriatic Arthritis

Rheumatoidlike arthritis accompanied by psoriasis of skin and nails; usually mild, with intermittent flare-ups. Affects men and women equally, onset is between ages thirty and thirty-five.

Symptoms:
Skin lesions usually precede arthritic component, but with full syndrome, lesions and arthritis occur together. Also general malaise, fever, and the eyes can also be affected.

ExRx:
Immobilization through splints or bed rest protects affected joints and reduces pain from movements. When pain subsides, practice ROMs, stretching, strengthening, and low-impact exercises. Avoid overexposure to sun. Practice such circulatory or aerobic exercises as water exercise, swimming, walking, and intersperse with seated exercises, for example cycling and rowing.

Reiter's Syndrome

An immune disorder that is a milder form of polyarthritis usually affecting men between the ages of twenty and forty. May be related to sexually transmitted or intestinal infections. Arthritic symptoms follow these diseases in weight-bearing joints and last from two to four months.

Symptoms:
Frequent and difficult urination with pus, mucus, and discharge from penis, painless ulcers on penis, and groin pain. Also, muscle wasting around arthritic joints, accompanied by joint swelling and skin lesions.

ExRx:
Doctor-prescribed corticosteroid therapy; recovery in two to sixteen weeks, with a 50% chance of recurring attacks. Do extra warm-ups with an emphasis on ROM exercises, followed by stretching and strengthening, especially for affected joint areas. Then, regular, moderate aerobic exercise performed with good posture techniques to preserve joints. Maintain good posture throughout the day. (For rehab, see Meta Rx, pp. 364–366.)

RHEUMATOID ARTHRITIS

This autoimmune disorder is a chronic inflammatory and potentially crippling disease that attacks the joints of the hands, arms, and feet and the surrounding ligaments, muscles, tendons, and blood vessels. Affects 6.5 million Americans, and can occur at any age. Women, ages thirty to sixty constitute 75% of sufferers; 10% are totally disabled. There is no cure or prevention, but you can manage the symptoms and slow down the progress of the disease while you regain strength and relieve pain. Different from osteoarthritis (see p. 307), which is a muscle and bone disorder linked to the aging process.

Symptoms:
Initially, unpredictable and spontaneous flare-ups and remissions of such nonspecific symptoms as fatigue, malaise, loss of appetite, and low-grade fever. Later, joint stiffness, swelling, and tenderness in fingers, wrists, knees, elbows, and ankles especially after inactivity and when rising in the morning. Eventually, joints ache even at rest. There are a variety of other symptoms: carpal tunnel syndrome, numbness, tingling, weakness in feet and hands, jaw pain (TMJ), and related earaches. Also, such cardio, pulmonary, and eye problems as pericarditis and iridocyclitis.

ExRx:
Aspirin and anti-inflammatory medications help relieve joint pain. Use ice packs for acute pain, moist heat if it is mild. Extra sleep (eight to ten hours) and frequent rest periods between activities help restore strength and relieve pain. Perform any activity or exercise slowly, at your own pace, and take frequent rests in between movements. Change your posture frequently from prone to seated to standing to distribute the work load over as many body areas as possible to maximize energy use and minimize pain. Use medication to help promote mobility and avoid too much inactivity. Use hot baths and showers at bedtime, in the morning (and throughout the day as needed) to reduce the need for medications. Practice postural correction techniques often—not only as a muscle-strengthening exercise, but also to reduce the pressure on joints in any position. Practice these postural exercises while walking, standing, sitting, or lying down. Sleep on your back on a firm mattress. Despite its painfulness, exercise is important and will help you overcome pain by increasing the muscle strength and flexibility around affected joints and by improving blood circulation. Use assisted-exercise techniques and single- or isolated-limb and single-digit exercises to limit the stress on other joints. Depending on the severity, joint reconstruction and replacement may be necessary.

JACK STUPP

DIAGNOSIS: RHEUMATOID ARTHRITIS

In 1980, at age fifty-four, Jack Stupp was diagnosed with rheumatoid arthritis and hospitalized with over twenty swollen joints. Five months later, confined to a wheelchair and taking twenty pain-killers daily, he was released and told not to exercise, as his doctors believed that exercise would worsen his condition. He was forced to use heavy gloves to open jars and a stick with a comb on the end because he couldn't lift his arms high enough to comb his hair. Doctors told him he would spend the rest of his life that way, and for the next three years he did.

In 1983, Jack went to Las Vegas for a trade show, then headed down to Arizona for a little rest and relaxation. There, he heard about a health resort called the Canyon Ranch and decided to give it a try. For three days he "sat around" taking steambaths, to no avail, then decided to go home. A fitness director found out about his decision and offered to work with him one-on-one. Jack decided to give it a try.

He checked into the Canyon Ranch, where the fitness director started him off with light stretches in a swimming pool, where the buoyancy of the water took some of the pressure off his joints. Five days later, he tried to go on a walk, his first in over three years, but couldn't even make it one-tenth of a mile. After two more weeks in the pool, Jack led the Canyon Ranch daily two-mile walk. In addition to the stretching, Jack credits his remarkable recovery to Arizona's dry climate and the stress-free environment.

Jack left his wheelchair in Arizona and returned to Toronto. His doctor there told him not to get too excited because Toronto's humidity and Jack's stressful lifestyle would bring back the pain and swelling. Three weeks later, Jack could still walk, but not as well, so he went back to the Canyon Ranch for two more weeks. For the next ten years, Jack would make three to four such trips a year. Each time he discontinued his exercises when he returned home.

Then, in 1990, Jack was diagnosed with spinal stenosis—a portion of his spine had closed, causing problems with his legs—so he underwent an operation to open his spine up.

SCLERODERMA

A degenerative, fibrotic (causing overgrowth of scar tissue), and occasionally inflammatory disease of connective tissues.

Symptoms:
Begins with Raynaud's disease (see p. 409), which manifests as white, blue, and reddish discoloration of the fingers and toes when they are exposed to cold, which can lead to ulcers and gangrene. Later, chronic ulcerations, pain, stiffness, and swelling of fingers and toes, as well as thickening and tightening of skin on face (including unnatural pinching of mouth and muscle contractures), esophagitis (inflammation of the esophagus), bowel movement difficulties, kidney and related high blood pressure problems, and hand debilitation. Also, gastrointestinal (e.g. diarrhea, bloating after meals) and respiratory

During 1992 he had a total knee replacement, and in 1993 he had the other knee replaced.

Six months after having his second knee replaced, Jack attended a ten-day seminar in Cancun, Mexico led by motivational speaker Anthony (Tony) Robbins. Each day, Jack attended meetings that lasted from ten a.m. to four a.m., and sat in pain. Every few hours the seminar organizers played what Jack calls "jump music" and the participants all got up and jumped and stretched for a few minutes to keep their minds alert and bodies comfortable. Jack sat and watched during these periods. But on the fifth day, he got up and jumped like he hadn't since he was first hospitalized thirteen years prior. When Jack told Tony this, Tony agreed that "movement will change your state" and took Jack on stage in front of 1,200 people.

On the last night of the seminar, the organizers set up a "fire-walk," forty feet of red-hot coals for the participants to walk across. Jack looked at it and thought, "Yeah, right," to himself, then ended up going ahead. He said his legs have since "turned around completely." Afterward, Jack flew straight to Arizona from Cancun and did a power aerobics class for the first time in his life—at age sixty-six. He also started an intense weight-training program and continued stretching.

This time when Jack returned to Toronto, he continued to exercise and now exercises for three hours daily—an hour of stretching, forty-five to sixty minutes of treadmill fast walking, and an hour of weights (on a three-day split). When he started weight training at the Canyon Ranch, his bench press max was forty pounds. At present, at the age of seventy, on the days he works his chest, Jack does three sets of twelve reps at 165 pounds.

Jack speaks across the country at schools and hospitals and has become a source of inspiration for people nationwide. He plans to open his first gym in a chain he is starting called Women's Fitness Club of Canada. Sixteen years ago, Jack Stupp was confined to a wheelchair and a life of inactivity. Look at him now!

problems (e.g. irregular heartbeat and shortness of breath).

ExRx:
No cure; treat the various symptoms to preserve normal body functions and reduce complications. Practice face and mouth stretching exercises and protect yourself from cold with warm clothing—keep mittens by your refrigerator to remove ice cubes and other cold items. Avoid skin infections because they will heal very slowly. Be cautious of sharp objects, keep your nails trimmed, and use exercise gloves. Keep skin dry of sweat but moisturized, and protected against abrasion and blistering. If you notice any foot or hand skin soreness, stop the activity and check your skin. Practice circulatory and aerobic exercises to increase the blood flow to hands and feet to prevent Raynaud's. For the same

reason, quit smoking cigarettes, which causes reduced blood flow. (For rehab, see Chapter Sixteen, Cardio Rx, and Chapter Seventeen, Psyche Rx)

SEXUAL DISORDERS RX

Psychological stress lies at the center of many sexual disorders, which is why this topic is part of the Psyche-Immune chapter. The body's reaction to stress is to secrete the chemical "cortisol," which suppresses the production of sex hormones. Stress also causes the constriction of peripheral arteries, thereby decreasing blood flow to your genitals and inhibiting sexual arousal.

SEXUAL THERAPY EXERCISES

Specific aerobic, strengthening, stretching, relaxation, and cardio exercise can help improve sexual performance and reduce symptoms related to sexual disorders. The recommended exercises for sexual therapy are aerobic exercises for increased endurance, blood flow, and production of endorphins. Strengthening exercises for the midriff, the abs, and buttocks, and Kegel exercises (see pp. 380–382) are also recommended because aerobic and continuous motion exercises such as walking and cycling increase the blood flow to genitalia.

By strengthening the muscles used in the sex act, both men and women gain better control of themselves and avoid or reduce their chances of having a sexual disorder. Exercise also brings better blood flow to the genitalia, strengthening the blood vessels that serve this area. It helps stimulate hormone production. If men accumulate too much excess fat, it converts their sex hormone, testosterone, into the female sex hormone, estrogen, which can flatten a man's libido. Sexual desire decreases, as does the firmness of erections. Testicles may even atrophy. Weight reduction (by exercise *and* diet) can reverse this process.

Similar to underexercising, overexercising can impede healthy sexuality. It can suppress a woman's menstrual cycle and estrogen flow. Many professional or competitive women athletes don't ovulate. During peak training periods, exercise can shrink a woman's vagina, and dry out and thin its lining. Overexercising can also make a man too exhausted to have an erection.

Because many sexual problems arise from a poor body image, reducing your body fat can help improve your self-image. This, in turn, can improve your sex life because you feel better about yourself, which makes you more open to possibilities, and, ultimately, makes you more desirable.

AROUSAL AND ORGASMIC DISORDERS

With an arousal disorder, a woman cannot reach or maintain the physical responses of sexual excitement, for example vaginal lubrication, blood vessel congestion in the genitalia, and the swelling of the external genitalia. With an orgasmic disorder, intense anxiety, depression, relationship problems, psychological disturbances, stress, fatigue, or drug and alcohol abuse inhibits a woman's ability to experience sexual orgasm.

Symptoms:
Little or erratic response to sexual stimulation.

ExRx:
Lower trunk-bending and stretching exercises, including Kegel exercises (pp. 380–382) and pelvic tilt exercise (see p. 203).

IMPOTENCE

The inability of a man to reach or maintain an erection sufficient to complete sexual intercourse. In primary impotence, a man has never achieved a sufficient erection. In secondary impotence (the more common and less serious), the man has achieved erections in the past, despite a present disability. Affects all age groups, but is more common with advancing age. Personal feelings of guilt, fear, inadequacy, interpersonal conflicts of preference, lack of communication, and ignorance of sexual functions are all contributing factors.

Symptoms:
Inability to achieve a full erection, combined with anxiety, sweating, palpitations, and sometimes extreme depression.

ExRx:
Practice sexual foreplay "games" that restrict full sexual activity, but encourage having fun, experiencing pleasure, and improving communication. Exercise with a partner. Aerobic exercises improve blood flow to the genitalia and reduce a stress response. Strengthening exercises in the lying-down position (e.g. abdominal and lower back) can also be helpful. In some cases, a counselor may also be helpful.

PAINFUL SEXUAL INTERCOURSE

This is usually a female physical problem rather than a psychological barrier. The physical problems range from an intact hymen to an acute infection of the vagina, bladder, or anal area.

Symptoms:
From mild aches to severe pain during and after sexual intercourse.

ExRx:
For psychological problems, practice sensory-control exercises. Also, deemphasize full sexual intercourse, instead focusing on fun, arousal, and foreplay. Kegel exercises can also help in strengthening and conditioning the genital area (see pp. 380–382).

PREMATURE EJACULATION

Inability by a man to control the ejaculation reflex during sexual intercourse. Occurs in all men of all age groups and most are quite healthy. This condition is completely reversible.

Symptoms:
A man is unable to prolong foreplay; he ejaculates before or as soon as penetration occurs.

ExRx:
Practice Kegel exercise (pp. 380–382), in addition to lower abdominal, and pelvic tilt exercises to strengthen and improve lower back, hip, abdominal, and pelvic muscles. Insight therapy, behavioral techniques, and practice sessions with a sex therapist are recommended.

VAGINISMUS

Spasms of lower vaginal muscles usually caused by fear of sexual penetration.

Symptoms:
Vaginal pain upon partial penetration by a male's penis.

ExRx:
Tense and relax pelvic muscles while a doctor or physical therapist inserts a graduated series of dilators into the vagina. (Also see Kegel exercises, pp. 380–382.)

WRIST, HAND, AND FINGER INJURIES RX

Wrist, hand, and finger injuries are part of the Psyche-Immune chapter because the exercise prescriptions for these injuries should be done as slowly and carefully and in a relaxed position. Any type of wrist, hand, or finger pain that lasts more than two weeks should be seen by an orthopedist, preferably a wrist and hand specialist.

Wrist, hand, and finger injuries most often result from falls that occur during skating, rollerblading, horseback riding, bicycling, and skiing or from frequent snap-and-twist motions caused by swinging at an object in such sports as bowling, rowing, and weight lifting. Also, overuse injuries such as carpal tunnel syndrome and ulnar tunnel syndrome can be caused by gripping objects, for example handle bars, racquet handles, sticks, and bats for too much time or with too much pressure.

The key to protecting yourself from the damaging and debilitating effects of hand, finger, and wrist injuries is early detection and immediate cessation of the aggravating activity. Also, you should learn to fall properly, avoiding outstretched hands.

Those therapeutic and rehab exercises used for fingers, hand, and wrist injuries can also be used for therapy and rehab for joint damage caused by arthritis.

GENERAL REHABILITATION GUIDELINES AND PROCEDURES

PHASE I: FOR ACUTE INJURIES

1. After surgery, the physical therapist will use either active- or passive-assisted exercise. Passive will consist of four to six major range of moving the injury body area in the four ranges of motion: flexion extension, supination, and pronation.
2. After you are able to move the injured area unassisted, the physical therapist will supervise unassisted ROMs and then isometric exercises on the muscles that are connected to the injured body area.

PHASE II: FOR MODERATE TO SEVERE INJURIES

1. When you are able to move the injured body area and you can do isometric exercises with your own strength and without undue pain, begin Phase II exercises.
2. Phase II exercises (bend/extend, flexion) are those that let you bend and strengthen the body area through the full range of its motion.

PHASE III: FOR MILD INJURIES

These involve dynamic exercises to strengthen muscles as well as stretch them through a full range of motion. They also involve regaining balance and motor-sensory pronation. After this phase in completed, you may begin the three levels of preventive and conditioning exercises in Part Two.

WEIGHT-LOADING EXERCISES

The amount of weight that you add depends on your own body weight and on your muscle strength and size. Here are the general guidelines. In general, do not use any weights until your doctor or physical therapist says that it is okay. Weight-loading exercises can then be added in Phase II and III of the rehab schedule.

WEIGHT LOAD/REPETITION SCHEDULE

	LOAD	REPETITIONS
Phase I	No weight	Determined by MD or PT
Phase II	See schedule	1–5
Phase III	See schedule	6–12

WEIGHT-LOADING SCHEDULE
USE FOR PHASES II AND III

	AMOUNT OF WEIGHT		
TYPE OF WEIGHT	SMALL FRAME	MEDIUM FRAME	LARGE FRAME
Hand-held	0–¼ lbs.	¼–½ lbs.	½–1 lbs.
Ankle	0–½ lbs.	½–1 lbs.	1–5 lbs.

ACUTE WRIST, HAND, AND FINGER INJURIES RX

COLLES FRACTURE

A crack or break of the lower radius bone in the forearm. The most common wrist fracture in adults over age thirty. Caused by contact sports and falling accidents.

Symptoms:
Pain, swelling, tenderness, deformity on the thumbside of the lower forearm.

ExRx:
A comminuted fracture (in which the bones are broken into small fragments) is difficult to heal without a cast or surgical attachment to hand (e.g., placing pins in the bones and attaching a rod between them). Because the cast leaves the hand, fingers, and forearm free to exercise, Phase I can begin for these parts. When the cast is removed, Phase I exercises for the wrist can begin. There is three to six months of rehabilitation and conditioning exercises before the injured wrist can be used in sports play.

FINGER DISLOCATIONS

A finger bone is forced out of position at the joint and often includes ligament sprain. Caused by a direct blow to the end of the finger.

Symptoms:
Popping sensation, pain, tenderness, loss of mobility, and deformity of joint.

ExRx:
Immobilize and apply ice, but do not try to realign the finger yourself as it may be broken. Seek medical attention instead. Doctor may realign joint and/or splint for three weeks. Six to twelve weeks are needed for recovery and rehab. Begin Phase I Rehab with a doctor's approval and continue through each phase of rehab.

HOOK OF HAMATE FRACTURE

A break in the hamate bone located over the wrist crease on the outside of the wrist. Caused by a single blow (i.e. the impact of the handle of a bat, racquet, or stick, or a karate chop), or by repetitive impact in golf, cycling, and so forth.

Symptoms:
Pain and tenderness of the outer edge or heel of the hand, weakened grip, and numbness in the little finger.

ExRx:
Surgery is usually essential and about four weeks in a cast. Hand, finger, thumb, and forearm exercises can begin one week into the cast-wearing period. Phase I Rehab for wrist begins after cast is removed and progresses through Phases II and III for four to six weeks of rehab.

JAMMED FINGER (FINGER SPRAIN)

A stretch or tear of finger ligaments or a tearing off of a portion of the joint bone caused by a bending back or a direct blow to finger (e.g. by a ball hitting a finger or the impact of a fall).

Symptoms:
Pain, swelling, and loss of finger movement.

ExRx:
Immobilize finger, seek medical attention, and apply ice for twenty minutes at a time. Doctor will prescribe plastic splint for one to two weeks and, afterward, allow you to "buddy tape" the injured finger to a healthy one during rehab period. If bone is torn (avulsion fracture), surgery is necessary, followed by finger immobilization for three weeks, then a protective splint for another three weeks. Hand and wrist Rx rehabilitation can take twelve weeks.

MALLET FINGER

The ripping away of the tendon that extends to the front end of the finger from the bone to which it is attached. Caused by a direct hit (e.g. by a baseball) that bends back your fingertip. Unless treated, this injury can cause permanent deformity.

Symptoms:
Pain on last finger joint and inability to move it.

ExRx:
Immobilize, apply ice, and seek medical attention. Doctor will splint finger, which will remain splinted for six to eight weeks. If a portion of finger joint (bone/cartilage) is torn, surgery is necessary to reattach, followed by up to twelve weeks of rest, and then hand and wrist Rx rehabilitation exercises begin. You should "buddy tape" injured finger to adjoining healthy one for extra protection when you return to sports play.

METACARPAL FRACTURE

Cracks or breaks of the bones at the base of the fingers. The two most common are the thumb and little finger fractures. Caused by punching too hard or by a forceful bending back of the fingers in a fall (common in field and court sports and in skiing, skating, and gymnastics).

Symptoms:
Extreme pain when moving thumb and thickening of the fifth knuckle.

ExRx:
Immobilize hand and finger with arm sling, get medical attention, apply ice for twenty minutes at a time. Immobilize little finger or thumb for six to eight weeks or three to six weeks, if surgery has been performed. Then begin hand and wrist Rx rehabilitation exercises.

SCAPHOID BONE FRACTURE (CARPONAVICULAR FRACTURE)

A crack or break of the scaphoid bone (located between the wrist and forearm bone); caused by an outstretched arm that forcefully bends up and back. Occurs most often in young athletes engaged in contact sports.

Symptoms:
Pain and tenderness in the crater between the two thumb tendons especially when your thumb is pulled backward; also swelling, bruising, and loss of mobility of the hand and wrist.

ExRx:
Apply ice lightly until you get medical assistance. Thumb must be immobilized by either a short- or long-arm (i.e. over the elbow) cast. Hand, finger, and forearm exercises can begin while the arm is still in a cast.

THUMB SPRAIN (SKIER'S THUMB)

An overstretching or tear of the ligaments that connect the metacarpal bone to the first thumb bone. Common injury when a skier falls because pole strap pulls the thumb back too far.

Symptoms:
Pain, tenderness, swelling, and bruising around the lower thumb joint.

ExRx:
Mild and moderate sprains require three weeks immobilization followed by hand and wrist Rx rehabilitation. Severe sprains (i.e. ruptures) are surgically repaired and require eight to twelve weeks of recovery, including wearing a protective thumb splint.

WRIST DISLOCATION

A dislocation of the ulna bone in which two or more of the eight wrist bones (carpals) press against one another, causing them to pop in and out. This is caused by a fall that overbends the hand backward or forward.

Symptoms:
Lump at the wrist and palm or knuckle side of hand; pain, swelling, tenderness, and loss of motion in the wrist and hand.

ExRx:
Immobilize the injured wrist, and put that arm in a sling. Seek medical attention for nonsurgical treatment. For first-degree (mild) and second-degree (moderate) injuries, begin Phase I for hand, fingers, thumb, and forearm, when pain permits, which is usually about one week after injury. Use ice for swelling and soreness from exercise sessions. For third-degree injuries (severe), recovery can take three to six months.

WRIST SPRAIN

A stretch or tear of ligaments around the wrist holding together either the radius and ulna bones or the eight carpals. Caused by a forceful backbend of the hand (e.g. a fall).

Symptoms:
Immediate pain over wrist joint, swelling within an hour.

ExRx:
First, rest and ice; for first-degree (mild) and second-degree (moderate) sprains begin Phase I or II rehab; for third-degree injuries, (severe) a splint is required, which can be removed after one week to begin Phase I

exercises. If the swelling continues, keep each exercise session short, but frequent. Recovery time is one week for mild; six to twelve weeks for moderate to severe.

Overuse Wrist and Hand Injuries

Carpal Tunnel Syndrome

A common form of wrist nerve entrapment, which is caused by a buildup of pressure on the median nerve that passes through the tunnel underneath the wrist. It is often the result of the excessive use of the wrist in such activities as cycling, typing, and holding too tightly on to exercise rails and handles. Occurs most often in middle-aged women usually with no readily apparent cause.

Symptoms:
Numbness, tingling, and pain in the fingers; often grows worse during the night. Sometimes accompanied by weakness in the thumb.

ExRx:
For mild to moderate symptoms, cease the aggravating activity; rest and ice. Seek medical attention. Doctor will prescribe anti-inflammatories, splinting, and sometimes cortisone injections. Rest hands and wrists for one to two weeks and wear a wrist splint, day and night. As therapy, avoid grasping, twisting, and flexing; slow down repetitive activities, shake out hands, and dangle your arms by your sides. For severe symptoms, surgery may be necessary. When nonsurgical, begin Phase II exercises as soon as the pain subsides. Continue for about two weeks, along with rest, ice, and splinting. After surgery, within one week begin with gentle ROM exercises for hand, fingers, thumb, and forearm. After about two weeks, when the stitches are removed from your wrist, start Phase I exercises and progress through Phases II and III for the next four to six weeks. Use Phase III exercises for mild wrist injuries. Practice hand, wrist, and forearm strengthening exercises such as wrist curls with light weights (i.e., up to two pounds) and wrist rolls with the weight attached to the end of a rope that is tied to a roll-up stick.

Softening of Lunate Bone (Kienböck's Disease)

Results when blood supply to the wrist is cut off. Caused by repeated shocks to the lunate bone, which is in the middle of the wrist.

Symptoms:
Gradual increase of pain, stiffness, weakness, and loss of movement in wrist and hand.

ExRx:
Rest and ice; seek medical attention. For mild or moderate cases, practice Phase II Rehab exercises. In severe cases, surgery will be necessary. Within one week after surgery, begin hand, finger, thumb, and forearm exercises. In about four weeks, after the cast is removed, start Phase I exercises on the wrist.

Tendinitis of the Finger and Hand (Flexor Tendinitis)

An inflammation of tendons that run from the forearm across the wrist and hand to the fingers. Caused by repetitive unaccustomed use such as forceful bending as in baseball pitching and golf club swinging.

Symptoms:
Gradual swelling, soreness, and stiffness in fingers and palm, sometimes difficulty in straightening the fingers.

ExRx:
Doctor will prescribe anti-inflammatories, rest, ice, and splinting for three to five days. Mild cases will recover in three to five days, severe injuries take up to one month. Immediate care can eliminate long-term rehab. Start with the hand and finger rehab phase consistent with the severity of the injury.

ULNAR TUNNEL SYNDROME ("HANDLE BAR PALSY")

An irritation of the ulnar nerve that runs along the heel or little finger side of your hand. Frequently caused by gripping handle bars for too long.

Symptoms:
Tingling and numbness in the little finger and ring finger, finger weakness, and loss of coordination.

ExRx:
Prevent by wearing padded gloves and reducing the amount of time you grip handle bars to one hour or less per day or five hours per week. Also, frequently change the pressure on your hands and their position by changing the grip and height of the bars. To rehab, cease the irritating activity. The longer that nerves remain inflamed, the greater danger of scar tissue building up a loss of motor control and sensation in your hand. Use rest and ice for mild to moderate symptoms; surgery is the only solution for severe conditions. Use the same rehab procedure as with carpal tunnel syndrome (p. 462).

WRIST GANGLION CYST

A concentration of synovial fluid under the skin around the wrist; usually caused by a wrist tendon injury.

Symptoms:
Lump with little or no pain, which can progress into greater pain and loss of motion to the wrist and hand.

ExRx:
Rest and ice with gentle compression and splinting will help for mild to moderate symptoms. For severe, you may need to have the fluid drained and wrist splinted. Thereafter, begin with rehab Phase II exercises.

WRIST TENDINITIS

An inflammation of the two flexor tendons that pass over the underside of the wrist from the forearm to the hand and fingers. Caused by repeated wrist bends in such activities as rowing, kayaking, shot put, tennis, bowling, and so forth.

Symptoms:
Local pain and difficulty gripping, also a cracking sensation in tendons.

ExRx:
Rest and ice; cease the irritating activity. Splinting may be needed. Start rehab Phase II for seven to ten days. If surgery is needed, begin ROMs and strengthening exercises for hand, fingers, thumb, and forearm, while still in the cast. After the cast is removed, begin Phase I exercises for the wrist.

WRIST-THUMB TENDINITIS (DE QUERVAIN'S DISEASE)

An inflammation of the abductor and extensor tendons linking the wrist to the thumb. Can be caused by the snapping of the wrist in repetitive throwing and racquet play.

Symptoms:
Hurts to make a "thumbs-up" signal, local swelling, tenderness, and pain in the wrist and thumb.

ExRx:
Cease the aggravating activity. For mild to moderate injuries, rest and ice, thumb splinting, anti-inflammatories; begin Phase II exercises (usually within first week) and continue for five to fourteen days. Severe cases may require surgery. After surgery, start Phase I exercises after about two weeks when cast is removed; continue four weeks of rehab.

Wrist, Hand, and Finger Exercises

Phase I Wrist and Hand Assisted ROMs are used after wrist and/or hand surgery and are done with a physical therapist and when you are relatively pain-free. Phase II Wrist and Hand Personal ROMs are used for moderate or severe wrist and/or hand injuries. If you have been exercising at Phase I, start Phase II when you are able to move your wrist or hand by yourself. Phase III Wrist and Hand Exercises are used for mild to moderate wrist and/or hand injuries. Start Phase III when you can do Phase II without pain. Phase III exercises can be repeated two to three times per day. You should add more weight or resistance after you can do thirty repetitions pain-free. Increase the weight by only 10% (at the maximum) each time you successfully reach thirty repetitions with the prior weight. When you increase the weight, start again with ten repetitions, building up to thirty.

Phase I: Wrist and Hand Assisted ROMs (With a Physical Therapist)

Practice these ROMs for severe injuries and after surgery. Your physical therapist will lead you through passive- and active-assisted ROM exercises.

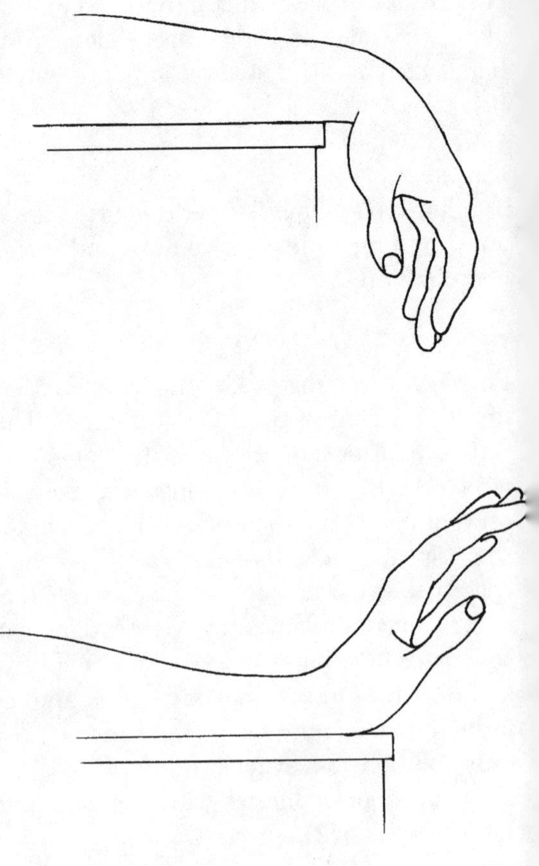

Wrist Raises ROM

Phase II: Wrist and Hand ROMs

Wrist Raises ROM (Dorsi Flexion/ Palmar Flexion)

- Rest your forearm on a table, palm down, hand and wrist hanging off the edge, fingers relaxed
- Bend your hand as far as possible upward, then downward
- On each hand, repeat five times, building up to thirty

Wrist Turns ROM (Radial Deviation/ Ulnar Deviation)

- Rest your forearm on a table, palm facing in, hand and wrist hanging off the edge, with your fingers extended
- Keep the heel of your hand (i.e. the bottom edge of your palm) on the table as you bend your hand as far upward as possible, then back downward
- On each hand, repeat five times, building up to thirty

Wrist Rotation

- With your arm extended out in front of you and slightly bent at the elbow, rotate your wrist in a circle, clockwise, five times building up to thirty
- Repeat the same number of rotations counterclockwise
- Repeat on the other hand

Wrist Turn (Pronation/Supination)

- Rest your forearm on a table, palm facing down
- Turn your wrist so that the back of your hand touches the table, then back to palm down position
- On each hand, repeat five times, building up to thirty

Fist and Finger Stretch Out

- Bend your elbow and prop it up on your hip or on a table top so that your forearm is vertically suspended in the air
- Slowly make a fist and hold it for a moment
- Then, slowly straighten and spread out your fingers
- On each hand, repeat five times, building up to thirty

Hand Squeeze

- Rest your arm on the table by propping it on your elbow; raise your forearm to a comfortable height that you can hold in position with palm up
- Squeeze an ace bandage or crumpled washcloth, repeating the same moves as for the fist and finger stretch out
- On each hand, repeat five times, building up to thirty

Finger Play

- Rest your arm on the table by propping it on your elbow and bend your arm, palm facing you
- With your thumb, proceed to touch your other four fingers, pushing the two together as hard as you can

- On each hand, repeat five times building up to thirty

Finger Palming

- Prop your elbow up and raise your fore-arm, palm facing out
- Touch the top of your palm with the tips of your fingers
- Pull your thumb back as you slightly arch your wrist at the end of each movement
- Hold for a moment, then stretch your fingers straight out in a right angle with your hand
- Repeat on the other hand
- Repeat on each hand five times building up to thirty

PHASE III: WRIST AND HAND EXERCISES

Wrist Raises ROM with Weights (Dorsi Flexion/Palmar Flexion

- Holding a small weight in your hand, rest your forearm on a table, palm-side down, hand and wrist hanging off the edge; make sure you do not overgrip the weight
- Bend your hand as far as possible upward, then downward
- On each hand, repeat five times building up to thirty

Wrist Turns ROM with Weights (Radical Deviation/Ulnar Deviation)

- Holding a small weight (¼ pound) in each hand, rest your forearm on a table, palm-side in, hand and wrist hanging off the edge
- Keep the heel of your hand on the table as you bend your hand as far upward as possible, then back downward
- On each hand, repeat five times, building up to thirty

HAND WEIGHT SCHEDULE FOR FOREARM

Small	⅛–½ lb.	tuna can
Medium	½–1 lb.	soup can
Large	1–5 lbs.	hardcover book

Towel Twist (Vertical)

- Sit or stand; hold a towel vertically out in front of you, one fist at head height, the other fist at chest level
- Twist each fist clockwise, then counter-clockwise
- Change your grip from thumbs up to thumbs down
- Release your grip of the towel with each twist, but do not let the towel fall
- Alternating hands, do five twists building up to thirty

Broomstick Roll-Up

- Tie a medium weight (½ lb.) to the end of a three-foot rope; tie the other end of the rope to a stick

- Grip the stick with both hands, palms down in the first stage, arms shoulder-width apart (the hanging weight should be in the center)
- Turn the stick by bending your wrists upward
- Do five to fifteen repetitions
- Next, lower the weight by bending your wrists downward for the same number of turns
- Repeat the exercise series with your palms up five to fifteen times

Tennis Ball Squeeze

- Stand or sit
- Rest your arm on the table by propping it on your elbow
- Squeeze a tennis- or rubber ball
- Repeat on each hand five times building up to thirty

Fist and Finger Stretch Out

- Wind a rubberband around the outside of your fingers, approximately in line with your knuckles
- Slowly make a fist; hold
- Next, slowly stretch and straighten out your fingers
- Repeat five to fifteen times on each hand.

RELAXATION EXERCISES

You can learn to relax your body with these long-term and short-term exercise techniques.

PROGRAM 1: LONG-TERM TECHNIQUES

1. Adopt a relaxed posture. Whenever you get a chance, rest your body. Avoid sitting on the edge of your seat, standing in lines, or lying with your head propped in awkward positions.
2. Slow down your pace. When you notice you are rushing about, losing track of things, getting tired easily, slow down your pace and use deliberate, continuous, and controlled movements.
3. Seek out and do exercises and activities that bring you joy and make you feel less competitive. The choice is an individual one. One person's chore is another person's treat.
4. Pace your daily activities and take short exercise breaks. The more stressed-out you feel, the more frequent your breaks should be—normally ten minutes every hour, but sometimes fifteen minutes or even a half hour may be necessary to restore your equilibrium.
5. Relax when you feel pain or pressure. Don't let pain mount up because it will, if it's not attended to.
6. Avoid longer bouts of pain by relaxing in the wake of smaller episodes.
7. Practice the appropriate relaxation exercise for overall or specific body area symptoms.

PROGRAM 2: DEEP-BREATHING EXERCISES

For anxiety and panic attacks and other severe stress, do deep breathing to counteract rapid shallow breathing and rapid heart rate, which is the Psyche-Immune equivalent of a muscle spasm.

Breath Control

The purpose of the following three exercises is to take control of your exaggerated, out-of-control (hyperventilation) breathing and heartbeat by breathing deeply and rhythmically, slowing down the pace of your breathing and relaxing your whole body in the process.

Controlled Breathing Exercise

- Slowly, breathe in through your nose counting one and two and three and so on as long as you can; mentally note how many counts you achieve
- Hold a brief second
- Breathe out through your mouth, taking as many counts as you did to breathe in
- Repeat exercise one to six times
- Repeat again
- If your symptoms persist, practice another set of breathing control exercises until you have normalized your breathing rate

Diaphragmatic or Stomach Breathing

Expand your capacity for staying relaxed by developing an expanded breathing capacity. As you continue to practice breath control, expand your stomach by pushing it out as you breathe in. This allows your lungs to fill with more air and slow down your rate of breath even further (up to five seconds per breath). A slower breathing rate also slows down your heartbeat.

Paper Bag Breathing

If your panic attack or hyperventilation is severe, practice breathing into a paper bag or cupped hands. Do not use a plastic bag! You are using a paper bag to increase the level or carbon dioxide that has been reduced because of overbreathing. The bag lets you rebreathe the carbon dioxide-laden air you just breathed out.

- Hold an empty paper bag tightly over your nose and mouth with both hands, leaving no holes for leakage
- Breathe in and out for a maximum of ten breaths until the unpleasant sensation of overbreathing ceases

Program 3: Deep Muscular Relaxation

Similar to deep-breathing exercises, these tension-release exercises can help bring exaggerated muscle tension under control by making your muscles tense even further through isometric contraction in order to help it fully release.

Moderately tense muscles can be relaxed by doing regular stretching and strengthening exercises, but severely tense muscles will not fully relax even from regular exercise. They need special tension-release exercises.

Practice the following set of tension-release exercises for one to five seconds of tension and the same amount of muscle relaxation. For example, if you tense a muscle group for three seconds, relax the same muscle group for another three seconds before moving on.

In this series, you will be tensing and relaxing the muscle groups of your body starting at the extremities of your hands, arms, shoulders, legs, thighs, buttocks, lower back, chest, neck, eyes, forehead, scalp, and face. Continue breathing through each contraction.

Practice these relaxation exercises in either the lying-down or seated position (except where specified). You can also practice these exercises in a series or a select body area whenever you feel muscles becoming tense.

Hands

- Clench both your fists with your knuckles facing out
- Hold for a count of one to six seconds
- Breathe in and out slowly
- As you breathe out, slowly release the grip of your fingers and let the blood circulate to your fingertips as you feel your hands grow heavier for another set of three to six seconds
- Repeat on each hand one to three times

Arms and Biceps

- Bend your arms at the elbow
- Keep your hands loose, tighten your biceps, hold for one to six seconds
- Relax your biceps as you lower your arm to the straightened-out position
- Repeat on each arm one to three times

Arms and Triceps

- Straighten your arm fully, tightening your tricep
- Hold for one to six seconds
- Release
- Repeat one to three times

Shoulders

- Shrug your shoulders, raising them as if to touch your ears
- Hold for one to six seconds
- Release
- Repeat one to three times

Feet

- Scrunch your toes together
- Hold for one to six seconds
- Release
- Repeat one to three times

Front Leg

- Flex your feet downward by pointing your feet away from your body
- Try to make your feet parallel to your legs
- Hold for one to six seconds
- Release
- Repeat one to three times

Back of Legs

- Flex your feet upward
- Press your heels down
- Hold for one to six seconds

- Release
- Repeat one to three times

Thighs

- Tighten the front of your thighs by pressing your knees down
- Hold for one to six seconds
- Release
- Repeat one to three times

Buttocks

- Squeeze your buttocks together
- Hold for one to six seconds
- Release
- Repeat one to three times

Lower Back

- In a lying-down position, flatten and press the small of your back into the floor
- Hold for one to six seconds
- Release
- Repeat one to three times

Chest

- Breathe in as you tighten your chest muscles
- Hold for one to six seconds
- Release
- Repeat one to three times

Neck

- Tilt your head back pointing your chin up
- Hold for one to six seconds
- Release
- Continue breathing
- Release mouth and jaw
- Pucker your lips and clench your teeth
- Hold for one to six seconds
- Release
- Repeat one to three times

Eyes

- Squeeze your eyelids together
- Hold for one to six seconds
- Continue breathing
- Release
- Repeat one to three times

Forehead

- Raise your eyelids
- Wrinkle your forehead
- Hold for one to six seconds
- Continue breathing
- Release
- Repeat one to three times

Scalp

- With your hands flat on the sides of your head, push your ears back, smoothing out the lines in your forehead

- Hold for one to six seconds
- Release
- Repeat one to three times

Face

- Scrunch all your facial muscles together—eyes tight, lips to nose
- Hold for one to six seconds
- Release
- Repeat one to three times

Please note: The head, neck, and back are the areas where muscle tension usually starts. Selectively practice ROMs and stretching exercises to relieve the tension as soon as possible.

INDEX

Page numbers in *italics* refer to illustrations.

Gary Yanker is the author of 14 books and over 100 original articles on health, business, and political topics. He has published in a smany as 14 languages and in over 60 countries. His columns and series articles have appeared in *The New York Times*, *American Health*, *Reader's Digest*, and *Woman's Day*. He holds a joint J.D./M.B.A. degree from Columbia University, and a B.A. in American Government from Georgetown University. Yanker has served as an adjunct professor on Intellectual Property at the University of Arizona, Loyola Marymount University, and Rutgers University. He was selected as a Reader's Digest Distinguished Speaker and is a member of of Phi Beta Kappa and the National Business Honor Society (Beta Gamma Sigma).